T0227022

Vulvovaginal Dermatology

Guest Editor

LIBBY EDWARDS, MD

DERMATOLOGIC CLINICS

www.derm.theclinics.com

Consulting Editor
BRUCE H. THIERS, MD

October 2010 • Volume 28 • Number 4

SAUNDERS an imprint of ELSEVIER, Inc.

W.B. SAUNDERS COMPANY
A Division of Elsevier Inc.

1600 John F. Kennedy Boulevard • Suite 1800 • Philadelphia, PA 19103-2899

http://www.theclinics.com

DERMATOLOGIC CLINICS Volume 28, Number 4
October 2010 ISSN 0733-8635, ISBN-13: 978-1-4377-2443-1

Editor: Carla Holloway
Developmental Editor: Jessica Demetriou

Dermatologic Clinics (ISSN 0733-8635) is published quarterly by Elsevier Inc., 360 Park Avenue South, New York, NY 10010-1710. Months of publication are January, April, July, and October. Business and editorial offices: 1600 John F. Kennedy Blvd., Suite 1800, Philadelphia, PA 19103-2899. Customer service office: 11830 Westline Drive, St. Louis, MO 63146. Periodicals postage paid at New York, NY, and additional mailing offices. Subscription prices are USD 317.00 per year for US individuals, USD 474.00 per year for US institutions, USD 371.00 per year for Canadian individuals, USD 568.00 per year for Canadian institutions, USD 434.00 per year for international individuals, USD 568.00 per year for international institutions, USD 148.00 per year for US students/residents, and USD 214.00 per year for Canadian and international students/residents. International air speed delivery is included in all *Clinics* subscription prices. All prices are subject to change without notice. **POSTMASTER:** Send address changes to *Dermatologic Clinics*, Elsevier Health Sciences Division, Subscription Customer Service, 3251 Riverport Lane, Maryland Heights, MO 63043. **Customer Service: 1-800-654-2452 (U.S. and Canada); 314-447-8871 (outside U.S. and Canada). Fax: 314-447-8029. E-mail: journalscustomerservice-usa@elsevier.com (for print support); journalsonlinesupport-usa@elsevier.com (for online support).**

Reprints. For copies of 100 or more, of articles in this publication, please contact the Commercial Reprints Department, Elsevier Inc., 360 Park Avenue South, New York, New York 10010-1710. Tel.: (212) 633-3813; Fax: (212) 462-1935; Email: repritns@elsevier.com.

The *Dermatologic Clinics* is covered in *MEDLINE/PubMed (Index Medicus)*, *Current Contents/Clinical Medicine, Excerpta Medica, Chemical Abstracts,* and *ISI/BIOMED.*

Printed and bound in the United Kingdom
Transferred to Digital Print 2011

Contributors

CONSULTING EDITOR

BRUCE H. THIERS, MD
Professor and Chairman, Department of Dermatology and Dermatologic Surgery, Medical University of South Carolina, Charleston, South Carolina

GUEST EDITOR

LIBBY EDWARDS, MD
Chief of Dermatology, Southeast Vulvar Clinic, Carolinas Medical Center, Charlotte, North Carolina

AUTHORS

YAA AMANKWAH, MB, ChB
Assistant Professor, Department of Obstetrics, Gynecology and Newborn Care, The Ottawa Hospital, University of Ottawa, Ottawa, Ontario, Canada

GRACE D. BANDOW, MD
Associate Pathologist, Dermatopathology; Director of Gynecologic Skin Pathology, Dermpath Diagnostics, Port Chester; Instructor of Clinical Dermatology, Department of Dermatology, Columbia University, New York, New York

JENNIFER BEECKER, MD
Division of Dermatology, University of Ottawa, The Ottawa Hospital, Civic Campus, Ottawa, Ontario, Canada

F. WILLIAM DANBY, MD, FRCPC
Adjunct Assistant Professor of Surgery (Section of Dermatology), Dartmouth Medical School, Hanover; Danby & Margesson, Manchester, New Hampshire

LIBBY EDWARDS, MD
Chief of Dermatology, Southeast Vulvar Clinic, Carolinas Medical Center, Charlotte, North Carolina

DEANA FUNARO, MD, FRCPC, FAAD
Clinical Professor, Vulvar Disease Division, Department of Dermatology, CHUM, University of Montreal, Quebec, Canada

ALLISON GODDARD, MD
Resident, Division of Dermatology, Loyola University School of Medicine, Maywood, Illinois

VLADA GROYSMAN, MD, FAAD
Assistant Professor, Department of Dermatology, University of Alabama at Birmingham, Birmingham, Alabama

HOPE HAEFNER, MD
Professor, Department of Obstetrics and Gynecology, The University of Michigan Hospitals, Ann Arbor, Michigan

MAI P. HOANG, MD
Associate Professor of Pathology, Dermatopathology Unit, Department of Pathology, Massachusetts General Hospital, Harvard Medical School, Boston, Massachusetts

CHRISTINA LAM, MD
Department of Dermatology, CHUM, University of Montreal; Dermatology Clinic, St-Luc Hospital, Montreal, Quebec, Canada

LYNETTE J. MARGESSON, MD, FRCPC
Adjunct Assistant Professor of Surgery (Section of Dermatology) and Obstetrics and Gynecology, Dartmouth Medical School, Hanover; Danby & Margesson, Manchester, New Hampshire

GINAT W. MIROWSKI, DMD, MD
Adjunct Associate Professor, Department of Oral Surgery Medicine Pathology, Indiana University School of Dentistry, Indianapolis, Indiana

RUTH MURPHY, PhD, MBChB, FRCP
Consultant Dermatologist and Paediatric Dermatologist, Department of Dermatology, Queens Medical Centre, Nottingham University Teaching Hospitals, Nottingham, United Kingdom

CLARE PIPKIN, MD
Assistant Professor, Department of Dermatology, Duke University, Durham, North Carolina

BETHANEE J. SCHLOSSER, MD, PhD
Assistant Professor, Departments of Dermatology and Obstetrics and Gynecology, Northwestern University, Chicago, Illinois

MARIA ANGELICA SELIM, MD
Associate Professor of Pathology and Dermatology; Director of Dermatopathology Unit, Department of Pathology, Duke University Medical Center, Durham, North Carolina

KRISTEN M.A. STEWART, MD
Dermatologist, Department of Dermatology, Naval Health Clinic New England, Newport, Rhode Island

ARUNA VENKATESAN, MD
Resident Physician PGYII, Department of Dermatology, Stanford Hospital and Clinics, Redwood City, California

Contents

functioning. Patient education is also important and is facilitated by patient brochures providing assurance that vulvodynia is a real disease.

Contact dermatitis of the vulva is common, with irritant contact dermatitis occurring more frequently than allergic contact dermatitis. Patients with chronic vulvar dermatoses are at greater risk and should continually be reassessed for possible contact dermatitis. Comprehensive and specific questioning about hygiene practices and product use is necessary to elicit a history of contactant use. Patch testing is required to identify relevant contact allergens, the most common of which include medicaments, preservatives, and fragrances. Patient education and follow-up are essential in optimizing treatment and preventing recurrence of vulvar contact dermatitis.

Lichen sclerosus (LS) is an inflammatory skin disease predominantly affecting the anogenital region. If untreated, progressive sclerosis results in scarring with distortion of the normal architecture. LS occurs more commonly in women than men but may occur in all age groups, including adolescents and prepubertal children. Its exact prevalence is unknown, but estimates range from 1:60 to 1:1000. In this article, LS is discussed in detail with respect to disease management in adults and children, risk of malignancy, and association with other diseases.

Vulvovaginal lichen planus is a chronic condition characterized by complex mucocutaneous findings. Patients may be asymptomatic or may have severe pain and itching. Findings vary from erythema, erosions, and white striae to severe scarring. Goals of treatment are to relieve symptoms and to minimize potential scarring. A multidisciplinary approach is advised for patients with widespread involvement to maximize treatment success (dermatologists, gynecologists, dentists, physical therapists, ophthalmologists, gastroenterologists, urologists, neurologists, anesthesiologists, psychologists, and psychiatrists).

The concept of vaginitis is widely accepted. Most physicians assume that vaginitis represents an infection, with nearly all vaginal complaints diagnosed as Candidiasis, bacterial vaginosis, or trichomonas. However, like the mouth, the vagina is covered with squamous epithelium, and therefore affected by various dermatoses. Some dermatoses prominently affect mucous membranes, such as lichen planus, pemphigus vulgaris, cicatricial pemphigoid, and blistering forms of erythema multiforme. In addition, some dermatoses affect only the vagina, including desquamative inflammatory vaginitis and atrophic vaginitis. The diagnosis and management of these

Dermatologic Clinics

FORTHCOMING ISSUES

January 2011

Tropical Dermatology
Scott Norton, MD and
Aisha Sethi, MD,
Guest Editors

April 2011

Mohs Surgery
Allison T. Vidimos, RPh, MD,
Christine Poblete-Lopez, MD,
and Christopher Gasbarre, DO,
Guest Editors

July 2011

Autoimmune Blistering Disease: Part I
Dédée F. Murrell, MA, BMBCh, FAAD, MD,
Guest Editor

RECENT ISSUES

July 2010

Innovative Therapeutics
Ted Rosen, MD,
Guest Editor

April 2010

Epidermolysis Bullosa: Part II – Diagnosis and Management
Dédée F. Murrell, MA, BMBCh, FAAD, MD,
Guest Editor

January 2010

Epidermolysis Bullosa: Part I – Pathogenesis and Clinical Features
Dédée F. Murrell, MA, BMBCh, FAAD, MD,
Guest Editor

RELATED INTEREST

Dermatologic Clinics April 2006 (Vol. 24, Issue 2)
Women's Dermatology
Kathryn Schwarzenberger, MD, *Guest Editor*
www.derm.theclinics.com

Preface
Vulvovaginal Dermatology

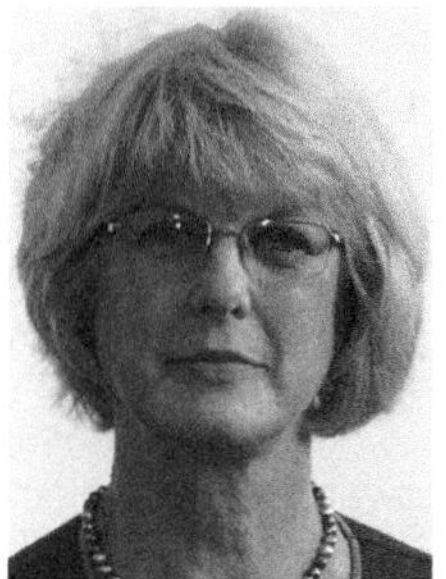

Libby Edwards, MD
Guest Editor

Vulvovaginal dermatology generally runs below the radar for the average dermatologist. Certainly, the vulva is covered with skin, so that skin diseases that affect extragenital areas can affect the vulva as well. Therefore, dermatologists are well armed to deal with vulvar dermatoses.

However, the vagina is also covered with squamous epithelium, an area rarely examined by the dermatologist. In addition, dermatoses are atypical in appearance when occurring on skin folds, including the vulva. Finally, chronic symptoms such as burning, dyspareunia, and pruritus do not fall into the area of any specific specialty. Nonetheless, dermatologists have the expertise to rule out both skin disease and infection as a cause of symptoms and make a diagnosis. The patient can then be treated or referred for treatment, whether that be physical therapists, pain management specialists, gynecologists, psychologists, or neurologists. This issue of *Dermatologic Clinics* is designed to provide information about these nondermatologic diseases with skin symptoms, as well as to inform the clinician of the differences in diagnosis and therapy of dermatoses on vulvovaginal skin, and to discuss noninfectious abnormalities of the vagina. Vulvology is a recently recognized new area of medicine. Interestingly, it is not a subspecialty of any particular specialty, although gynecologists are usually the clinicians first consulted by women with vulvar symptoms. Over the past nearly 30 years, I have watched vulvar dermatology grow from the very few American vulvologists, Peter Lynch, Maria Turner, Marilynne McKay, and Stephanie Pinkus, to a still small but increasing number of extremely bright, creative, and caring dermatologists, many of whom have contributed to this *Dermatologic Clinics* volume. These include some of us few old-timers such as Lynne Margesson and Bill Danby, as well as some of these younger, talented dermatologists including Kristen Stewart, Grace Bandow, Bethanee Schlosser, Clare Pipkin, Deana Funaro, Jennifer Beecker, and Vlada Groysman. Ruth Murphy and Ginat Mirowski are almost old-timers, and Ginat is expert in both vulvar and oral dermatology. Aruna Venkatesan is a dermatology resident who, when in medical school, was one of the most talented clinicians of any age or experience who has ever spent time in my office learning vulvovaginal dermatology. Collaboration with other specialties, especially gynecology, pathology, physical therapy, psychology, and pain management, is crucial to both the diagnosis and therapy of vulvar diseases. Hope Haefner and Yaa Amankwah are gynecologists who have added their knowledge and experience to this issue. Hope is as adept at vulvar dermatology as any vulvar dermatologist; she regularly holds my hand with difficult cases, and she adds her gynecologic and surgical skills to my patients as well. We are joined by dermatopathologist Angelica Selim, who beautifully describes the new classification of dermatoses fashioned by dermatologists Peter Lynch and Micheline Moyal-Barracco for the International Society for the Study of Vulvovaginal Disease (ISSVD).

No discussion of the people who have added to the specialty of vulvology would be complete

Dermatol Clin 28 (2010) xi–xii
doi:10.1016/j.det.2010.08.012
0733-8635/10/$ – see front matter

without acknowledging the enormous contribution of the ISSVD. In addition to the new classification of vulvar dermatoses, the standardization of terminology of dermatoses, classification of vulvar intraepithelial neoplasia, and classification of vulvar pain have been enormous contributions to the field of vulvovaginal medicine. The ISSVD was formed 40 years ago to standardize terminology among specialties and countries, to share experience and promote understanding of vulvovaginal disease, and to foster friendships among specialties and countries. Members of the ISSVD, both individually and as a group, are transforming the care of women with chronic vulvovaginal symptoms. My gratitude and affection for these members and these authors are enormous.

Libby Edwards, MD
Southeast Vulvar Clinic
Carolinas Medical Center
4335 Colwick Road, Suite D
Charlotte, NC 28211, USA

E-mail address:
ledwardsmd@aol.com

Therapeutic Principles in Vulvovaginal Dermatology

Jennifer Beecker, MD

KEYWORDS

- Vulvovaginal therapy • Anticandidal therapy
- Vaginal corticosteroids

The management of chronic vulvovaginal symptoms is a challenge that requires attention to several unique issues. Vulvovaginal diseases are often multifactorial. Successful treatment requires attention to all aspects of the disease. Often these components need to be addressed simultaneously; however, this is not difficult with an organized approach. Much like a complete approach to other chronic dermatologic diseases, such as atopic dermatitis, patients must be educated about the disease and daily skin care; the primary disease and also secondary infections must be treated, adverse effects must be anticipated; and rescue care for acute flares must be offered. The goal of treatment of chronic vulvovaginal disease is often control, not cure.

GENERAL MEASURES

There are several general measures that are essential for the successful treatment of any vulvovaginal disease. Despite adequate diagnosis and treatment, patients may fail to improve if these fundamentals are not addressed. These include educating patients about the nature of their disease, addressing psychosexual issues, stopping irritants, using appropriate vehicles for medications, anticipating and treating iatrogenic disease, prescribing estrogen when appropriate, and having a rescue plan for acute symptoms.

Education

Symptoms of vulvovaginal disease are common, yet women are often unaware of this fact and feel isolated with their problems. Patients commonly feel embarrassed discussing their problems and, therefore, often have many concerns that are unaddressed. Many have fears that their symptoms represent cancer, sexually transmitted disease, or infidelity.[1] These topics should be discussed as directly as possible, because patients may not volunteer their fears. It is a good idea to ask patients what they think their problem is, to get an idea of their concerns so that they can be addressed immediately. Vulvovaginal disease can significantly interfere with sexual function and intimacy as well as overall disposition. Frustration and depression are common and can contribute to a pain syndrome, if present. It is important to take the time to support patients. In addition, counseling is important for patients and their partners. Involving the partner from the first visit is ideal. Resources with accurate information are helpful because there are many myths on the Internet and elsewhere. Referring patients to the International Society for the Study of Vulvovaginal Disease (www.ISSVD.org) is suggested because there are educational resources available that are up to date, and may help women feel less alone in their disease.[1,2] The National Vulvodynia Association (www.NVA.org) is another excellent resource for patients. In the author's experience, referring patients to support groups is not helpful, because many of the people participating are unhappy and not supportive in a positive way. Handouts are a great idea, because there is

Division of Dermatology, University of Ottawa, 737 Parkdale Avenue, Ground Floor East, The Ottawa Hospital, Civic Campus, Ottawa, Ontario K1Y 4E9, Canada
E-mail address: jbeecker@rogers.com

Dermatol Clin 28 (2010) 639–648
doi:10.1016/j.det.2010.07.001

often an enormous amount of information to absorb at the initial encounter, and patients are able to review the information again at home.

An important part of the educational process is management of patients' expectations. Vulvovaginal disease is often chronic, and the aim of care is control, not cure, for most diseases. This needs to be explained clearly to patients, followed up by a comprehensive care plan of how patients will get better, but not necessarily cured of their disease.

Psychosexual Issues

It is well known that depression can occur in conjunction with almost all chronic pain syndromes.[3] Depression can also alter pain perception.[3] For successful treatment of vulvovaginal disorders, depression or any other psychological issues must be addressed. As discussed previously, counseling is imperative for most patients. Sex therapy or couples counseling is often helpful as well. In addition, the use of antidepressants is encouraged. Fortunately, the tricyclic class of antidepressants has the advantage of also treating chronic pain and producing sedation to prevent nighttime scratching.[3] If tricyclics are ineffective at treating the depressive symptoms, however, other classes of antidepressants can be considered (discussed later).

Irritant and Allergic Contact Dermatitis

Vulvovaginal disease often has multiple concurrent etiologies, and it is imperative to consider allergic contact dermatitis in all patients. Irritant and allergic contact dermatitis are often not the primary problems but secondary complications. Irritant contact dermatitis is common, because vulvar skin is inherently more sensitive than other skin areas and has weak barrier function.[4,5] Diseased vulvar skin is often even more prone to irritation. Irritants are substances or practices that would create irritation in most people if used often enough or left on the skin long enough. Irritant contact dermatitis is nonimmunologic.[6] Alternatively, allergic contact dermatitis requires prior sensitization to an allergen and constitutes an immunologic memory T-cell response on re-exposure to that allergen. This can result in an inflammatory cutaneous reaction.[4,7,8] In vulvar irritant and allergic contact dermatitis, some patients only have sensory irritation, with no detectable skin change.[4,9]

Irritants include strong irritants, such as topical mediations for genital warts that cause an acute reaction, and weaker irritants that have a more cumulative effect (**Table 1**). Weaker irritants include moisture, friction, vaginal discharge, urine feces, soaps/cleansers, feminine wipes or sprays, douches, sanitary pads, creams, semen, lubricants, and spermicides.[1,4,9] Aggressive washing with wash cloths is another common cause of irritation, as is overly frequent washing, often out of fear of odor or concern that poor hygiene is the cause of the symptoms. In addition, use of a hair dryer to dry the vulva after bathing should be discouraged as this can cause chapping and irritation.

Allergic contact dermatitis is less common than irritant contact dermatitis, but is still common (**Table 2**). The incidence of vulvar contact dermatitis has been reported to vary from 20% to 30%.[4,10] In a recent study of 50 women with vulvar pruritus, 8 patients (16%) had one or more relevant positive allergic reactions. The relevant allergens were usually cosmetics, preservatives, and medicaments.[10] In another study, 47% of patients with lichen simplex chronicus had positive patch tests.[11] Although it is not clear whether or not the allergic contact dermatitis triggered the lichen simplex chronicus or if the allergy was secondary

Table 1
Common vulvar irritants

Physical irritants	Excessive washing, wash cloths, hair dryers, sanitary pads, tight clothing
Hygiene products	Soaps and cleanser, powders, douches, perfumes, deodorants, bubble bath/oils/salts, depilatory creams, adult or baby wipes
Body fluids	Sweat, vaginal secretions (normal or abnormal), urine, feces, semen
Medicaments	Antifungal creams, topical antibacterial agents, over-the-counter anti-itch creams
Lubricants and contraceptives	Spermicides, condoms, diaphragms, lubricants

Table 2
Common vulvar contact allergens (cosmetics, preservatives, and medicaments)

Topical anesthetics (eg, benzocaine)	Chlorhexidine (eg, in K-Y Jelly [Johnson & Johnson])
Topical antibiotics (eg, neomycin) Perfumes	Latex (eg, latex condoms)
Preservatives (in creams, prescription creams, hygiene products, and nail polish)	Topical antifungal medications (eg, imidazoles and nystatin)
Topical steroids	

to treatments used for the lichen simplex chronicus, it is important to recognize and treat both problems concurrently. If no dermatitis is present, it is unlikely that allergic contact dermatitis is playing a role.[12]

Some of the more significant allergens implicated in vulvar allergic contact dermatitis include topical anesthetics, ethylenediamine, topical antibiotics, fragrances, antifungal creams, and topical steroids. Benzocaine is a common allergen found in many over-the-counter anti-itch creams, including Vagisil, which is a specifically marketed for vaginal and vulvar symptoms and commonly tried by women before they present to a physician.[4,8] Ethylenediamine is found in generic Mycolog or Kenacomb cream. Neomycin is another common culprit found in antibacterial creams.[4] Fragrance is ubiquitous in hygiene products. Nystatin, imidiazoles, and corticosteroids are known sensitizers, as are the preservatives in their cream vehicles.[4,8] Corticosteroid allergy should be considered in anyone not improving with a steroid-responsive disease.[13]

Allergic contact dermatitis is diagnosed by patch testing. Patch testing should be considered in all patients presenting with vulvar dermatoses or pruritus. It should always be performed when a patient is not responding to therapy as expected. Most patients with vulvovaginal problems present to their physician only after trying several home remedies. They have often tried several over-the-counter creams, cleansers, and antifungal and antibacterial treatments.[14] It is important to have a high index of suspicion for both irritant and allergic contact dermatitis. General measures suggested for all patients include only washing once a day with plain water and fingertips; stopping all products used on the vulva or vagina (including over-the-counter and prescription products); not using panty liners or pads; and avoiding spermicides, condoms, and some lubricants, such as K-Y Jelly, which has chlorhexidine and preservatives (Astroglide and vegetable oil are acceptable).[7,9] Avoiding tight clothing, such as jeans, is helpful. If an emollient is needed, plain petrolatum used just after bathing is safe and effective.[7,15] These instructions should be given to patients in a handout if possible. General instructions for patients to decrease irritant and allergen exposure include

Stop all products used on vulva and vagina
Avoid sanitary pads, use tampons
Avoid spermicides, condoms, and K-Y Jelly (vegetable oil or Astroglide are acceptable)
Wear loose clothing.

Vehicles

When at all possible, topical creams or gels should be avoided when treating vulvovaginal disease because they tend to sting and burn, causing further irritation to the area. In addition they contain more preservatives and additives than ointments do and therefore have more potential for causing irritant or allergic contact dermatitis.[13] Ointments should be used for topical treatment, even if they require compounding. Sometimes oral treatment is preferred to avoid any manipulation or further irritation to the area or for severe disease.

Anticipate Adverse Events and Iatrogenic Disease

Vulvovaginal candidiasis and contact dermatitis are common complications when treating vulvovaginal disease. Many of the treatments used to treat vulvovaginal disease, such as antibiotics, corticosteroids, and estrogen, predispose patients to vulvovaginal candidiasis.[16–18] A prudent approach is to use antifungal prophylaxis during treatment. Oral fluconazole (150 mg weekly) is a good choice rather than a topical antifungal to avoid the risk of irritant or allergic contact dermatitis.[7] The presciber must be mindful of the risk of medication interactions with oral fluconazole.

It is impossible to completely remove the risk of allergic contact dermatitis, but using ointments rather than creams decreases the risk of preservative allergy, because creams contain more preservatives.[13] Careful prescribing, asking patients to avoid self-treatment, and having a high index of suspicion when patients are recalcitrant or flaring help minimize the possibility of allergic contact dermatitis from complicating vulvovaginal disease.

Estrogen Replacement

Estrogen deficiency can make any vulvovaginal problem worse, and it can sometimes be the primary problem. Estrogen maintains the tissue of the vagina and introitus, and without it, these tissues become atrophied, dry, and fragile.[4] There are many causes of low estrogen, including medications (oral contraceptive pills and tamoxifen), menopause, the postpartum period, and breastfeeding.[4] Estrogen-deficient patients are particularly susceptible to trauma from normal activities, scratching, or irritants. All patients should be evaluated for estrogen deficiency and estrogen replaced in those who are deficient. This is essential for the successful treatment of their vulvovaginal condition (discussed later).

Rescue Medications

Most patients with vulvovaginal disease have acute exacerbations of their symptoms at times. It can alleviate patient anxiety to have a rescue plan with techniques/tools and medications that patients can turn to when they have acute worsening of their condition. Cold compresses kept in the refrigerator (not the freezer, to avoid frostbite) are ideal for patients to use to alleviate pain or pruritus. Cool water soaks act similarly by hydrating the tissue and, therefore, temporarily sealing small cracks and fissures in the skin.[7] Patients can soak for 10 to 15 minutes up to 2 times a day, pat the area dry, and then gently cover the area with plain petrolatum to seal in the moisture and create some barrier protection. Petrolatum is irritant- and preservative-free, is inexpensive, and has minimal risk of causing any secondary problems.[8] Patients should be cautioned that soaking too often may be counterproductive because it can dry out the tissues and cause irritation in itself.[7]

Topical xylocaine is helpful relief for acute symptoms as well as to facilitate sexual intercourse or even micturition.[7,19] It can be applied 30 minutes before intercourse. Unfortunately, a frequent side effect is burning and stinging from both the 2% xylocaine gel and 5% xylocaine ointment, which limits its use in many patients.[7] In the authors' recent experience, success was found with a dental formula of lidocaine powder 10%, prilocaine power 10%, and tetracaine power 4% compounded into a gel.

Nightime sedation is a key part of a rescue plan. Many vulvovaginal patients have poor sleep secondary to itch or pain. Patients who can sleep often have poor quality sleep because they are scratching in their sleep, and this also prevents the improvement of their condition. Lack of quality sleep can contribute to depression and difficulties coping with pain or itch.[20,21] Dermatologists are often most comfortable using sedating antihistamines, such as diphenhydramine or hydroxyzine hydrochloride, to assist sleep. If these medications are not successful, or if patients are scratching in their sleep, tricyclic antidepressants, such as amitrityline or doxepin, are often more effective for sedation because they induce deeper sleep for a longer period of time. This may help decrease scratching during sleep and improve sleep quality.

Lastly, patients experiencing an exacerbation of their condition must be seen and evaluated for the cause of the flare. Infections and allergic contact dermatitis are common causes of flares; thus, a timely history, physical examination, appropriate cultures, and treatment often can truncate an acute flare quickly.

SPECIFIC MEDICATIONS

Corticosteroid Therapy

Topical corticosteroid therapy

Topical corticosteroids are the mainstay of treatment of many vulvovaginal diseases, including lichen sclerosus, lichen planus, and other pruritic diseases. The modified mucous membranes are relatively steroid resistant, and often potent or superpotent corticosteroids, such as clobetasol proprionate, are required for successful treatment.[7] A common error in treating vulvar diseases is using a topical steroid that is not potent enough for too little period of time. It is rare to see atrophy of the modified mucous membranes of the vulva. It is important to demonstrate to patients exactly where the ointment is to be applied, so that the corticosteroid is not causing side effects on areas that are not steroid resistant, such as the hair-bearing labia majora, crural crease, perianal skin, and medial thighs.[7,13] If topical steroid is needed in these nonresistant areas, a less potent steroid is considered and patients should be followed closely for side effects. Adverse effects from topical steroids applied to these nonsteroid-resistant areas include atrophy of the skin, striae (which are permanent), steroid rosacea/dermatitis, erythema, candidiasis, exacerbation of condylomata accuminata, epidermal cysts, and, rarely, systemic absorption.[13] Although iatrogenic Cushing syndrome can develop with less than 50 g per week of topical clobetasol,[13,22,23] far less than 1 g per week is used on the vulva. Systemic absorption has been reported from mucosal application as well,[24] but this is generally not a clinical problem except in infants overtreated under diaper occlusion. This again emphasizes the importance of demonstrating the proper technique of application and the amount of topical ointment to be applied, which is typically far smaller than a pea. In most cases, 30 g of clobetasol propionate ointment should last longer than 6 months.[2,25] In addition, all patients using potent or ultrapotent steroids on the vulva should be followed closely and examined at least monthly.[7,19,23] If there are any concerns or adverse events, hypothalamus-pituitary-adrenal (HPA) axis testing can be performed.[22,23]

Ointments are the preferred vehicle in the vulvovaginal area as creams and gels tend to sting and burn and have more preservatives in them.[7,13] Anecdotally, it has been the authors' experience that the Temovate brand (Dermovate in Canada) seems better tolerated on the vulva than the clobetasol propionate generic ointment; however, this has not been reported or published elsewhere.

Many studies have shown that once-a-day dosing of topical corticosteroids is adequate for most dermatologic diseases.[2,26] Pharmokinetic studies have shown measurable plasma levels of clobetasol propionate 48 hours after a single application of ointment.[27] Twice-daily dosing could be considered in resistant disease, however, because studies of severe resistant psoriasis show slight superiority of multiple daily applications compared with once-daily applications.[28]

Once a patient's condition has stabilized, the frequency of application can be decreased, or the potency of the steroid can be decreased. Many vulvovaginal diseases require chronic maintenance therapy. One option is to decrease the frequency to every other day and then, if the remission is sustained, continue to decrease the frequency. If patients' disease returns at any point, they are titrated back up to the dose or frequency that was effective.[25] Some diseases, such as lichen sclerosus, are not curable, and patients who have that disease must remain on minimal dosing for ongoing control. It has been the authors' experience that ultrapotent steroids 3 times a week on the vulva for chronic maintenance therapy have minimal risk of side effects.[7] Sometimes using plain petrolatum on the days steroid is not applied is helpful because of the emollient effect, and it also keeps the routine of applying topicals daily. It is often harder for patients to remember to apply medication 2 or 3 times a week rather than daily application.

Intravaginal corticosteroid therapy

Intravaginal topical corticosteroids are used for treatment of lichen planus or desquamative inflammatory vaginitis.[29–31] There are no commercially available intravaginal corticosteroids available, but hydrocortisone acetate 25-mg rectal suppositories are used off label. Other options include compounding a 500-mg hydrocortisone suppository or using topical corticosteroid ointment with an applicator. These are typically used once daily before bed, and titrated down in frequency or potency as soon as possible.[31] The absorption of topicals is greater in the vagina than on the vulva, but little is known about the optimal frequency or potency to limit systemic absorption.[31] Patients must be monitored frequently for side effects and the signs and symptoms of Cushing disease, and physicians must have a low threshold for HPA testing. It is reasonable to consider HPA testing in patients who use potent intravaginal corticosteroids (clobetasol or hydrocortisone 500-mg suppositories) more than 3 times a week.[19,23]

Intralesional corticosteroid therapy

Intralesional corticosteroids are especially helpful for thick plaques (eg, lichenification), which are not penetrated well by topical therapies; stubborn areas that are not responding to topicals; areas with deep inflammation (eg, hidradenitis suppurativa); patients with poorly controlled pruritus; or patients with questionable compliance. Depending on the problem, up to two 1-mL injections of triamcinolone acetonide (10 mg/mL) can be used, ideally with a 30-gauge needle. Generally the 10-mg/mL dosing is used if the desired effect is thinning of the lesion. Sometimes only 0.1 mL is needed, for example, in the case of a small but thickened scar. When the anti-inflammatory effect is more desired, as is the case of cysts, the triamcinolone can be diluted further to 3.3 mg/mL using injectable saline.[7] If repeat injections are needed, these are generally done at 6-week intervals. The main side effects of intralesional corticosteroids can include atrophy and hypopigmentation.[7,13]

Systemic corticosteroid therapy

Systemic corticosteroids are usually reserved for severe cases, for example, severe erosive lichen planus, and are used to get the condition under control so that patients can then tolerate topical agents. Often short courses, usually 2 to 4 weeks, are used using 40 to 60 mg per day of oral prednisone.[19] There is no need to taper if the treatment is less than 2 weeks in duration.[32] Topical corticosteroids should be started before the oral prednisone is stopped to prevent flaring during the transition time. An alternative to oral prednisone is intramuscular triamcinolone acetonide (60–80 mg). The effect of this lasts approximately 1 month.[32] The side effects of systemic steroids make it an unacceptable treatment for long-term therapy of vulvovaginal conditions.[19]

Topical Calcineurin Inhibitors

Pimecrolimus and tacrolimus are immunomodulators that block the release of inflammatory cytokines from T lymphocytes in the skin while promoting cutaneous innate host defenses.[33] They are approved as second-line therapies for atopic dermatitis and are used off label for many other dermatologic disorders, including vulvovaginal disease. Tacrolimus comes as an ointment and pimecrolimus as a cream. They are approximately equivalent to a midpotency topical corticosteroid.[34] The main advantage of topical calcineurin inhibitors is they do not have the side effects topical corticosteroids do, such as atrophy of the skin and HPA axis suppression. Several small studies suggest benefit in many vulvovaginal disorders; however, their use is limited on the vulva by their common side effect of stinging and burning, which is more pronounced on eroded skin.[33,35–38] Keeping the tube of medication cool in the refrigerator sometimes helps alleviate some of the stinging, but it cannot be tolerated by many patients. In addition, there are concerns about calcineurin inhibitors increasing the risk of progression to cancer. Vulvovaginal diseases (eg, lichen sclerosus and erosive lichen planus) have a small but real risk of progression to squamous cell carcinoma (SCC). There is concern that calcineurin inhibitors may inhibit immunocompetent cells, which normally survey the skin and prevent premalignant cells from developing into cancers.[39,40] There are case reports where there was likely a causal relationship between the use of topical tacrolimus and the development of SCC on the gentials.[39,41]

Currently, topical pimecrolimus and tacrolimus are considered second-line agents for the treatment of many steroid-responsive vulvovaginal dermatoses when topical corticosteroids cause side effects or the area is steroid resistant.[33,37,40,41] Patients should not use these agents if they have a compromised immune system or an active skin infection.[34,41]

Antifungal Therapy

Topical antifungal therapy

Women with vulvovaginal diseases commonly experience vulvovaginal candidiasis as a complication of their treatment. Corticosteroids, estrogen, and antibiotics all predispose patients to vulvovaginal candidiasis.[16–18]

Patients with chronic or unresponsive candidiasis should undergo culture, because management failure is more often due to misdiagnosis than medication failure. Before starting any antifungal treatment for vulvovaginal *Candida* infection, it is imperative to obtain a culture. Many patients with vulvar symptoms have been labeled as having vulvovaginal candidiasis for months and sometimes years, in the absence of documented infection.[42] Often there is another diagnosis other than candidiasis to explain the vulvar symptoms. In addition, it is important to determine the species and sensitivities, because some species may be resistant to first-line treatments. In one study, more than 20% of *Candida* isolates were resistant to fluconazole.[16]

Most topical antifungal preparations are available only as creams, which are inherently irritating to the vagina and vulva. When possible, oral treatment can be prescribed to avoid exposing the vulva to more irritants. An alternative to systemic treatment is nystatin ointment or vaginal tablets, the most soothing topical anticandidal agents. It can be used nightly for 2 weeks.[43]

Candida albicans is the most frequently isolated yeast from the vagina and tends to be sensitive to all azoles and nystatin (a polyene).[7,16] In recent studies, *Candida glabrata* is the second most common isolate from vaginal cultures and is known to have resistance to the entire class of azoles and polyene antifungal agents.[16,44] Generally, nonalbicans *Candida* infections are asymptomatic, but when treatment is desired, intravaginal boric acid tablets (600 mg) can be compounded and used daily for 2 to 3 weeks. Patients should be advised to use this vaginally only, because it is toxic if ingested orally. Another treatment for nonalbicans *Candida* is flucytosine topically. It might be more efficacious than boric acid, but there are no randomized studies to show this. It is more expensive than boric acid. Flucytosine is compounded to form ointment in tube applicators. A 5-g dose is used nightly for 14 days.[44]

Systemic antifungal therapy

Systemic treatment or prophylaxis for yeast infection is often preferred over topical treatment because it eliminates the potential for further irritation to the vulva. Prophylaxis to prevent vulvovaginal candidiasis is often needed when treating patients with vulvar disease. Antiyeast prophylaxis should be considered when an antibiotic is prescribed in patients with chronic vulvovaginal issues. In addition, antifungal medications can be prescribed for the first few weeks when estrogen replacement is instituted. There is a highly significant relationship between the use of estrogen and the occurrence of vulvovaginal candidaisis.[16,17] Once the vagina is fully estrogenized, *Candida* becomes less of a problem.[7] For antibiotic and corticosteroid therapy, the prophylaxis should be considered for the duration of the treatment, but this needs to be individualized for each patient.

If there is evidence of vaginal *Candida* infection, a single dose of oral fluconazole (150 mg) can be given.[45] In more complicated or resistant cases, another option for treatment is fluconazole given in 3 doses of 150 mg at 72-hour intervals.[46] If there is significant vulvar involvement, more doses may be needed, or a topical may be used concurrently on the vulva.[7] In recurrent vulvovaginal candidiasis, defined as four or more symptomatic attacks in a 12-month period, fluconazole (150 mg) can be given weekly to maintain remission after the first 3 doses have been given to induce disease remission.[18] One drawback of using oral fluconazole is its many interactions with other drugs. Fluconazole is the only medication with Food and Drug Administration approval for vulvovaginal candidiasis.[7] Itraconazole and, less so, terbinafine, are useful orally as well.

Antibiotic Therapy

In dermatology, antibiotics are often used for their anti-inflammatory effects as well as their antimicrobial action.[47]

Topical antibiotics

The most common topical antimicrobial agents used in vulvovaginal diseases are clindamycin (2% cream) and metronidazole gel. Both are useful to treat group B streptococcus (GBS), keeping in mind that these bacteria can be a normal colonizer of the vagina and only occasionally cause infections.[31] A 5-g dose is inserted into the vagina nightly for 7 days. An alternative is clindamycin ovules (100 g for 3 days). Clindamycin is also used to treat desquamative inflammatory vaginitis, and in this case it is used more for its anti-inflammatory action. The treatment is more chronic in nature, and often several weeks are needed before improvement is noted. Close follow-up is warranted because relapse is not uncommon.[32,48–50] *Clostridrium difficile* infection is a rare side effect.[51]

In addition to its use in GBS, metronidazole (0.75% gel) is used to treat bacterial vaginosis at a dosage of 5 g daily (one applicator is inserted into the vagina nightly for 5 days).[43]

In general, it is best for patients to avoid over-the-counter topical antibiotics, in particular those containing neomycin. Many of these antibiotics are known potent sensitizers and the risk of allergic contact dermatitis is high.[52]

Systemic antibiotics

Systemic antimicrobials are preferred to topical therapy in patients with chronic vulvovaginal symptoms to limit irritants and allergens affecting the vulvovaginal area. Topical antibiotics tend to come as gels or creams, which are inherently more irritating to the vulva and vagina. The risk of allergic contact dermatitis can make the use of oral metronidazole and oral clindamycin more appealing. Metronidazole (500 mg twice daily for 7 days) or clindamycin (300 mg twice daily for 7 days) can be used for bacterial vaginosis.[45] Metronidazole is also the treatment for trichomoniasis.[45] Bacterial vaginitis should be cultured and the antibiotic chosen by sensitivities. GBS can often be treated with penicillin V potassium, amoxicillin, ampicillin, or clindamycin but often relapses immediately.[31]

Estrogen Therapy

Estrogen deficiency can make any vulvovaginal problem worse and sometimes can be the primary cause of the disorder (discussed previously). There are several different methods of estrogen delivery, including topical intravaginal cream, intravaginal tablets, estrogen-releasing vaginal ring, and oral replacement therapy.[53] It has been the author's experience that estradiol-17β cream (Estrace) is better tolerated than conjugated equine estrogen cream (Premarin), although the latter is less expensive. Both are dosed 3 times a week intravaginally at night. Vaginal tablets (Vagifem) are sometimes more acceptable to patients who find the creams irritating and messy, and treatment with 17β-estradiol vaginal tablets has been shown equivalent to conjugated equine estrogen vaginal cream for atrophic vaginitis.[54] Other trials have found that women seemed to favor the estradiol-releasing ring (Estring), followed by the vaginal tablets, and then the cream.[53] Choosing a method of delivery that patients find acceptable may increase compliance and improve treatment outcomes. None of these methods resulted in appreciable systemic estradiol levels.[54] Systemic estrogen is another option; however, some women may find they need topical estrogen as well.

There is a significant relationship between the use of estrogen and *Candida* infection.[16,17] Oral fluconazole (150 mg weekly) for the first few 5 weeks of estrogen therapy or, alternatively, nystatin ointment or an azole cream coadministered in the same applicator as the estrogen helps ameliorate this risk.[7]

Psychoactive Medications

Vulvovaginal dieases are often complicated by pain and itching, and often this results in poor sleep as well. Central nervous system medications that have been shown to help these symptoms, when caused by neuropathic pain or itching, include tricyclic antidepressants (eg, amitriptyline), neuroleptics (eg, gabapentin), analgesics for neuropathy (eg, pregabalin), and selective norepinephrine reuptake inhibitors (SNRIs), such as venlafaxine. These medications can help with the sleep disorder, pain, and depressive symptoms that often accompany vulvovaginal disease.[55] Tricyclic antidepressants, such as amitriptyline or doxepin, are often dosed at night because they are sedating and benefit patients who are up at night with pain of itch. They create a deeper level of sleep than antihistamines do, and, therefore, people are less likely to scratch in their sleep. They also help with depression, but if patients are depressed, counseling should be prescribed as well.[7] Gabapentin and pregabalin are also indicated for neuropathic pain but are less sedating.[56] SNRIs (eg, venlafaxime) can help with pain and depression as well.[3] The medication choice should be based on patients' predominant symptoms, whether or not pain, itch, sleep disturbance, depression, or a combination of these. All of these medications are best started at very low doses and titrated up slowly to effect.

Other Techniques/Tips

Pelvic floor muscle physiotherapy has been shown to help when vulvodynia is present as a primary or secondary condition.[57] Physiotherapy has the added bonus of one-on-one time with a professional familiar with vulvovaginal problems. This provides an outlet for patients to discuss their problem outside of counseling and somewhat normalizes their situation so they do not feel as isolated because of their disease.

Constipation can complicate vulvovaginal symptoms. It can be helpful to ask if constipation is an issue, and if it is, address dietary changes, such as increasing fluids and fiber, and recommend and prescribe stool softeners when needed.

Smoking is a risk factor for cancer and has been shown a factor in vulvar intraepithelial neoplasia, also known as SCC in situ or Bowen disease. In one study, women who smoked had more extensive disease and were also more likely to have persistent disease after treatment.[58] Patients who smoke and have vulvar disease should, therefore, be counseled to stop, because this may put them at higher risk for their disease to be complicated by cancer.

Recalcitrant Problems

If vulvovaginal patients fail to improve, several factors should be considered. The first is adherence. Studies of dermatology patients using topical therapies have shown that adherence is poor at best in most patients.[59,60] It is easy to see how nonadherence could occur: for example, patients may be alarmed by warnings on the package of steroids or calcineurin inhibitors and not want to use them. Another barrier to adherence could be elderly or obese patients who may have difficulty with application of topical medications.

The second factor to be considered in recalcitrant vulvovaginal disease is the possibility of allergic contact dermatitis. This can be acute, subacute, chronic, or irritant contact dermatitis from the prescribed treatment or something a patient is using at home.

If a vulvovaginal problem is resistant to treatment, the general measures (discussed previously) should be addressed, such as educating patients about the nature of their disease, addressing psychosexual issues, stopping irritants, using appropriate vehicles for medications, anticipating and treating for iatrogenic disease, prescribing estrogen when appropriate, and having a rescue plan for acute symptoms. Associated symptoms, such as constipation, should be addressed. Patients do not improve unless these general measures are attended to simultaneously.

Lastly, always consider an incorrect initial diagnosis or that a new disease may have developed if there is lack of response to therapy. Have a low threshold for rebiopsy to rule out Paget disease or malignant transformation. Think about possible systemic disease that may have developed that may need systemic control, such as diabetes mellitus or Crohn disease, because local factors are less effective.

SUMMARY

Vulvovaginal disease, like many dermatologic diseases, tends to be chronic. Similar to treatment of diseases like atopic dermatitis, chronic vulvovaginal disease requires a multifaceted approach, often addressing multiple issues concurrently. General principles apply to all vulvovaginal patients and must be considered in each patient for treatment to be ultimately successful. The goal of treatment is often control, not cure.

REFERENCES

1. Margesson LJ. Vulvar disease pearls. Dermatol Clin 2006;17:20–7.

2. ACOG Practice Bulletin No. 93: diagnosis and management of vulvar skin disorders. Obstet Gynecol 2008;111(5):1243–53.
3. Bair MJ, Robinson RL, Katon W, et al. Depression and pain comorbidity: a literature review. Arch Intern Med 2003;163(20):2433–45.
4. Margesson LJ. Contact dermatitis of the vulva. Dermatol Ther 2004;4(2):145–55.
5. Britz MB, Maibach HI. Human cutaneous vulvar reactivity to irritants. Contact Dermatitis 1978;5: 375–7.
6. Stotnicki-Grant S. Allergic contac dermatitis versus irritant contact dermatitis. Discussion paper prepared for The Workplace Safety and Insurance Appeals Tribunal, 2008.
7. Edwards L. Principles of therapeutics for vulvovaginal disease. In: Black MM, Ambros-Rudolph C, Edwards L, et al, editors. Obstetric and gynecologic dermatology. 3rd edition. London: Mosby; 2008. p. 369–77.
8. Rietschel RL, Fowler JF. The pathogenesis of allergic contact hypersensitivity. In: Rietschel RL, Fowler JF, editors. Fischer's contact dermatitis. 5th edition. Philadelphia: Lippincott Williams and Wilkins; 2001. p. 1–7, 175, 193–5, 203–10, 236.
9. Managing common vulvar skin conditions. The vulva is subject to a range of skin problems, many of them inadvertently self-inflicted. Harv Womens Health Watch 2008;16(3):3–5.
10. Utas S, Ferahbas A, Yildez S. Patients with vulval pruritis: patch test results. Contact Dermatitis 2008;58:296–8.
11. Lewis FM, Shah M, Gawkrodger DJ. Contact sensitivity in pruritus vulvae: patch test results and clinical outcome. Am J Contact Dermat 1997;8:137–40.
12. Lucke TW, Fleming CJ, McHenry P, et al. Patch testing in vulvar dermatoses: how relavent is nickel? Contact Dermatitis 1998;38:111.
13. Warner MR, Camisa C. Topical corticosteroids. In: Wolverton SE, editor. Comprehensive dermatologic drug therapy. 2nd edition. Philedelphia: Elsevier; 2007. p. 595–624.
14. Nyirjesy P, Weitz MV, Grody MH, et al. Over-the-counter and alternative medicines in the treatment of chronic vaginal symptoms. Obstet Gynecol 1997;90(1):50–3.
15. Sideri M, Origoni M, Spinaci L, et al. Topical testosterone in the treatment of vulvar lichen sclerosus. Int J Gynaecol Obstet 1994;46:53–6.
16. Bauters TG, Dhont MA, Temmerman MI, et al. Prevalence of vulvovaginal candidiasis and susceptibility to fluconazole in women. Am J Obstet Gynecol 2002;187(3):569–74.
17. Dennerstein GJ, Ellis DH. Oestrogen, glycogen and vaginal candidiasis. Aust N Z J Obstet Gynaecol 2001;41(3):326–8.
18. Sobel JD. Management of patients with recurrent vulvovaginal candidiasis. Drugs 2003;63(11): 1059–66.
19. Moyal-Barracco M, Edwards L. Diagnosis and therapy of anogenital lichen planus. Dermatol Ther 2004;17:38–46.
20. Tsuno N, Besset A, Ritchie K. Sleep and depression. J Clin Psychiatry 2005;66(10):1254–69.
21. Wirz-Justice A. Sleep deprivation in depression: what do we know, where do we go? Biol Psychiatry 1999;46(4):445–53.
22. Ohman EM, Rogers S, Meenan FO, et al. Adrenal suppresion following low-dose topical clobetasol propionate. J R Soc Med 1987;80:422–4.
23. Gonzalez-Moles MA, Scully C. Vesiculo-erosive oral mucosal disease-management with topical corticosteroids: 920 protocols, monitoring of effects and adverse reactions, and the future. J Dent Res 2005;84(4):302–8.
24. Pramick M. Cushing's syndrome caused by mucosal corticosteroid therapy. Int J Dermatol 2009;48(1): 100–1.
25. Neill SM, Tatnall FM, Cox NH. Guidelines for the management of lichen sclerosus. Br J Dermatol 2002;147(4):640–9.
26. Lagos BR, Maibach HI. Frequency of application of topical corticosteroids: an overview. Br J Dermatol 1998;139:763–6.
27. Pierard GE, Pierard-Franchimon C, Ben Mosbah T, et al. Adverse effects of topical corticostreroidd. Acta Derm Venereol Suppl (Stockh) 1989;69:26–30.
28. Fredriksson T, Lassus A, Bleeker J. Treatment of psoriasis and atopic dermatitis with halocinonide cream applied once and three times daily. Br J Dermatol 1980;102:575–7.
29. Anderson S, Kutzer S, Raymond HK. Treatment of vulvovaginal lichen planus with vaginal hydrocortisone suppositories. Obstet Gynecol 2002;100(2):359–62.
30. Sobel JD. Treatment of vulvovaginal lichen lanus with vaginal hydrocortisone suppositories. Curr Infect Dis Rep 2002;4(6):507–8.
31. Edwards L. Vaginitis. In: Black MM, Ambros-Rudolph C, Edwards L, et al, editors. Obstetric and gynecologic dermatology. 3rd edition. London: Mosby; 2008. p. 301–16.
32. Wolverton SE. Systemic corticosteroids. In: Wolverton SE, editor. Comprehensive dermatologic drug therapy. 2nd edition. Philedelphia: Elsevier; 2007. p. 127–61.
33. Goldstein AT, Thaci D, Luger T. Topical calcineurin inhibitors for the treatment of vulvar dermatoses. Eur J Obstet Gynecol Reprod Biol 2009;146(1): 22–9.
34. Lin AN. Topical calcineurin inhibitors. In: Wolverton SE, editor. Comprehensive dermatologic drug therapy. 2nd edition. Philedelphia: Elsevier; 2007. p. 672–89.

35. Kelekci HK, Uncu HG, Yilmaz B, et al. Pimecrolimus 1% cream for pruritus in postmenopausal diabetic women with vulvar lichen simplex chronicus: a prospective non-contolled case series. J Dermatolog Treat 2008;19(5):274–8.
36. Sarifakioglu E, Gumus II. Effciacy of topical pimecrolimus in the treatment of chronic vulvar pruritus: a prospective case series—a non-controlled, open-label study. J Dermatolog Treat 2006;17(5):276–8.
37. Lonsdale-Eccles AA, Velangi S. Topical pimecrolimus in the treatment of genital lichen planus: a prospective case series. Br J Dermatol 2005;153(2):390–4.
38. Volz T, Caroli U, Ludtke H. Pimecrolimus cream 1% in erosive oral genital lichen planus–a prospective randomized double-blind vehicle-controlled study. Br J Dermatol 2008;159(4):936–41.
39. Langeland T, Engh V. Topical use of tacrolimus and squamous cell carcinoma on the penis. Br J Dermatol 2005;152(1):183–5.
40. Bunker CB, Neill S, Staughton RC. Topical tacrolimus, genital lichen sclerosus, and risk of squamous cell carcinoma. Arch Dermatol 2004;140(9):1169.
41. Ormerod AD. Topical tacrolimus and pimecrolimus and the risk of cancer: how much cause for concern? Br J Dermatol 2005;153(4):701–5.
42. Cooper SM, Wojnarowska F. Anogenital (non-venereal) disease. In: Bolognia JL, Jorizzo JL, Rapini RP, editors. Dermatology. 2nd edition. Spain: Elsevier; 2008. p. 1059–74.
43. Edwards L. The diagnosis and treatment of infectious vaginitis. Dermatol Ther 2004;17:102–10.
44. Sobel JD, Chaim W, Nagappan V, et al. Treatment of vaginitis caused by *Candida glabrata*: use of topical boric acid and flucytosine. Am J Obstet Gynecol 2003;189(5):1297–300.
45. The Center for Disease Control and Prevention. Diseases characterized by vaginal discharge. Sexually transmitted diseases treatment guidelines 2006. The Center for Disease Control and Prevention. Available at: http://www.cdc.gov/std/treatment/2006/vaginal-discharge.htm#vagdis3. Accessed September 1, 2009.
46. Sobel JD, Weisenfel HC, Martens M, et al. Maintenance fluconazole therapy for recurrent vulvovaginal candidiasis. N Engl J Med 2004;351:876–83.
47. Ashourian N, Cohen PR. Systemic antibacterial agents. In: Wolverton SE, editor. Comprehensive dermatologic drug therapy. 2nd edition. Philedelphia: Elsevier; 2007. p. 39–74.
48. Murphy R, Edwards L. Desquamative inflammatory vaginitis: what is it? J Reprod Med 2008;53(2):124–8.
49. Murphy R. Desquamative inflammatory vaginitis. Dermatol Ther 2004;17(1):47–9.
50. Sobel JD. Desquamative inflammatory vaginitis: a new subgroup of purulent vaginitis responsive to topical 2% clindamycin therapy. Am J Obstet Gynecol 1994;171(5):1215–20.
51. Milstone EB, McDonald AJ, Scholhamer CF. Pseudomembranous colitis after topical application of clindamycin. Arch Dermatol 1981;117(3):154–5.
52. Wetter D, Davis M, Yiannias J, et al. Patch test results from the Mayo Clinic Contact Dermatitis Group, 1998–2000. J Am Acad Dermatol 2005;53 (3):416–21.
53. Suckling JA, Kennedy R, Lethaby A, et-al. Local oestrogen for vaginal atrophy in postmenopausal women. Cochrane Database Syst Rev 2006;2:CD001500.
54. Rioux JE, Devlin C, Gelfand M, et al. 17(beta)-estradiol vaginal tablet versus conjugated equine estrogen vaginal cream to relieve menopausal atrophic vaginitis. Menopause 2000;7(3):156–61.
55. Poleshuck EL, Bair MJ, Kurt Kroenke K, et al. Pain and depression in gynecology patients. Psychosomatics 2009;50:270–6.
56. Edwards L. New concepts in vulvodynia. Am J Obstet Gynecol 2003;189(3S):S24–9.
57. Glazer HI. Dysesthetic vulvodynia. Long term follow-up after treatment with surface electromyomgraphy-assisted pelvic floor muscle rehabilitation. J Reprod Med 2000;45(10):798–802.
58. Khan AM, Freeman-Wang T, Pisal N, et al. Smoking and multicentric vulval intraepithelial neoplasia. J Obstet Gynaecol 2009;29(2):123–5.
59. Feldman S, Camacho F, Krejci-Manwaring J, et al. Adherence to topical therapy increases around the time of office visits. J Am Acad Dermatol 2007;57(1):81–3.
60. Hodari KT, Nanton JR, Carroll CL, et al. Adherence in dermatology: a review of the last 20 years. J Dermatolog Treat 2006;17(3):133–5.

A Histologic Review of Vulvar Inflammatory Dermatoses and Intraepithelial Neoplasm

Maria Angelica Selim, MD[a,*], Mai P. Hoang, MD[b]

KEYWORDS

• Vulva • External genitalia • Dermatitis • VIN
• ISSVD classification

Currently, urogenital complaints are among the most common problems encountered by family practitioners, gynecologists, and dermatologists.[1,2] When a patient suffering from a vulvar disorder presents to the health care system, there are 3 elements to be considered: (1) the patient's sociocultural background that affects how she perceives the disease often leading to delay in seeking care or self-treatment, (2) the clinical presentation of the disease, and (3) the clinical setting of this evaluation, as there is not a single medical specialist trained to care for the spectrum of diseases occurring in this anatomic location.

In response to the intricacy of vulvar disorders, the International Society for the Study of Vulvovaginal Disease (ISSVD) was created to facilitate the exchange between clinicians and pathologists involved in the care of these patients. Often, the "diagnosis" on a biopsy result is not the name of a disease, but rather a description of the microscopic findings. For the average clinician, this is sometimes unhelpful. In an attempt to allow the clinician to benefit from a nondiagnostic biopsy, the ISSVD recently developed a histologic classification of inflammatory vulvar disorders that allows for the generation of a differential diagnosis based on microscopic findings (**Table 1**). This can be extremely useful when correlated with a clinical differential diagnosis. The ISSVD has also proposed a clinically relevant histologic classification for vulvar intraepithelial neoplasia (VIN) (**Table 2**).[3,4]

This article uses the multidisciplinary approach proposed by ISSVD. After a brief review of the embryology and anatomy of the vulva, various biopsy techniques are discussed. The latter act as a preamble to a review of the histology of vulvar inflammatory dermatoses and intraepithelial neoplasm.

VULVAR EMBRYOLOGY AND ANATOMY

Until the 12th week of gestation, the external genitalia of both sexes are indistinguishable, also called undifferentiated stage. However, the formation of the external genitalia is the end result of events that begin during embryonic week 4 in the mesodermal structure lateroventral to the cloacal plate. Immediately ventral to the plate, the genital tubercle is formed by 2 paired elevations of the ectoderm. The genital tubercle evolves into the clitoris. Directly lateral to the cloacal plate, the same process forms 2 parallel urogenital folds.

[a] Dermatopathology Unit, Department of Pathology, Duke University Medical Center, PO Box 3712, Durham, NC 27710, USA
[b] Dermatopathology Unit, Department of Pathology, Massachusetts General Hospital, Harvard Medical School, 55 Fruit Street, Warren 820, Boston, MA 02114, USA
* Corresponding author.
E-mail address: selim001@mc.duke.edu

Dermatol Clin 28 (2010) 649–667
doi:10.1016/j.det.2010.07.005

Table 1
Modified version of the 2006 ISSVD classification of vulvar dermatoses: pathologic subsets and their clinical correlates

Spongiotic pattern	Eczematous dermatitis (atopic, contact, and allergic)
Acanthotic pattern	Lichen simplex chronicus (primary and secondary) Psoriasis Reiter's syndrome
Lichenoid pattern	Lichen sclerosus Lichen planus
Dermal sclerosis pattern	Lichen sclerosus
Vesiculobullous pattern	Bullous pemphigoid Cicatricial pemphigoid Pemphigoid gestationis Pemphigus vulgaris Pemphigo vegetans
Acantholytic pattern	Hailey-Hailey disease Darier's disease Acantholytic dermatosis of the vulvocrural area
Granulomatous pattern	Crohn's disease Melkersson-Rosenthal syndrome
Vasculopathic pattern	Aphthous ulcers Behcet's disease Plasma cell vulvitis

Data from Lynch PJ. 2006 International Society for the Study of Vulvovaginal Disease classification of vulvar dermatoses: a synopsis. J Low Genit Tract Dis 2007; 11(1):1–2; and Lynch PJ, Moyal-Barracco M, Bogliatto F, et al. 2006 ISSVD classification of vulvar dermatoses: pathologic subsets and their clinical correlates. J Reprod Med 2007;52(1):3–9,110.

Table 2
Old and new classification of VIN lesions

Old Classification	New Classification
VIN I	No cancer precursor
(Classic) VIN II/III	Usual VIN (uVIN) Warty VIN Basaloid VIN Mixted (warty-basaloid)
(Well-) differentiated VIN III/VIN simplex	Differentiated VIN (dVIN)

Abbreviation: VIN, vulvar intraepithelial neoplasia.

The medial urogenital fold will become the labia minora, the more lateral urogenital fold becomes the labia majora. The urogenital sinus, into which the vagina opens, enlarges and becomes the vestibule of the external genitalia lined by endodermal epithelium.

The vulva lies within the anterior perineal triangle limited anteriorly by the mons pubis and posteriorly by the perineum, whereas the crural folds and hymen\hymeneal ring represent the lateral and medial limits respectively. The labia majora, the most external structures of the vulva, are 2 thick skin folds that are fused anteriorly to form the mons pubis and blend posteriorly in the perineum. They are derived from ectodermal tissue. The lateral aspect is covered by dry keratinized hair-bearing skin with sweat glands and the medial aspect by a moist partially keratinized modified mucous membrane. Medial to the labia majora are the labia minora, 2 thin-pigmented skin folds. They anteriorly fuse around the clitoris forming the prepuce above and frenulum below and they posteriorly fuse leading to the formation of the fourchette. Modified mucous membrane covers the labia minora with numerous apocrine glands; prominent ectopic sebaceous glands can be seen especially in the medial aspect of these skin folds. The Hart's line is located at the base of the medial aspect of the labia minora, limited between the modified mucosa of the labia minora and the mucosa surface of the vestibule. The vestibule, the innermost portion of the vulva, extends from the Hart's line to the hymen. Multiple structures open to this space, including the urethra and Skene glands (paraurethral glands lateral to the urethra) in the anterior portion of the vestibule and the Bartholin glands or major mucus-producing vestibular glands in the posterior lateral aspect, at the 5 and 7 o'clock positions.

DIAGNOSTIC PROCEDURE: THE BIOPSY

The evaluation of a patient starts with a thorough clinical history and careful physical examination. During this process, a differential diagnosis is created, and the confirmation or elimination of potential diagnoses may rely on tests that can be performed in the physician's office. One of such procedures is a tissue biopsy. To help the pathologist specifically address the patient's major diagnostic dilemmas, a series of considerations need to be addressed before performing the actual procedure. First, consider the type of lesion or extent of the process to ensure the correct selection of the biopsy procedure: shave versus punch or excisional biopsy. Second, take into account the purpose of the biopsy—histologic analysis, microbiology culture, or direct immunofluorescence tests, to determine the type of fixative in which one needs to transfer the specimen. And third, write a thorough clinical history including questions on the requisition form submitted with the specimen. The latter will empower the pathologist to render the best interpretation.

The choices of biopsy techniques include shave biopsy or snip with curved iris scissors, punch biopsy, and excisional biopsy. If the suspected disease involves the epidermis/mucosa and superficial dermis/submucosa (eg, contact dermatitis, lichen planus) or it is a polypoid lesion, a shave biopsy or snip with curved iris scissors may be selected. Pigmented lesions should not be sampled with these procedures because the base of the lesion is the key in defining the biologic potential of the melanocytic proliferation and it is frequently not represented in a shave. The classical shave biopsy, predominantly performed on lesions on the dry hair-bearing skin, is performed by gently pinching the skin with fingers into a tense fold and then shaving the lesion with a number 15 scalpel blade or razor blade. The sample should be obtained with a cut parallel to the surface with a depth into but not through the dermis. One advantage of the shave biopsy is a rapid and good cosmetic result, without the need of sutures. There are, on the other hand, disadvantages to be considered, including scar if the biopsy was performed too deep and the possibility that a deeper process can be missed. A technical variation of the shave biopsy is the snip by curved iris scissors. This procedure renders excellent results when the lesion is in extremely thin non–hair-bearing skin that cannot be easily held for a shave biopsy. The procedure consists of tenting the skin with a 5-0 or 6-0 suture, and, when the suture lifts the skin, cutting through the base with a curved iris scissor.

A punch biopsy samples epidermis/squamous epithelium, dermis/submucosal, and subcutaneous tissue. This technique should be selected to sample tumors, ulcers, inflammations with deep components that extend to the subcutis or deep submucosal, and some pigmented lesions. The biopsy is obtained by twisting the punch instrument up to the hub. The sample that remains attached at the base should be carefully lifted with forceps or a needle to avoid producing crush artifact, and then cut at the base with scissors. Sutures are used to close the defect depending on the size of the punch instrument. The advantage of a punch biopsy is the possibility to sample deeper tissue with good cosmetic and quick healing when sutured. The disadvantages include the limited size of the sample and its depth, which is limited to the length of the cylinder.

An incisional biopsy includes the entire skin up to the subcutaneous tissue. It is the preferred procedure when large-vessel vasculitis and panniculitis are in the differential diagnosis. An excisional biopsy should be entertained to remove pigmented lesions that are highly concerning for malignant melanoma.

After choosing the type of biopsy, selecting the area to sample is of paramount importance for the diagnosis. If the patient has an ulcer, the biopsy should be taken from the border of the lesion/edge of the ulcer and not in the necrotic center. If the biopsy is part of the workup of a blistering disorder, 2 punch biopsies should be performed: one at the edge of the blister for histologic examination and a second biopsy at nonaffected perilesional skin for direct immunofluorescence studies. A third punch biopsy can also be performed in structural disorders leading to blistering disease for electron microscopy.

Selecting the transportation medium is another important step. If a biopsy is performed for routine histology examination, the sample should be fixed in formalin in a 1:10 ratio (tissue:formalin). If a biopsy is done for direct immunofluorescence, molecular studies for gene rearrangement when lymphoma is in the differential diagnosis, or cultures, then saline-soaked gauze without preservatives is the transport of excellence with prompt delivery of the tissue to the laboratory. Michelle/Zeus media and glutaraldehyde fixative are used to preserve tissue for direct immunofluorescence studies and electron microscopy, respectively.

VULVAR DERMATITIS

The classification of histologic patterns of vulvar diseases was intended to be used as an aid to the differential diagnosis of these disorders.

Spongiotic Pattern

Eczematous dermatitis is a common condition that can affect the vulva of all ages.[5–10] The clinical determination of underlying causes can be difficult and the histologic features are similar regardless of the underlying etiology; thus, clinical pathologic correlation is essential.[9] Irritant contact dermatitis and allergic contact dermatitis are the 2 common forms of exogenous dermatitis seen in the vulva. An allergic type is a cell-mediated response to sensitizing agents such as nickel or rubber and the irritant type is related to exposure to chemical or physical agents.

The clinical feature is erythematous papules and plaques associated with pruritus, dryness, or burning (**Fig. 1**).[5] There can be pain and dyspareunia.[6] A superficial scale crust is frequently seen. Irritant contact dermatitis is more common than allergic contact dermatitis. It develops within minutes to hours and is typically localized to the area of exposure.[11] Patients with atopic dermatitis are more likely to develop allergic contact dermatitis.[12] Rubbing and scratching in response to pruritus result in superimposed changes of lichen simplex chronicus.

Histopathologically, eczematous dermatitis is characterized by intercellular edema or spongiosis within the epidermis and a dermal infiltrate of lymphocytes and occasional eosinophils (**Fig. 2**). Intraepidermal vesicles can be seen in the acute phase. Mild hyperkeratosis is seen in the subacute phase. Epidermal hyperplasia and minimal spongiosis are seen in the chronic phase. When acute inflammation is seen within the stratum corneum, periodic acid-Schiff (PAS) and tissue Gram stains should be performed to exclude fungal and bacterial infection, respectively.

Atopic dermatitis

Atopic dermatitis, the most common form of endogenous dermatitis, is a chronic dermatitis that affects individuals with a personal or family history of atopic diathesis (eczema, asthma, allergic seasonal rhinitis). The disease typically begins in childhood with decreased frequency with age. Vulvar involvement can be seen in women with atopic dermatitis.[13] Dryness and scaliness may be the only signs. Superimposed changes of lichen simplex chronicus, such as lichenification and excoriations, can be seen.

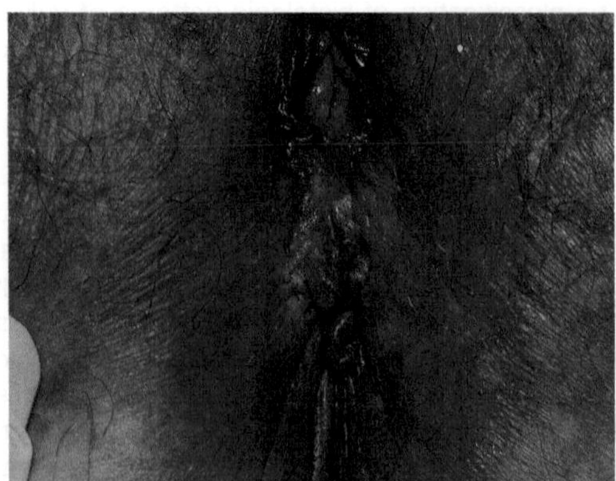

Fig. 1. Red, edematous, excoriated plaques of eczematous dermatitis are characteristic of localized atopic dermatitis and contact dermatitis. (*Courtesy of* Libby Edwards, MD, Charlotte, NC.)

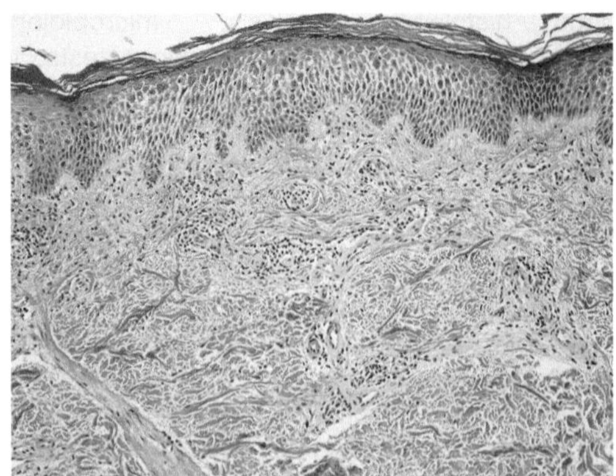

Fig. 2. Hyperkeratosis, epidermal spongiosis, and superficial dermal inflammatory infiltrate are characteristics of a subacute spongiotic dermatitis (hematoxylin-eosin, original magnification ×100). (*Courtesy of* Mai P. Hoang, MD, Boston, MA.)

The histologic findings can be nonspecific, namely epidermal hyperplasia and focal spongiosis. Mast cells and eosinophils may be identified within the superficial dermis.

Acanthotic Pattern

Lichen simplex chronicus

Lichen simplex chronicus denotes a characteristic skin response of repeated rubbing and/or scratching that often involves the vulva.[14,15] Lichen simplex chronicus often presents as thickened and erythematous scaly plaques. Associated excoriation and hyperpigmentation are often seen. The lesion is usually solitary and often affects the labia majorus. A biopsy is not necessary for lichen simplex chronicus. Histologically, it is characterized by hyperkeratosis, epidermal acanthosis, hypergranulosis, and superficial dermal fibrosis. The coarse, vertically oriented superficial dermal collagen bundles are less prominent in the vulva.[15]

Psoriasis

Psoriasis is a multifactorial chronic relapsing dermatosis diagnosed in about 5% of women presenting to a dermatologist with persistent vulvar symptoms. The classical clinical presentation consists of well-demarcated red to salmon-colored plaques with silver scale present in the extensor surfaces of the extremities, sacral region, and scalp (**Fig. 3**). When the vulva and perineum are involved, they usually are associated with classic lesions in other parts of the body. Trauma, infection, and drugs can trigger psoriasis; this event is also known as Koebner phenomenon. The latter occurs in a fifth of the patients, and the involvement of the vulva exposed to friction may

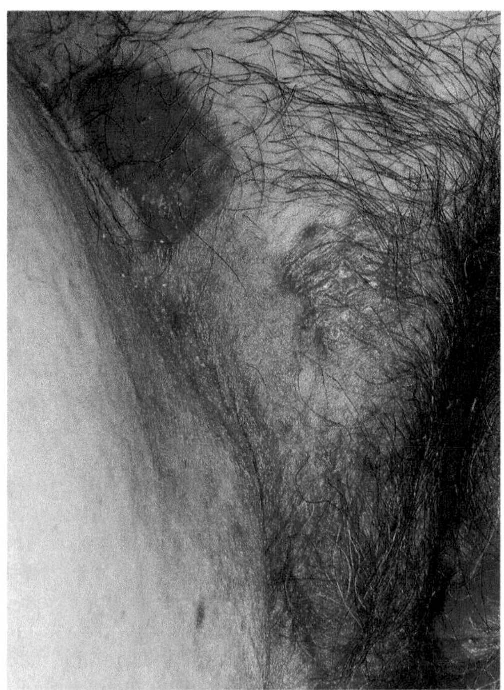

Fig. 3. Well demarcated, thickened, scaling, red plaques are classic for psoriasis and correlate with the microscopic picture of acanthosis. (*Courtesy of* Libby Edwards, MD, Charlotte, NC.)

partially reflect this phenomenon. Psoriasis in external genitalia has a predilection for hair-bearing areas like mons pubis and labia majora. When the flexural folds and anogenital region are affected, also known as inverse psoriasis, the lesions present as well-demarcated, thin erythematous plaques without significant scale owing to the moisture in the region.[16] These lesions can be differentiated from eczema, especially seborrheic dermatitis, because of the intense erythema and the well-demarcated borders; however, cases with overlapping features can be encountered and they are called "sebopsoriasis." Painful intergluteal and perianal fissuring are complications with high morbidity. Commonly, the diagnosis is established when typical lesions are detected in other parts of the body. Other helpful diagnostic clues seen in 30% of patients with psoriasis consist of nail involvement in the form of pitting, "oil drop spots" (red-brownish discoloration of the nail plate), or onycholysis (nail bed psoriasis leading to lifting of the nail plate).

The histologic changes of psoriasis evolve over time.[17,18] Dilatation of superficial dermal blood vessels is the earliest histologic change. Parakeratosis and epidermal hyperplasia develop over time. Lesions in hair-bearing skin show characteristic features of a fully developed psoriatic lesion, such as (1) stratum corneum with confluent parakeratosis with collection of neutrophils (Munros microabscesses); (2) epidermal psoriasiform hyperplasia with evenly elongated rete ridges associated with hypogranulosis, Kogoj microabscesses (collection of neutrophils in epidermis), mitotic activity, and thinning of the surprapapillary plate; and (3) papillary dermis with tortuous vessels associated with perivascular lymphocytic and neutrophilic infiltrate (**Fig. 4**). Lesions in non–hair-bearing skin have reduced parakeratotic surface and more spongiosis. Coexistence of infections (eg, staphylococcal infection or candida), contact dermatitis (owing to application of creams, disinfectants, and so forth), or lichen simplex chronicus secondary to scratching may affect the histologic presentation.

Reiter syndrome

Reiter syndrome is a seronegative spondyloarthropathy with cutaneous erythematous plaques that occur following a bacterial infection. Two types of infection that predispose to Reiter syndrome are "endemic" and "epidemic."[19] The endemic type is often caused by *Chlamydia trachomatis*.[19] The epidemic type often follows outbreaks of enteric infections including *Shigella dysenteriae*, *Salmonella typimurium*, or *Yersinia enterolitica*.[19]

Vulvar involvement is rare and preferentially occurs in women with HIV infection.[20,21] The cutaneous lesions of Reiter syndrome or "keratoderma blennorrhagicum" begin as small erythematous macules that coalesce to form plaques with overlying scale-crust. These lesions resemble vulvar

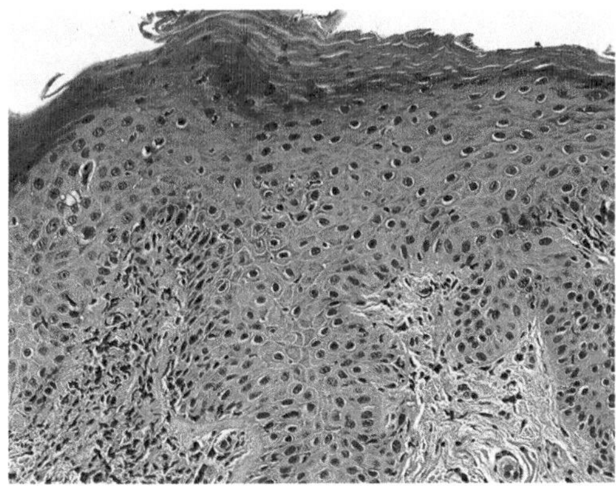

Fig. 4. In a case of inverse psoriasis, focal hypogranulosis with overlying parakeratosis containing neutrophils are noted (hematoxylin-eosin, original magnification ×200). (*Courtesy of* Mai P. Hoang, MD, Boston, MA.)

pustular psoriasis clinically.[20] Ulceration can be seen.[22] The histologic appearance is identical to that of psoriasis.

Lichenoid Pattern

Lichen sclerosus

Lichen sclerosus is a common chronic dermatosis involving the vulva. Although the etiology of lichen sclerosus is not known, autoimmunity and infectious and environmental etiologies have been implicated.[23,24] The term "lichen sclerosus" is now the preferred term and the suffix "et atrophicus" is no longer used.[25] It is occasionally associated with VIN of the differentiated type and squamous cell carcinoma.[26]

The clinical lesions of lichen sclerosus are typically white, scaly plaques with wrinkled or thinned appearance (**Fig. 5**). They are often symmetric and affect the labia minora, clitoris, prepuce, frenulum, perineal body, and vulvar vestibule. Other body regions such as the arms or trunk can be involved in approximately 20% of cases.[25] Superimposed changes of lichen simplex chronicus are often present owing to the intense pruritic nature of this lesion. Lichen sclerosus has a bimodal peak incidence affecting prepubertal girls and menopausal women.[25] Lichen sclerosus has a relapsing and remitting course with poor correlation between signs and symptoms.[24] The symptoms include dysuria, painful defecation, and rectal bleeding and may be mistaken as evidence of sexual abuse.[27] Of note, childhood lichen sclerosus and sexual abuse are not mutually exclusive: in a series of 42 cases of prepubertal lichen sclerosus, 28% presented with evidence of sexual abuse.[27]

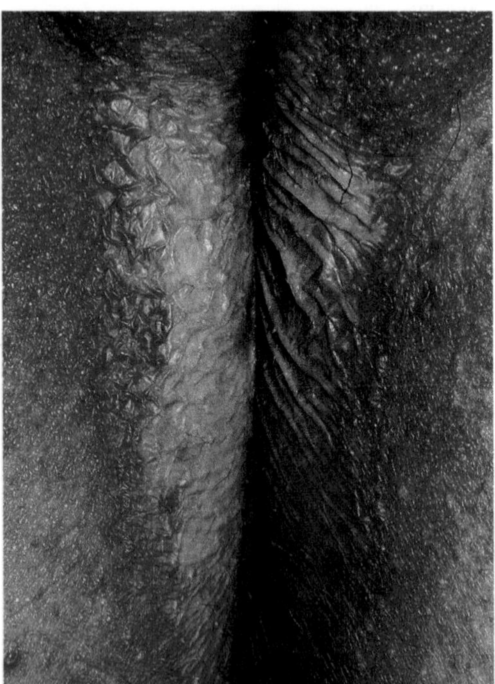

Fig. 5. A well-demarcated, hypopigmented, crinkled plaque is typical for lichen sclerosus. (*Courtesy of* Libby Edwards, MD, Charlotte, NC.)

The histologic appearance of lichen sclerosus is dependent on the age of the lesion and where the biopsy is taken. The early histologic features may be basal vacuolar alteration of the epidermis and occasional necrotic keratinocytes, or a bandlike infiltrate of lymphocytes and histiocytes in the superficial dermis, often mistaken as lichenoid dermatitis, such as lichen planus (**Fig. 6**A). The more established lesions show atrophic epidermis, superficial dermal edema, and/or sclerotic or hyalinized dermal collagen bundles. An inflammatory dermal infiltrate is seen below this superficial area of sclerosis (**Fig. 6**B). Often, parakeratosis and epidermal hyperplasia, changes of superimposed lichen simplex chronicus, are present as well. The histologic differential diagnosis of lichen sclerosus includes lichen planus and radiation dermatitis.

Lichen planus

Lichen planus is a chronic cell-mediated immune reaction affecting skin and mucous membranes. Although the physiopathology of this disease is not completely understood, altered antigen in basal keratinocytes triggered by viruses, drugs, or allogeneic cells may play a role in its development. Lichen planus presents with a wide range of clinical presentations: hypertrophic, atrophic, actinic, linear, zosteriform, erosive, and bullous types.[2,28–30] Half of the women affected by this papulosquamous disease have genital involvement. The disorder may persist for 1 to 2 years; however, the mucosal involvement may last longer. Hyperpigmentation is a common sequela, especially in African American patients. Lichen planus has been associated with immunodeficiency states, malignancies, cirrhosis, peptic ulcer, hepatitis C, hepatitis B, and ulcerative colitis, among others.

Clinically, vulvar lichen planus can take many forms, which creates frequent delays in the diagnosis. The genital lesions can be cutaneous, mucosal, or combined. Overwhelmingly, morphology on vulvovaginal surfaces is the erosive form, occurring only on the mucous membranes and modified mucous membranes. The cutaneous pattern has 2 presentations: the first form is the genital involvement as part of generalized cutaneous lichen planus and the second type is hypertrophic lichen planus. The

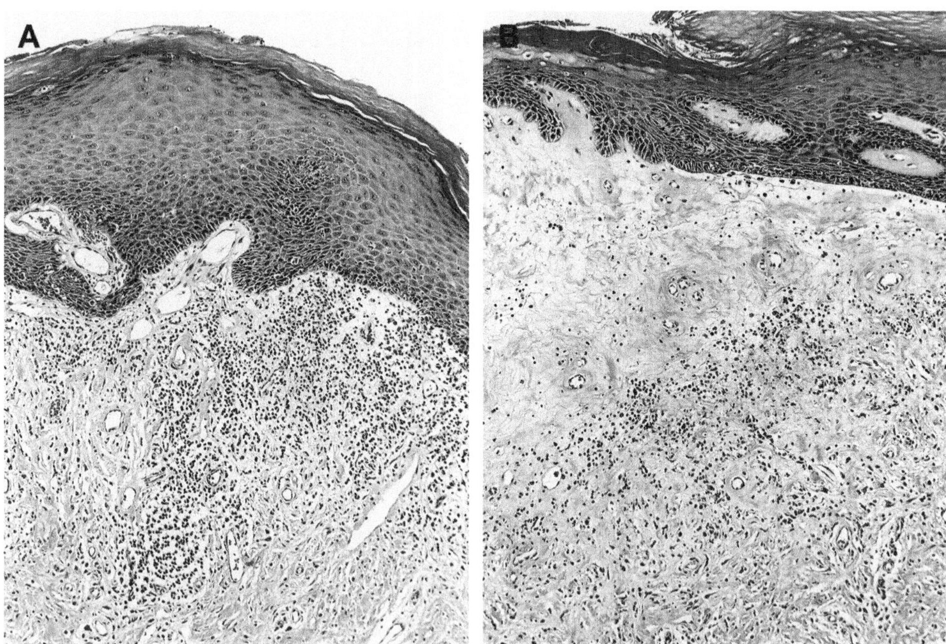

Fig. 6. (*A*) The early histologic features of lichen sclerosus are basal vacuolar alteration of the epidermis and occasional necrotic keratinocytes, and a bandlike infiltrate of lymphocytes and histocytes in the superficial dermis (hematoxylin-eosin, original magnification ×200). (*B*) The more established lesions show atrophic epidermis, superficial dermal edema, and/or sclerotic or hyalinized dermal collagen bundles. An inflammatory dermal infiltrate is seen below this superficial area of sclerosis (hematoxylin-eosin, original magnification ×100). (*Courtesy of* Maria Angelica Selim, MD.)

clinical lesions of the first group are well demarcated, erythematous to violaceous, flat-topped papules and plaques without scale involving labia minora and majora as well as mons pubis. No scar is formed when the lesions resolve. Surface changes may include fine white lines in oral lesions also known as Wickham striae. Hypertrophic lichen planus presents as hyperkeratotic white plaques. Although uncommon, it can be confused with a malignancy. Cutaneous lichen planus is frequently itchy, leading to superimposed lichen simplex chronicus and secondary infections that may mask the characteristic clinical and histologic findings. Mucosal lichen planus, like the cutaneous counterpart, has 2 types of presentations: reticulated and erosive lichen planus (**Fig. 7**).[31] Reticulated lichen planus acquired its name from the white lines running across an erythematous surface in the non–hair-bearing labial surface, similar to the changes seen in oral lichen planus. The erosive variant presents with bright red and eroded epithelium surrounded by reticulated white lacy plaques.[32] This is a very symptomatic lesion producing soreness, postcoital bleeding, dysuria, and dyspareunia. Over time, the scarring forms result in labial atrophy, clitoral phimosis, and narrowing of the introitus, ending in effacement of the normal anatomy of the vulva. The erosive lesions can affect the vagina and produce shortening or narrowing of this region. Erosive lichen planus is often indistinguishable from other erosive or bullous diseases such as cicatricial pemphigoid and pemphigus vulgaris, so that the reticulate oral lesions may be diagnostically helpful. The presence of lichen planus involving the oral-vaginal-vulvar mucosae is known as the vulvovaginal gingival syndrome.[33]

Histologic features characteristic of lichen planus include the presence of basal layer hydropic degeneration with Civatte body formation, a bandlike (lichenoid) infiltrate in the upper dermis by lymphocytes (**Fig. 8**A) with admixed plasma cells in mucosal lichen planus (**Fig. 8**B), and pigment incontinence (macrophages containing phagocytosed melanin). Step sections may be required to reach a final diagnosis because of the patchy nature of the changes and the superimposed secondary changes like lichen simplex chronicus and infections. Additional biopsies with multiple steps may be needed in the erosive presentation of lichen planus because of the extensive loss of epithelium. Accurate diagnosis is seminal, as erosive lichen planus can be treated with immunosuppressive therapy and the presence of chronic lichen planus in vulva is associated with a risk of developing squamous cell carcinoma.[34–36] Lichen

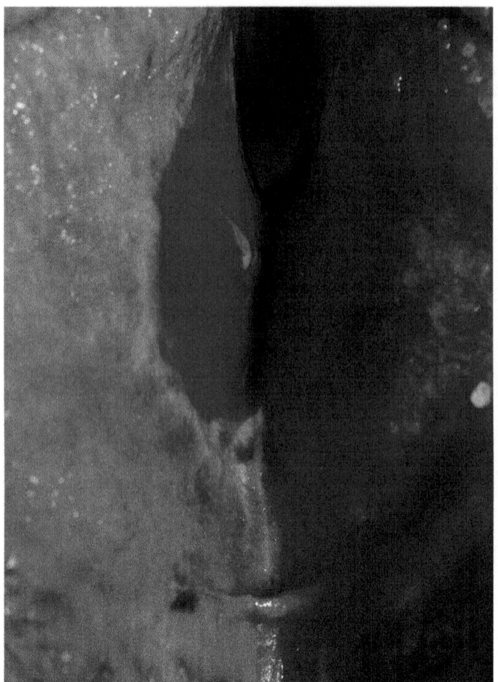

Fig. 7. Vestibular erosion is the most common presentation of vulvar lichen planus; the surrounding, irregular, and coalescing white linear papules are less common but classic and pathognomonic. (*Courtesy of* Libby Edwards, MD, Charlotte, NC.)

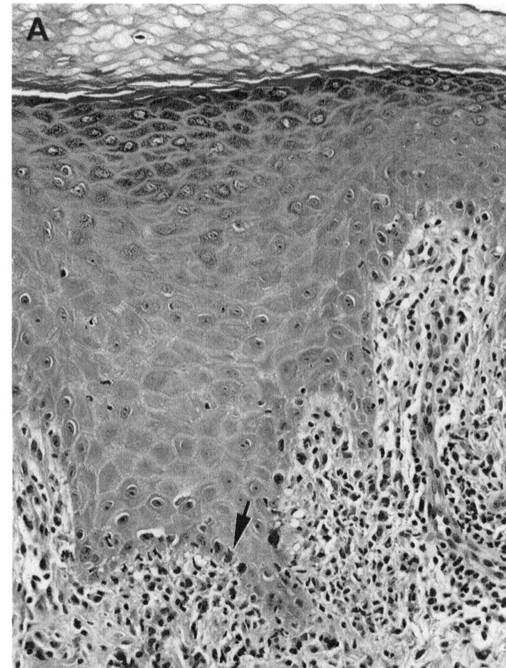

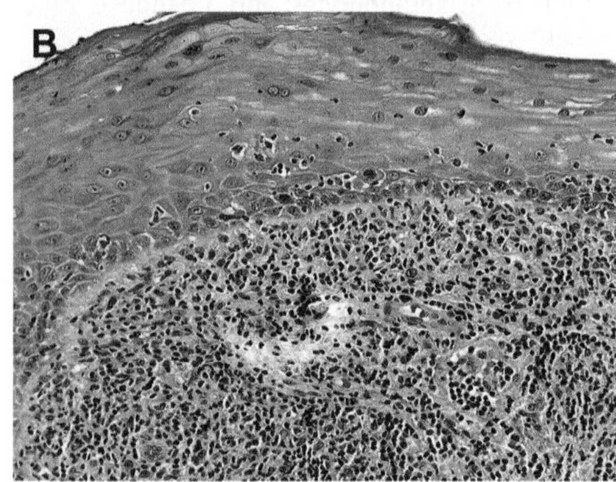

Fig. 8. (*A*) Hyperkeratosis, hypergranulosis, and vacuolar changes of the basal layer associated with Civatte bodies (*arrow*) is characteristic of lichen planus affecting hair-bearing skin (hematoxylin-eosin, original magnification ×200). (*B*) Mucosal lichen planus have similar histologic features with the characteristic plasma cells associated with lymphocytes in the inflammatory reaction (hematoxylin-eosin, original magnification ×200). (*Courtesy of* Maria Angelica Selim, MD.)

planus–like drug reaction may mimic the idiopathic type; however, eosinophils in the infiltrate would favor a drug reaction.

Vesiculobullous Pattern

Although essentially any bullous dermatosis can involve the vulva, the entities described in the following sections may be the first to be observed and biopsied by the gynecologist (see **Table 1**).[3,4] Definitive diagnosis of most bullous diseases requires clinicopathologic correlation.

Bullous and cicatricial pemphigoid

Bullous and cicatricial pemphigoid are subepidermal autoimmune bullous disorders. Although cicatricial pemphigoid is associated with scarring and mucosal involvement, bullous pemphigoid is not. Both are caused by autoantibodies against components of hemidesmosome and type VII collagen, resulting in damage of the basement membrane and subsequent loss of adhesion between the dermis and epidermis.[37] However, both can be the result of a drug hypersensitivity reaction.[38]

The lesions of bullous pemphigoid present initially as tense blisters on erythematous base on dry, keratinized skin, and without Nikolsky sign (detachment of the superficial epidermis from the underlying dermis when the examining finger is slid over the skin surface). Erythema and urticarial lesions can be prodromal changes. Trunk, groin, and flexural areas are commonly affected sites.[39,40]

Cicatricial pemphigoid has a predilection for mucosal sites such as conjunctivae and oral mucosa. The clinical lesions are similar to those of bullous pemphigoid on keratinzed surfaces, with the exception of associated scarring.[41,42] Nikolsky sign is seen. Cicatricial pemphigoid more commonly involves the modified mucous membranes and membranes of the vulva than bullous pemphigoid,[43] where lesions generally appear erosive rather than bullous, as the blisters quickly rupture on this thin and fragile skin (**Fig. 9**).

In both types of pemphigoid, the histology is characterized by a subepidermal vesiculation containing a variable numbers of eosinophils and neutrophils (**Fig. 10**A). Subepithelial scarring is seen in cicatricial pemphigoid. Direct immunofluorescence studies usually demonstrate a linear IgG (**Fig. 10**B) and C3 deposition at the basement membrane zone. Deposition of IgA and/or IgM may or may not be present.[44] Indirect immunofluorescence studies performed on salt split skin usually demonstrate that autoantibodies from the patient's serum are associated with the roof or epidermal side of the blister. Serum autoantibodies to the 230-kD BPAg1 and 180-kD BPAg2 can be demonstrated by immunoblotting, but this is usually not necessary.[45]

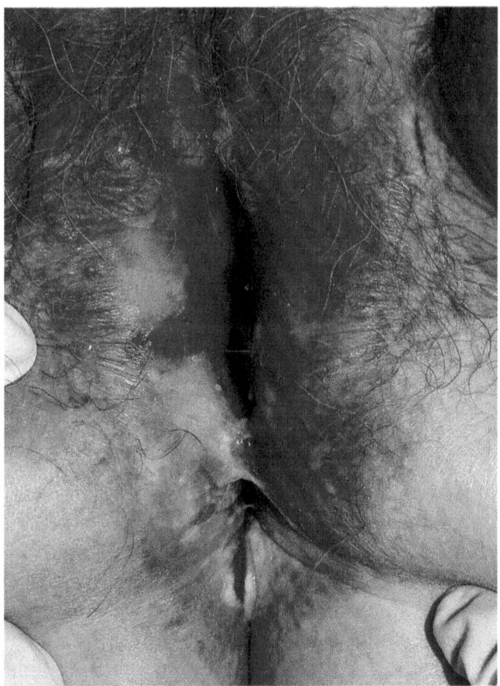

Fig. 9. Mucous membrane erosions with surrounding white epithelium and loss of vulvar architecture is typical but nonspecific for cicatricial pemphigoid, as well as for lichen planus and pemphigus vulgaris. (*Courtesy of* Libby Edwards, MD, Charlotte, NC.)

Pemphigus vulgaris and pemphigus vegetans

Pemphigus vulgaris, a rare acquired immunobullous disorder, is caused by autoantibodies against desmoglein 3, a 130-kD glycoprotein that is a component of desmosome.[46] Patients often present with painful mucosal erosions and/or flaccid bullae involving the mouth, nasal, or anogenital mucosa. Nikolsky sign is present. Vulvar involvement by pemphigus vulgaris typically present as erosions that can resolve with scarring.[47] In the pemphigus vegetans variant, hypertrophic or warty vegetations develop in association with the bullae. The localized and self-limited character of pemphigus vegetans distinguishes it from pemphigus vulgaris.

In pemphigus vulgaris, acantholysis results in intraepidermal blister with basilar cells aligned at the floor of the blister resembling a row of "tombstones." In addition to the mentioned histologic features, verrucous epidermal hyperplasia, intraepidermal eosinophilic microabscesses, and dermal infiltrate of lymphocytes and eosinophils are also seen in pemphigus vegetans.[48] In both pemphigus vulgaris and pemphigus vegetans, epidermal and intercellular IgG and C3 depositions are seen on direct immunofluorescence studies. Circulating autoantibodies to epidermal intercellular spaces can be detected with an indirect immunofluorescent method against monkey esophageal epithelium; and the titer correlates with the clinical activity of the disease. Although Hailey-Hailey disease, Darier disease, and acantholysis of the vulvocrural area are in the histologic differential for pemphigus, the direct immunofluorescence studies of these cases are negative.

Pemphigoid gestationis

Herpes gestationis is a vesiculobullous disease seen in pregnancy and with a strong association with HLA-DR3 and -DR4.[49] The autoantibodies bind to 180-kDa hemidesmosome antigen (BPAg2).[49]

The initial presentation, usually in the second trimester, includes severe pruritus and macular erythematous rash that leads to blistering and superficial ulcerations. The keratinzed surfaces of the vulva and pubic area may be involved in addition to the trunk and upper thigh. Spontaneous resolution follows soon after delivery, although it may occur during the late third trimester.

Histologic features include a subepidermal vesiculation and superficial dermal infiltrate of lymphocytes and eosinophils. Direct immunofluorescence studies demonstrate linear C3 deposition at the basement membrane zone. The main differential diagnosis is bullous pemphigoid, which is not associated with pregnancy.

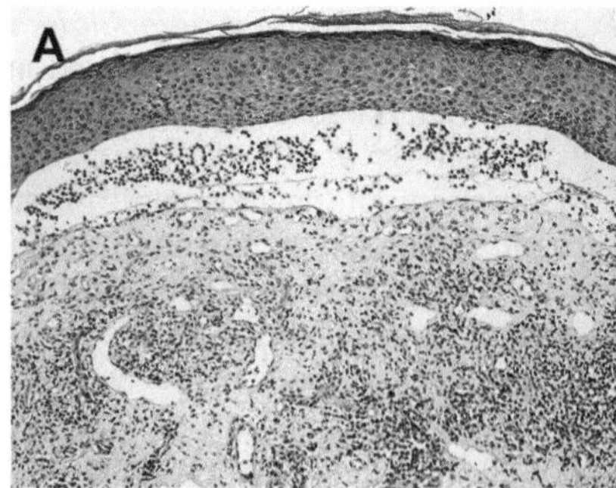

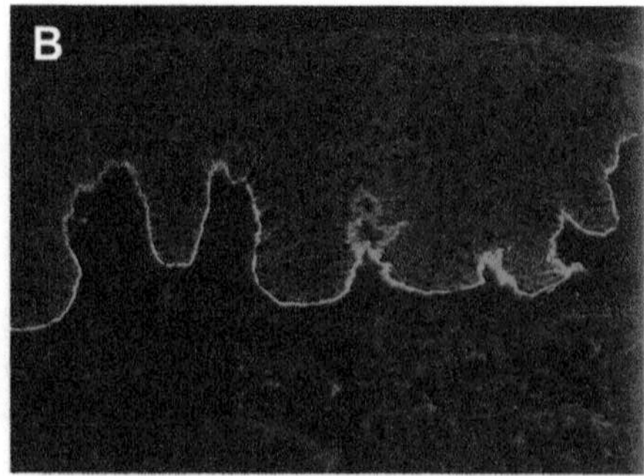

Fig. 10. (*A*) A subepidermal blister filled with numerous eosinophils is seen in a case of bullous pemphigoid (hematoxylin-eosin, original magnification ×100). (*B*) Direct immunofluorescence examination reveals strong linear IgG deposition at the basement membrane zone. (*Courtesy of* Mai P. Hoang, MD, Boston, MA.)

Linear IgA disease

The disease presents as clusters of annular lesions or "clusters of jewels" on lower abdomen, pelvic, inguinal, and genital areas. They are usually pruritic and become ulcerated and crusted within 24 hours. The eruption can be preceded by a bacterial or viral infection[50,51] or it is drug induced, often by vancomycin.[52]

A subepidermal blister containing neutrophils is seen. Direct immunofluorescence examination demonstrates a linear IgA deposition at the basement membrane zone. The antigen is a 97-kDa molecule, identical to the carboxyl terminal of 180-kDa (BPAg2), located at the basement membrane.[53]

Erythema multiforme (and blistering forms of Stevens-Johnson syndrome and toxic epidermal necrolysis)

Vulvar involvement has been reported in association with Stevens-Johnson syndrome and toxic epidermal necrolysis, which are more severe forms of erythema multiforme. Involvement of skin as well as mucous membrane with associated high fever characterizes this syndrome. Drug hypersensitivity is often the underlying cause.[54]

The disease can present at any age but is uncommon in childhood. The characteristic clinical lesion is a targetoid lesion (central zone of necrosis, blister, or erosion surrounded by erythema and edema) most frequently affecting the extremities in a symmetric distribution, with a strong mucosal predilection.

The histologic features can be varied depending on the age of the lesion. Erythema multiforme is characterized histologically by interface dermatitis with necrotic keratinocytes and prominent dermal infiltrate of lymphocytes and histiocytes.

Acantholytic Pattern

Hailey-Hailey disease

Hailey-Hailey disease is an autosomal dominant acantholytic genodermatosis whose pathogenesis is thought to involve mutations in a calcium pump, ATP2C1.[55] Intracellular junctions are thought to be weakened by dysregulation of calcium metabolism; however, one-third of patients have no family history of the disease.

Onset of the disease occurs during adolescence. There is predilection of the disease for flexural or intertriginous areas.[55] Isolated vulvar involvement has been reported.[56,57] The lesions start as tiny pruritic, linear/angular erosions in a background of white maceration that spread centrifugally to surrounding skin with associated crust and foul odor. Resolution can result in hypopigmentation but not scarring. Superinfection with *Candida albicans*, *Staphylococcus aureus*, and herpesvirus can be seen.[56,58]

Intraepidermal acantholysis involving the entire epidermis results in a "dilapidated brick wall" appearance. Direct immunofluorescence studies are negative.

Darier disease

Darier disease is an uncommon genodermatosis whose pathogenesis is thought to be a result of mutation of a gene on chromosome 12q encoding a calcium pump protein, ATP2A2.[59] Although it can be autosomal dominant, only half of the cases in a large series have a positive family history.[60]

The patients often present at puberty, but also can present later in life, with numerous hyperkeratotic papules usually distributed over the trunk. The disease has a seborrheic distribution and frequently involves the vulva. Localized vulvar presentation can be seen.[61,62] Nails tend to be thin, brittle, and dystrophic. Superinfection with bacteria, virus, or fungus is common.

Histologic sections show columns of parakeratosis and epidermal acanthosis with suprabasilar acantholysis. Characteristic corps ronds and grains, forms of dyskeratotic cells within the epidermis and stratum corneum, respectively, are usually present. In the differential diagnosis, Hailey-Hailey disease has more extensive acantholysis and warty dyskeratoma is a solitary and papillary lesion.

Acantholytic dermatosis of the vulvocrural area

Acantholytic dermatosis of the vulvocrural area often presents as papules that are smaller than 1 cm, solitary or grouped, and flesh colored.[63,64]

The histologic features of acantholytic dermatosis of the vulvocrural area are similar to those of Darier disease or Hailey-Hailey disease. They are namely intraepidermal acantholysis and scattered dyskeratotic cells including corps ronds and grains. However, direct immunofluorescence studies are negative. Acantholytic dermatosis of the vulvocrural area is often a solitary lesion, whereas Darier and Hailey-Hailey diseases are associated with a family history.

Granulomatous Pattern

Crohn disease

Cutaneous involvement by Crohn disease (CD) is a frequent extraintestinal tract manifestation that affects 20% to 40% of cases,[65] especially those suffering from colonic disease. Burgdorf[66] classified these lesions into 4 categories: (1) granulomatous cutaneous disease (including peristomal and perianal inflammation with sinus tract and fistulas as well as metastatic CD), (2) oral changes (eg, aphthae-like ulcers and cobblestoning), (3) nutrition-related changes (eg, acquired zinc deficiency), and (4) miscellaneous idiopathic markers (eg, pyoderma gangrenosum, erythema nodosum). Genital involvement, most frequently seen in the pediatric population, can occur either by direct extension of perineal disease or less frequently as metastatic CD, defined as granulomatous inflammation occurring distant to and separated from the gastrointestinal tract. Nearly one-third of the women suffering from CD have gynecologic features.[65] Perianal involvement with fistula formation is the most frequent manifestation of cutaneous CD (58%–76%).[67,68] Vulvar ulcers may be the initial manifestation in 25% of these patients.[69] Clinically, CD affecting vulva may appear as tender perivulvar "knifelike" ulcerations, fissures, skin tags, swelling, and sinus tracts leading to skin bridges and healing ending in severe scarring (**Fig. 11**). The severity of skin lesions does not always reflect the degree of activity of the bowel disease. The differential diagnosis includes foreign body giant cell reaction, hidradenitis suppurativa, sarcoidosis, tuberculosis, venereal diseases (lymphogranuloma venereum, granuloma inguinale, and syphilis), deep mycotic infection, and Melkerson-Rosenthal syndrome.

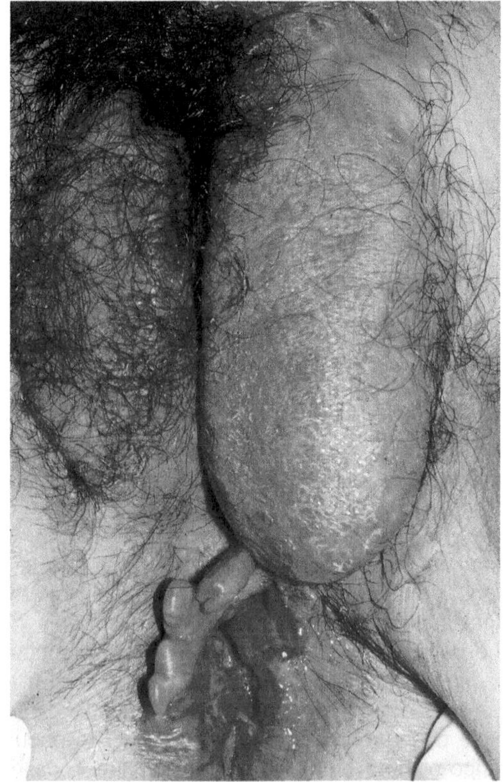

Fig. 11. Edema of the vulva and skin tags are typical findings in anogenital Crohn disease. (*Courtesy of* Libby Edwards, MD, Charlotte, NC.)

The characteristic histologic findings include the presence of noncaseating granulomas in dermis (**Fig. 12**). Special stains to rule out infection should be performed, including Ziehl-Neelson, periodic acid Schiff, and Gram stains.

There should be a high degree of suspicion for metastatic CD, especially in children suffering from genital and/or perirectal fissures, ulcers, hemorrhoids, skin tags, swelling, or chronic genital indurations and inflammation. Investigation for potential occult intestinal involvement is warranted.

Vasculopathic Pattern

Aphthous ulcer

Aphthae are ulcers affecting the mouth, and, less frequently, the genital region. Although the pathogenesis is unknown, it has been proposed that

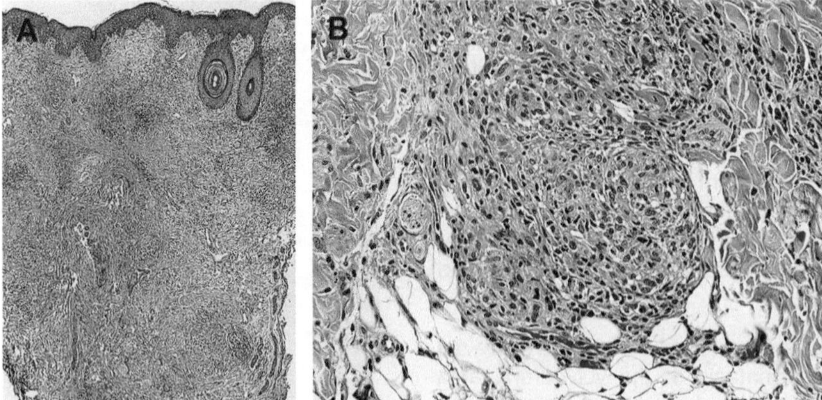

Fig. 12. (*A*) Dermal granulomas are seen in the dermis of patients with metastatic Crohn disease (hematoxylin-eosin, original magnification ×20). (*B*). The typical lesion is a noncaseating granuloma (hematoxylin-eosin, original magnification ×100). (*Courtesy of* Maria Angelica Selim, MD.)

these ulcerations are the result of formation of immune complex triggered by local injury or infection. The recurrent nature of the disease militates against an infection; however, in the first episode the patient should be investigated for infectious causes. Found primarily in young girls from 9 to 18 years of age, most patients with genital ulcers have concurrent or past oral ulcers. The occurrence of both oral and genital aphthae is called aphthae major.[70] These patients fail to show systemic involvement. When there is evidence of other organ involvement, then Behcet disease should be considered.[71] Aphthae in the genitalia present clinically as well-circumscribed round to oval ulcers of 1 to 3 cm with white to red fibrinous base and red borders. The most affected area is the modified mucous membranes of the vulva, although it can affect any area in the genitalia. The punched out appearance of the aphthae may raise concern for a chancre; aphthae lack the indurated, firm, painless base of the chancre. Other infectious ulcers to consider in the differential diagnosis display certain characteristics allowing its identification: chancroid is more irregular and shaggy, granuloma inguinale consists of eroded nodules with indurated borders or vegetations, and lymphogranuloma venereum ulcers are transient and painless but followed by significant lymphadenopathy.

A biopsy of an aphthous ulcer is the same as that seen in ulcers of Behcet disease (see the following section), showing nondiagnostic features with a shallow ulcer and acute and chronic inflammation. Special stains for infectious organisms are negative.

Behcet disease

Behcet disease is a systemic recurrent disease characterized by the clinical triad of oral ulcers, genital ulcers, and ocular inflammations. In 1990, the International Study Group for Behcet's Disease proposed clinical diagnostic criteria for this disorder.[72] Turkey has the highest incidence of this disease with more than 80 cases per 100,000 people, whereas the United States has fewer than 2 cases per 100,000 people.[73] The pathogenesis of this disorder is unknown; however, it has been postulated that vasculitis and autoimmune response may play a role in this disorder. Behcet disease evolves with flare ups and remissions affecting young adults.[74] Aphthous stomatitis is the initial manifestation in most of the cases and may precede other manifestations by several years. Classically, the patient suffers for 10 days with a painful, nonscarring circular ulcer involving the oral mucosa not fixed to the bone (buccal mucosa, tongue, and lip). Genitoanal ulcers are more painful, larger, and deeper than oral lesions.[71] Ulcerations in the vulva may be so deep that they can lead to fenestration and gangrene. Complex aphthosis or aphtha major, lesions affecting only the oral area and genitalia, is considered to be a *form fruste* of this disease. Among cutaneous lesions that can be present simultaneously to the ulcers are purpuric lesions secondary to vasculitis, erythema nodosum, and neutrophilic processlike pyoderma gangrenosum, sterile vesiculopustules, and Sweet syndrome–like lesions.[75] Pathergy, lesions occurring after trauma, is a diagnostic criterion for this disorder. Ocular manifestations range from the classic posterior uveitis to anterior uveitis, glaucoma, and cataracts. Other organs may be affected and manifest as gastrointestinal signs and symptoms mimicking inflammatory bowel disease, arthritis, and vascular disease that ranges from occlusive arterial disease to venous thrombosis and even aneurysm. Advanced stages of the disease may include neurologic manifestations like acute meningitis, nerve palsies, or meningoencephalitis. The latter is associated with poor prognosis.

Frequently, the histologic features are nonspecific. Early lesions include superficial ulcer with neutrophilic-rich acute inflammatory response. The biopsy may show evidence of lymphocytic or neutrophilic vasculitis with damage of the vessels leading to fibrin deposition and thrombosis. However, in view of the presence of an ulcer, it is difficult to ascertain if this is a primary or secondary vasculitis. These vascular changes acquire relevance in nonulcerated biopsy. Pathergy lesions show vessels with neutrophilic infiltrate in the absence of fibrinoid changes, this constellation of histologic features has been named as pustular vasculitis or "Sweetlike vasculitis."

Plasma cell vulvitis (Zoon's vulvitis)

In 1957, Garnier described a rare benign chronic inflammatory condition characterized by erythematous plaques found in postmenopausal women.[76] The histologic findings parallel those described by Zoon in the foreskin in 1952.[77] Cases of this disease have been published under several synonyms: plasma cell vulvitis, Zoon's vulvitis, and vulvitis circumscripta plasmacellularis. In view of the involvement of multiple mucosal and cutaneous surfaces sharing the same histologic findings, the name of plasma cell orificial mucositis and idiopathic lymphoplasmacellular mucositis-dermatitis have been proposed.[78] Clinically it presents as one or multiple shiny, glazed, deeply erythematous patches and plaques with an orange hue and multiple purpuric "cayenne pepper spots" (**Fig. 13**).[79–81] These lesions are sharply demarcated, and often bilateral and symmetric, and tend to coalesce. Rarely, erosions and friability can be seen. Most of the patients are postmenopausal women; however, a wide age range (8–80 years) is seen in the literature. The most frequently affected areas are the inner face of the labia minora and periurethral mucosa, although lesions in the labia majora, clitoris, and fourchette have been published. The patients frequently complain of pruritus, burning, pain, and dyspareunia.[79,80] In the pediatric population, it has been described as a mimicker of child abuse.[82] The clinical differential diagnosis includes lichen planus, vulvar intraepidermal neoplasm, extramammary Paget disease and fixed drug reaction. A biopsy is mandatory for the correct diagnosis.

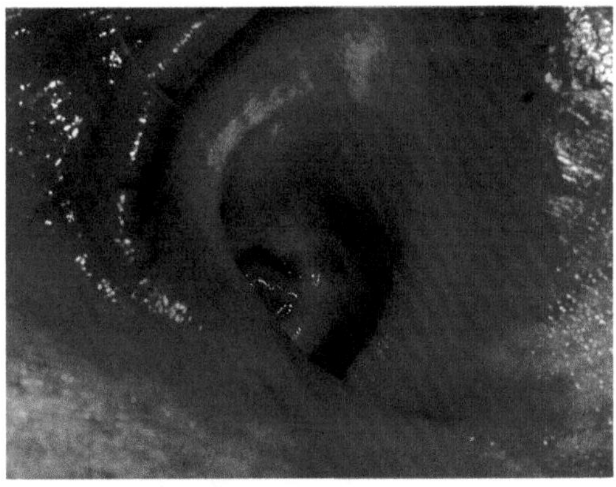

Fig. 13. Vulvitis plasmacellularis has a very characteristic feature of wel-demarcated dark redness or brown-red patches, most often in the vestibule. (*Courtesy of* Libby Edwards, MD, Charlotte, NC.)

Histologically, the epidermis is usually atrophic and moderately spongiotic (**Fig. 14**A). The keratinocytes acquire a lozenge or diamond shape. A dense, predominantly plasmacytic, infiltrate is seen in the dermis associated with vascular proliferation, erythrocytes extravasations, and hemosiderin deposition (**Fig. 14**B). The diagnosis of this disease can be a challenge, as not all of these criteria are present in the same histologic section. Virgili and colleagues[83] demonstrated that the percentage of plasma cells appears to be paramount in making this diagnosis. When the biopsy shows more than 50% of plasma cells in the infiltrate, this finding was sufficient. When the percentage was 25% to 50%, other criteria like epithelial atrophy and hemosiderin deposition were necessary to render this diagnosis. When the density of the plasma cells was less than 25%, this feature was attributed to mucosal site of involvement. Although the etiology of this disease is unknown, it has been postulated that trauma, virus, or an autoimmune response to an unidentified antigen may play a role. Its natural history consists of recurrent remissions and relapses of different lengths.

Squamous Cell Carcinoma and Premalignant Lesions (Vulvar Intraepithelial Neoplasm)

Squamous cell carcinoma (SCC) is the most frequent carcinoma arising in the vulva with an incidence of 1 to 2/100,000.[84] This tumor accounts for 3% to 5% of all gynecologic malignancies and 1% of all carcinomas in women.[84] Two types of vulvar SCC with their own premalignant lesions have been recognized. The most frequent type affects elderly patients, leading to the formation of well-differentiated keratinizing SCC in a background of lichen sclerosus and differentiated VIN (dVIN).[85] It is believed that this type of VIN is underreported based on the difficulties in recognizing the histopathologic changes and the short

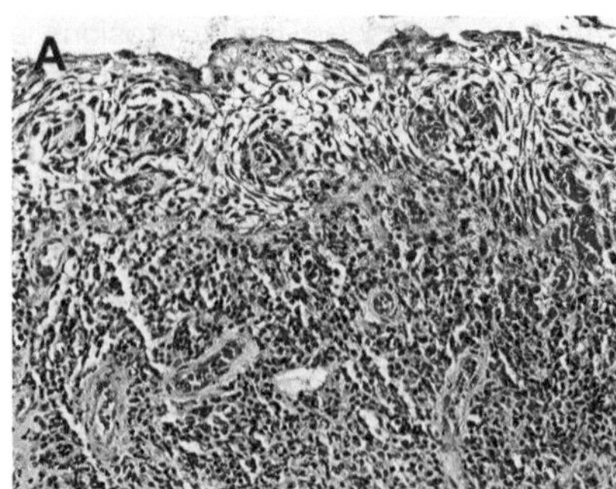

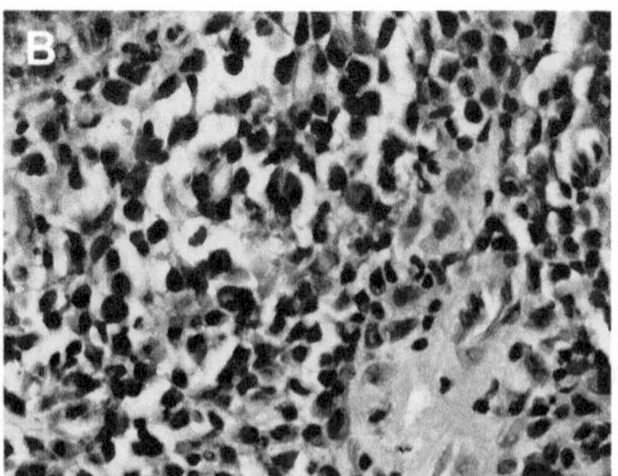

Fig. 14. (*A*) In plasma cell vulvitis, the epidermis is usually atrophic and spongiotic with lozenge or diamond-shaped keratinocytes (hematoxylin-eosin, original magnification ×100). (*B*) A dense predominantly plasmacytic infiltrate is seen in dermis associated with vascular proliferation, erythrocytes extravasations, and hemosiderin deposition (hematoxylin-eosin, original magnification ×400). (*Courtesy of* Maria Angelica Selim, MD.)

life span before transforming into an invasive SCC.[86,87] The second type occurs in younger women infected by high-risk HPV, especially types 16 and 18.[85,88] The SCC seen in these patients is frequently nonkeratinizing and is preceded by usual VIN (uVIN) of the warty and basaloid types. Approximately one-quarter of SCCs are associated with uVIN. These patients need a thorough cervical and perianal examination in view of the coexistence of multifocal human papilloma virus (HPV) infection affecting the cervix (22% of patients with uVIN have cervical intraepithelial neoplasia),[89] vagina, and anus.

In the 1960s, Abell[90] described the first case of dVIN under the name of "intraepithelial carcinoma of simplex type."[91] He coined this name to identify a highly differentiated vulvar carcinoma in situ that needed to be separated from the "intraepithelial carcinoma of Bowen's type," currently known as uVIN. The term "differentiated" was introduced in 1977 to underscore the differentiated nature of the morphologic features of this disease.[91] In the latest classification originated from ISSVD (see **Table 2**),[3,4] the term "VIN III, differentiated type" has been replaced by "VIN, differentiated type." The published incidence of this disease is approximately 2% to 5%; however, it is believe that this disease is underrecognized because of its difficult clinical and pathologic diagnosis.[91–95] It affects postmenopausal women (mean age of 67 years) and is associated with lichen sclerosus[91] and lichen planus. dVIN is commonly solitary, opposite to the multifocal nature of uVIN.[96] The etiology of dVIN remains unknown. Although HPV has been isolated in few cases, it is believed that it does not play a role in the genesis of dVIN.[95–98] Alteration of p53 has been proposed as an etiologic factor; however, Liegl and Regauer[99] suggested that these changes are secondary to ischemic stress. dVIN has a protean clinical presentation that ranges from a gray-white discoloration with a roughened surface, to an erythematous lesion with or without ulceration, to an ill-defined raised white plaque (**Fig. 15**). Sometimes, the lesion and symptomatology can be masqueraded by the background of lichen sclerosus[96] or lichen planus. Histologically, the epithelium is thickened with parakeratosis and atypical keratinocytes restricted to the basal and parabasal layers, whereas the superficial layers have normal maturation without evidence of viral infection (**Fig. 16**). At higher

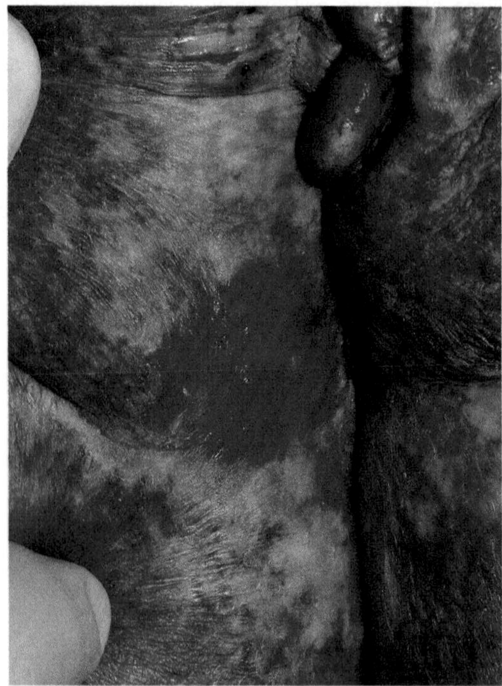

Fig. 15. Both red and white, thickened plaques within lichen sclerosus are typical of dVIN. (*Courtesy of* Libby Edwards, MD, Charlotte, NC.)

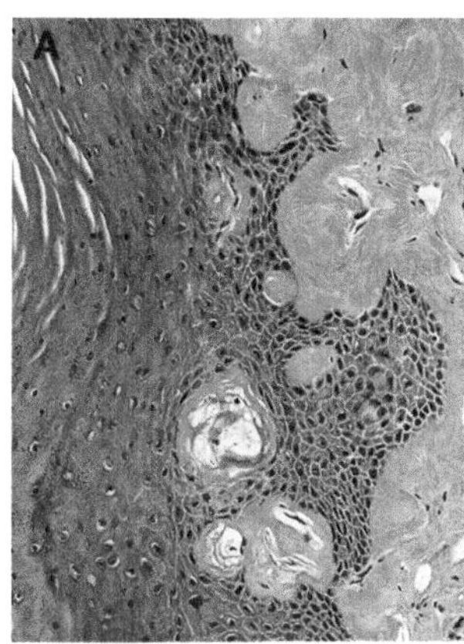
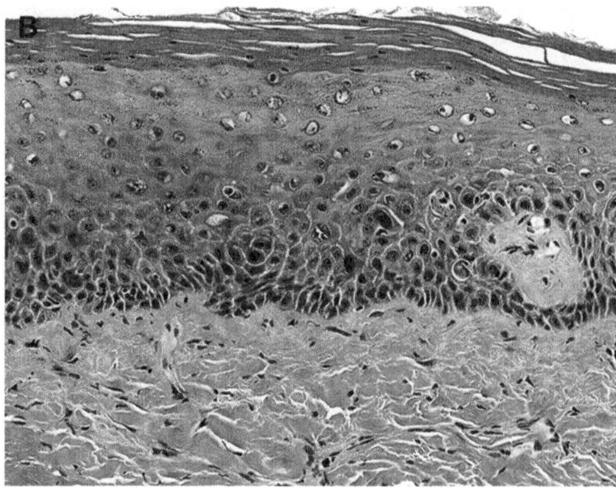

Fig. 16. (*A*) A background of lichen sclerosus without basal atypia is seen (hematoxylin-eosin, original magnification ×200). (*B*) Focally, atypical keratinocytes restricted to the basal and parabasal layers characteristic of dVIN were noted (hematoxylin-eosin, original magnification ×200). (*Courtesy of* Maria Angelica Selim, MD.)

power, nuclear changes of enlargement, pleomorphism, and hyperchromatism and mitoses are seen. dVIN is associated with keratinizing SCC, the pathway of carcinogenesis has not been elucidated. It has been proposed that because of the high proliferative activity in dVIN, it might be more likely to progress to invasive SCC than uVIN.[96,100,101] Thus, any suspicious lesion should be biopsied. The treatment of dVIN is recommended to be surgical to avoid evolution to SCC.

A myriad of terms have been used in the literature to describe what we presently know as uVIN. In the early 1990s, Bowen described "squamous intraepithelial lesions." Kaufman, in 1965, divided non-neoplastic forms from neoplastic vulvar diseases. He sub-classified the precancerous lesions into 3 categories: Queyrat erythroplasia, Bowenoid carcinoma in situ, and carcinoma simplex.[102] In 1976, ISSVD introduced the term of vulvar intraepithelial neoplasm (VIN). The latter was graded based on the degree of epithelium involvement; lower third of the epithelium VIN I, two-thirds of the epithelium VIN II, and the entire epithelial thickness VIN III. In view of the absence of clear evidence of a continuum of VIN lesions leading to vulvar carcinoma, ISSVD in 2003 decided to eliminate VIN I and merge VIN II and III into uVIN.[88]

In summary, VIN can present in 2 forms with different biologic behavior: uVIN and dVIN.[88,103] uVIN is divided into warty type previously described as Bowenoid disease and basaloid type that affects older population with higher tendency to invade. Tumors with both patterns, basaloid and warty, have been identified.[103] Both patterns are associated with high-risk HPV infection, especially HPV type 16. In clinical practice, no difference is made regarding patterns. The advantage of the latest ISSVD classification resides in the identification of uVIN and dVIN with extensive differences in clinicopathological behavior and malignant potential.

Worldwide, the incidence of uVIN is increasing with 5 of 100,00 women per year affected. This increase parallels the increase in HPV prevalence. It affects females in their 30s and 40s who usually are cigarette smokers and suffer from other manifestations of HPV infections, such as condylomata acuminate, and other viral infections, such as herpes viral infection and human immunodeficiency virus. The malignant progression of uVIN is estimated in less than 10%.[102] The classic clinical presentation consists of raised, well-demarcated asymmetrical whitish to erythematous plaques (**Fig. 17**). The most common locations in order of frequency are the labia

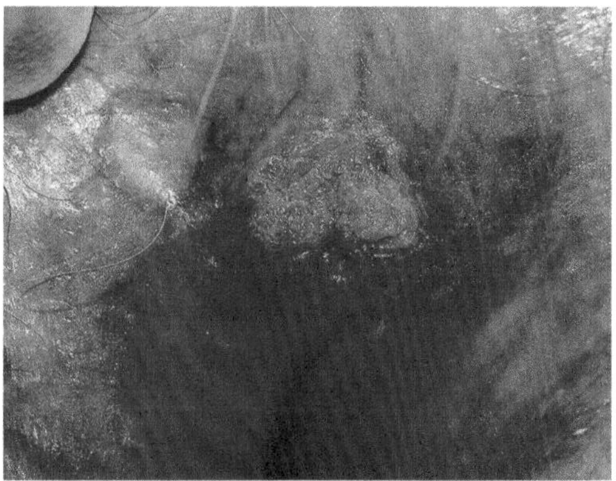

Fig. 17. uVIN of the warty type often resembles HPV infection, with a papillomatous surface. (*Courtesy of* Libby Edwards, MD, Charlotte, NC.)

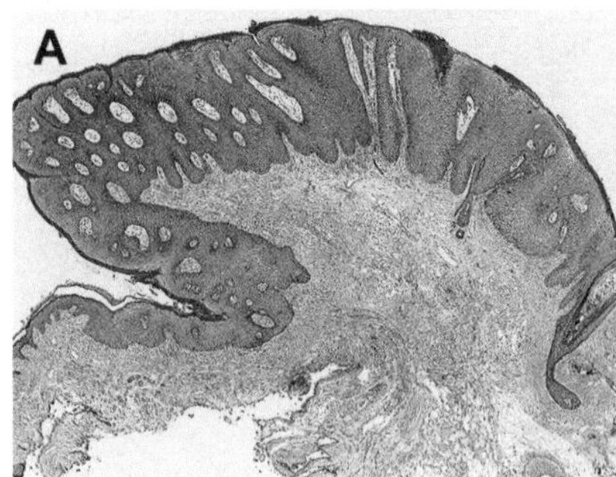

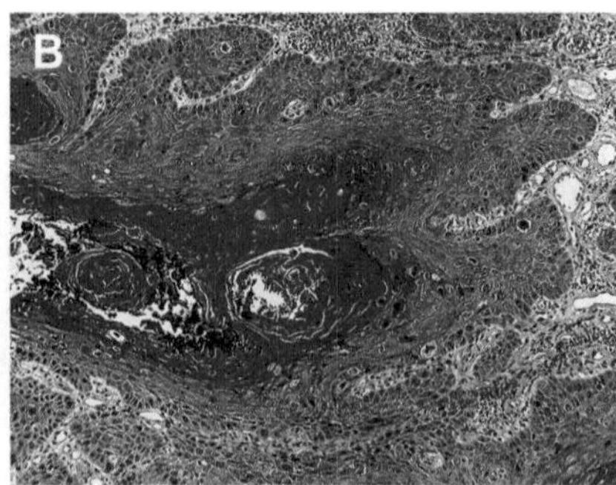

Fig. 18. (*A*) Histopathologically, uVIN presents as thickened epidermis associated with hyperkeratosis and/or parakeratosis with loss of polarity (hematoxylin-eosin, original magnification ×20). (*B*) High-power view shows koilocytes and keratinocytes with high nuclear-to-cytoplasmic ratio, nuclear hyperchromasia, irregular nuclear contours and mitosis at all levels of the epidermis (hematoxylin-eosin, original magnification ×40). (*Courtesy of* Maria Angelica Selim, MD.)

majora, the labia minora, and posterior fourchette. Multifocal involvement is noted in approximately 40% of the cases and decreases with the age of the patient.[91,95,104] Thorough examination of the vagina, cervix, and anus is pertinent in these patients, as 25% to 66% will suffer from intraepithelial or invasive squamous neoplasias.[90–94,105] The most common presenting symptom is pruritus, followed by pain, ulceration, and dysuria.[104]

Histopathologically, uVIN presents as thicken epidermis associated with hyperkeratosis and/or parakeratosis.[91] There is loss of polarity with high nuclear-to-cytoplasmic ratio, nuclear hyperchromasia, irregular nuclear contours, and mitosis at all levels of the epidermis (**Fig. 18**). Koilocytes, cells with clear or vacuolated cytoplasm that exhibit shrunken pyknotic nuclei, are numerous. In the warty pattern of uVIN, the surface shows a papillomatous quality. In the basaloid pattern, the surface is relatively flat with a diffuse proliferation of small, undifferentiated keratinocytes with a small amount of cytoplasm. Local conservative surgical removal of these lesions is considered. Local treatment with antiviral agents has been proposed. Imiquimod is also showing promising results; however, randomized controlled trials are needed to confirm the preliminary data.

REFERENCES

1. Foster DC. Vulvar disease. Obstet Gynecol 2002; 100(1):145–63.
2. Lewis FM, Shah M, Harrington CI. Vulval involvement in lichen planus: a study of 37 women. Br J Dermatol 1996;135(1):89–91.
3. Lynch PJ. 2006 International Society for the Study of Vulvovaginal Disease classification of vulvar dermatoses: a synopsis. J Low Genit Tract Dis 2007;11(1):1–2.
4. Lynch PJ, Moyal-Barracco M, Bogliatto F, et al. 2006 ISSVD classification of vulvar dermatoses: pathologic subsets and their clinical correlates. J Reprod Med 2007;52(1):3–9, 110.
5. Fischer G, Spurrett B, Fischer A. The chronically symptomatic vulva: aetiology and management. Br J Obstet Gynaecol 1995;102(10):773–9.
6. Fischer GO. The commonest causes of symptomatic vulvar disease: a dermatologist's perspective. Australas J Dermatol 1996;37(1):12–8.
7. Heller DS, Randolph P, Young A, et al. The cutaneous-vulvar clinic revisited: a 5-year experience of the Columbia Presbyterian Medical Center Cutaneous Vulvar Service. Dermatology 1997;195(1):26–9.
8. O'Hare PM, Sherertz EF. Vulvodynia: a dermatologist's perspective with emphasis on an irritant contact dermatitis component. J Women's Health Gend Based Med 2000;9(5):565–9.
9. Marren P, Wojnarowska F. Dermatitis of the vulva. Semin Dermatol 1996;15(1):36–41.
10. Fivozinsky KB, Laufer MR. Vulvar disorders in prepubertal girls. A literature review. J Reprod Med 1998;43(9):763–73.
11. Elsner P, Wilhelm D, Maibach HI. Multiple parameter assessment of vulvar irritant contact dermatitis. Contact Dermatitis 1990;23(1):20–6.
12. Leung DY. Pathogenesis of atopic dermatitis. J Allergy Clin Immunol 1999;104(3 Pt 2): S99–108.
13. Pincus SH. Vulvar dermatoses and pruritus vulvae. Dermatol Clin 1992;10(2):297–308.
14. Virgili A, Bacilieri S, Corazza M. Managing vulvar lichen simplex chronicus. J Reprod Med 2001;46(4):343–6.
15. O'Keefe RJ, Scurry JP, Dennerstein G, et al. Audit of 114 non-neoplastic vulvar biopsies. Br J Obstet Gynaecol 1995;102(10):780–6.

16. Farber EM, Nall L. Genital psoriasis. Cutis 1992; 50(4):263–6.
17. Cox AJ, Watson W. Histologic variations in lesions of psoriasis. Arch Dermatol 1972;106(4):503–6.
18. Ragaz A, Ackerman AB. Evolution, maturation and regression of lesions of psoriasis: new observations and correlation of clinical and histologic findings. Am J Dermatopathol 1979;1(3):199–214.
19. Armor B. Reiter's syndrome: diagnosis and clinical presentation. Rheum Dis Clin North Am 1998;24(4): 677–95.
20. Edwards L, Hansen RC. Reiter's syndrome of the vulva: the psoriasis spectrum. Arch Dermatol 1992;128(6):811–4.
21. Winchester R, Bernstein DH, Fischer HD, et al. The co-occurrence of Reiter's syndrome and acquired immunodeficiency. Ann Intern Med 1987;106(1):19–26.
22. Lotery HE, Galask RP, Stone MS, et al. Ulcerative vulvitis in atypical Reiter's syndrome. J Am Acad Dermatol 2003;48(4):613–6.
23. Meyrick Thomas RH, Ridley CM, et al. Lichen sclerosus et atrophicus and autoimmunity—a study of 350 women. Br J Dermatol 1988;118(1):41–6.
24. Ball SB, Wojnarowska F. Vulvar dermatoses: lichen sclerosus, lichen planus and vulval dermatitis/ lichen simplex chronicus. Semin Cutan Med Surg 1998;17(3):182–8.
25. Smith YR, Haefner HK. Vulvar lichen sclerosus: pathophysiology and treatment. Am J Clin Dermatol 2004;5(2):105–25.
26. Carlson JA, Ambros R, Malfetano J, et al. Vulvar lichen sclerosus and squamous cell carcinoma: a cohort, case control and investigational study with historical perspective: implications for chronic inflammation and sclerosis in the development of neoplasia. Hum Pathol 1998;29(9):932–48.
27. Powell J, Wojnarowska F. Childhood vulvar lichen sclerosus: an increasingly common problem. J Am Acad Dermatol 2001;44(5):803–6.
28. Edwards L. Vulvar lichen planus. Arch Dermatol 1989;125(12):1677–80.
29. Hammock LA, Barrett TL. Inflammatory dermatoses of the vulva. J Cutan Pathol 2005;32(9):604–11.
30. Lewis FM. Vulval lichen planus. Br J Dermatol 1998;138(4):569–75.
31. Kirtschig G, Wakelin SH, Wojnarowska F. Mucosal vulval lichen planus: outcome, clinical and laboratory features. J Eur Acad Dermatol Venereol 2005;19(3):301–7.
32. Mann MS, Kaufman RH. Erosive lichen planus of the vulva. Clin Obstet Gynecol 1991;34(3):605–13.
33. Eisen D. The vulvovaginal–gingival syndrome of lichen planus. The clinical characteristics of 22 patients. Arch Dermatol 1994;130(11):1379–82.
34. Dwyer CM, Kerr RE, Millan DW. Squamous carcinoma following lichen planus of the vulva. Clin Exp Dermatol 1995;20(2):171–2.
35. Franck JM, Young AW Jr. Squamous cell carcinoma in situ arising within lichen planus of the vulva. Dermatol Surg 1995;21(10):890–4.
36. Zaki I, Dalziel KL, Solomonsz FA, et al. The under-reporting of skin disease in association with squamous cell carcinoma of the vulva. Clin Exp Dermatol 1996;21(5):334–7.
37. Liu Z, Diaz LA. Bullous pemphigoid: end of the century overview. J Dermatol 2001;28(11): 647–50.
38. Vassileva S. Drug-induced pemphigoid: bullous and cicatricial. Clin Dermatol 1998;16(3):379–87.
39. Marren P, Wojnarowska F, Venning VA, et al. Vulvar involvement in the auto-immune bullous diseases. J Reprod Med 1993;38(2):101–7.
40. Urano S. Localized bullous pemphigoid of the vulva. J Dermatol 1996;23(8):580–2.
41. Frith P, Charnock M, Wojnarowska F. Cicatricial pemphigoid diagnosed from ocular features in recurrent severe vulval scarring. Two case reports. Br J Obstet Gynaecol 1991;98(5):482–4.
42. Chan LS, Ahmed AR, Anhalt GJ, et al. The first international consensus on mucous membrane pemphigoid: definition, diagnostic criteria, pathogenetic factors, medical treatment and prognostic indicators. Arch Dermatol 2002;138(3):370–9.
43. Ridley CM. Cicatricial pemphigoid of the vulva. Am J Obstet Gynecol 1985;152(7 Pt 1):916–7.
44. Korman NJ. Bullous pemphigoid. The latest in diagnosis, prognosis, and therapy. Arch Dermatol 1998;134(9):1137–41.
45. Lim HW, Bystryn JC. Evaluation and management of disease of the vulva: bullous diseases. Clin Obstet Gynecol 1978;21(4):1007–22.
46. Amagai M. Pemphigus: autoimmunity to epidermal cell adhesion molecules. Adv Dermatol 1996;11: 319–52.
47. Batta K, Munday PE, Tatnall FM. Pemphigus vulgaris localized to the vagina presenting as chronic vaginal discharge. Br J Dermatol 1999;140(5): 945–7.
48. Wong KT, Wong KK. A case of acantholytic dermatosis of the vulva with features of pemphigus vegetans. J Cutan Pathol 1994;21(5):453–6.
49. Schornick JK. Herpes gestationis. Dermatol Clin 1993;11(3):527–33.
50. Wojnarowska F, Frith P. Linear IgA disease. Dev Ophthalmol 1997;28:64–72.
51. Egan CA, Zone JJ. Linear IgA bullous dermatosis. Int J Dermatol 1999;38(11):818–27.
52. Klein PA, Callen JP. Drug-induced linear IgA bullous dermatosis after vancomycin discontinuance in a patient with renal insufficiency. J Am Acad Dermatol 2000;42(2 Pt 2):316–23.
53. Ishiko A, Shimizu H, Masunaga T, et al. 97-kDa linear IgA bullous dermatosis antigen localizes in the lamina lucida between the NC16A and carboxyl

terminal domain of the 180 kDa bullous permphigoid antigen. J Invest Dermatol 1998;111(1):93–6.
54. Huff JC, Weston WL, Tonnesen MG. Erythema multiforme: a critical review of characteristic diagnostic criteria and causes. J Am Acad Dermatol 1983;8(6):763–75.
55. Burge SM. Hailey-Hailey disease: the clinical features, response to treatment and prognosis. Br J Dermatol 1992;126(3):275–82.
56. Evron S, Leviatan A, Okon E. Familial benign chronic pemphigus appearing as leukoplakia of the vulva. Int J Dermatol 1984;23(8):556–7.
57. Wieselthier JS, Pincus SH. Hailey-Hailey disease of the vulva. Arch Dermatol 1993;129(10):1344–5.
58. Misra R, Raman M, Singh N, et al. Hailey-Hailey disease masquerading as candidiasis. Int J Gynaecol Obstet 1993;42(1):51–2.
59. Sakuntabhai A, Ruiz-Perez V, Carter S, et al. Mutation in ATP2A2, encoding a Ca^{2+} pump, cause Darier disease. Nat Genet 1999;21(3):271–7.
60. Burge SM, Wilkinson JD. Darier-White disease: a review of the clinical features of 163 patients. J Am Acad Dermatol 1992;27(1):40–50.
61. Barrett JF, Murray LA, MacDonald HN. Darier's disease localized to the vulva. Case report. Br J Obstet Gynaecol 1989;96(8):997–9.
62. Ridley CM, Buckley CH. Darier's disease localized to the vulva (correspondence). Br J Dermatol 1991; 98(1):112.
63. Chorzelski TP, Kudejko J, Jablonska S. Is papular acantholytic dyskeratosis of the vulva a new entity? Arch Dermatol 1984;6(6):557–60.
64. Wong T-Y, Mihm MC Jr. Acantholytic dermatosis localized to genitalia and crural areas of male patients: a report of three cases. J Cutan Pathol 1994;21(1):27–32.
65. Kingland CR, Alderman B. Crohn's disease of the vulva. J R Soc Med 1991;84(4):236–7.
66. Burgdorf W. Cutaenous manifestations of Crohn's disease. J Am Acad Dermatol 1981;5(6):689–95.
67. Ephgrave K. Extra-intestinal manifestations of Crohn's disease. Surg Clin North Am 2007;87(3):673–80.
68. Sandborn WJ, Fazio VW, Feagan BG, et al. AGA technical review on perianal Crohn's disease. Gastroenterology 2003;125(5):1508–30.
69. Martin J, Holdstock G. Isolated vulval oedema as a feature of Crohn's disease. J Obstet Gynaecol 1997;17(1):92–3.
70. Black M, McKay M, Braude P, et al. Obstetric and gynecologic dermatology. 2nd edition. London; Edimburh; New York; Philadelphia; St Lous; Sydney; Toronto: Mosby: International Limited; 2002.
71. Haidopoulos D, Rodolakis A, Stefanidis K, et al. Behçet's disease: part of the differential diagnosis of the ulcerative vulva. Clin Exp Obstet Gynecol 2002;29(3):219–21.
72. Criteria for diagnosis of Behçet's disease. International Study Group for Behçet's Disease. Lancet 1990;335(8697):1078–80 [No authors listed].
73. Jorizzo JL, Abernethy JL, White WL, et al. Mucocutaneous criteria for the diagnosis of Behçet's disease: an analysis of clinicopathologic data from multiple international centers. J Am Acad Dermatol 1995;32(6):968–76.
74. Mangelsdorf HC, White WL, Jorizzo JL. Behçet's disease. Report of twenty-five patients from the United States with prominent mucocutaneous involvement. J Am Acad Dermatol 1996;34(5 Pt 1): 745–50.
75. Magro CM, Crowson AN. Cutaneous manifestations of Behçet's disease. Int J Dermatol 1995; 34(3):159–65.
76. Garnier G. Benign plasma-cell erythroplasia. Br J Dermatol 1957;69(3):77–81.
77. Zoon JJ. [Differential diagnosis between chronic circumscribed benign plasmacellular balanitis and Queyrat's erythroplasia]. Ned Tijdschr Geneeskd 1952;96(38):2349–53 [in undetermined language].
78. Brix WK, Nassau SR, Patterson JW, et al. Idiopathic lymphoplasmacellular mucositis-dermatitis. J Cutan Pathol 2010;37(4):426–31.
79. McCreedy CA, Melski JW. Vulvar erythema. Vulvitis chronica plasmacellularis (Zoon's vulvitis). Arch Dermatol 1990;126(10):1352–3.
80. Yoganathan S, Bohl TG, Mason G. Plasma cell balanitis and vulvitis (of Zoon). A study of 10 cases. J Reprod Med 1994;39(12):939–44.
81. Li Q, Leopold K, Carlson JA. Chronic vulvar purpura: persistent pigmented purpuric dermatitis (lichen aureus) of the vulva or plasma cell (Zoon's) vulvitis? J Cutan Pathol 2003;30(9):572–6.
82. Albers SE, Taylor G, Huyer D, et al. Vulvitis circumscripta plasmacellularis mimicking child abuse. J Am Acad Dermatol 2000;42(6):1078–80.
83. Virgili A, Levratti A, Marzola A, et al. Retrospective histopathologic reevaluation of 18 cases of plasma cell vulvitis. J Reprod Med 2005;50(1):3–7.
84. Hacker NF. Vulvar cancer. In: Berek S, Hacker NF, editors. Practical gynaecologic oncology. 5th edition. Philadelphia: Lippincott Williams & Wilkins; 2000. p. 553–96.
85. van der Avoort I, Shirango H, Hoevenaars BM, et al. Vulvar squamous cell carcinoma is a multifactorial disease following two separate and independent pathways. Int J Gynecol Pathol 2006;25(1):22–9.
86. Fox H, Wells M. Recent advances in the pathology of the vulva. Histopathology 2003;42(3):209–16.
87. Sideri M, Jones RW, Wilkinson EJ, et al. Squamous vulvar intraepithelial neoplasia: 2004 modified terminology, ISSVD Vulvar Oncology Subcommittee. J Reprod Med 2005;50(11):807–10.

88. Monk BJ, Burger RA, Lin F, et al. Prognostic significance of human papillomavirus DNA in vulvar carcinoma. Obstet Gynecol 1995;85(5 Pt 1):709–15.
89. Lara-Torre E, Perlman SE. Vulvar intraepithelial neoplasia in adolescents with abnormal Pap smear results: a series report. J Pediatr Adolesc Gynecol 2004;17(1):45–8.
90. Abell MR. Intraepithelial carcinoma of epidermis and squamous mucosa of vulva and perineum. Surg Clin North Am 1965;45(5):1179–98.
91. Hart WR. Vulvar intraepithelial neoplasia: historical aspects and current status. Int J Gynecol Pathol 2001;20(1):16–30.
92. van Beurden M, ten Kate FJ, Smits HL, et al. Multifocal vulvar intraepithelial neoplasia grade III and multicentric lower genital tract neoplasia is associated with transcriptionally active human papillomavirus. Cancer 1995;75(12):2879–84.
93. Hampl M, Sarajuuri H, Wentzensen N, et al. Effect of human papillomavirus vaccines on vulvar, vaginal, and anal intraepithelial lesions and vulvar cancer. Obstet Gynecol 2006;108(6):1361–8.
94. Joura EA, Lösch A, Haider-Angeler MG, et al. Trends in vulvar neoplasia. Increasing incidence of vulvar intraepithelial neoplasia and squamous cell carcinoma of the vulva in young women. J Reprod Med 2000;45(8):613–5.
95. Preti M, van Seters M, Sideri M, et al. Squamous vulvar intraepithelial neoplasia. Clin Obstet Gynecol 2005;48(4):845–61.
96. Yang B, Hart WR. Vulvar intraepithelial neoplasia of the simplex (differentiated) type: a clinicopathologic study including analysis of HPV and p53 expression. Am J Surg Pathol 2000;24(3):429–41.
97. Medeiros F, Nascimento AF, Crum CP. Early vulvar squamous neoplasia: advances in classification, diagnosis, and differential diagnosis. Adv Anat Pathol 2005;12(1):20–6.
98. van de Nieuwenhof HP, Massuger LF, van der Avoort IA, et al. Vulvar squamous cell carcinoma development after diagnosis of VIN increases with age. Eur J Cancer 2009;45(5):851–6.
99. Liegl B, Regauer S. p53 immunostaining in lichen sclerosus is related to ischaemic stress and is not a marker of differentiated vulvar intraepithelial neoplasia (d-VIN). Histopathology 2006;48(3):268–74.
100. Roma AA, Hart WR. Progression of simplex (differentiated) vulvar intraepithelial neoplasia to invasive squamous cell carcinoma: a prospective case study confirming its precursor role in the pathogenesis of vulvar cancer. Int J Gynecol Pathol 2007;26(3):248–53.
101. Mulvany NJ, Allen DG. Differentiated intraepithelial neoplasia of the vulva. Int J Gynecol Pathol 2008;27(1):125–35.
102. Kaufman RH, Gardner HL. Intraepithelial carcinoma of the vulva. Clin Obstet Gynecol 1965;8:1035–50.
103. Scurry J, Wilkinson EJ. Review of terminology of precursors of vulvar squamous cell carcinoma. J Low Genit Tract Dis 2006;10(3):161–9.
104. McNally OM, Mulvany NJ, Pagano R, et al. VIN 3: a clinicopathologic review. Int J Gynecol Cancer 2002;12(5):490–5.
105. de Bie RP, van de Nieuwenhof HP, Bekkers RL, et al. Patients with usual vulvar intraepithelial neoplasia-related vulvar cancer have an increased risk of cervical abnormalities. Br J Cancer 2009;101(1):27–31.

Clinical Care of Vulvar Pruritus, with Emphasis on One Common Cause, Lichen Simplex Chronicus

Kristen M.A. Stewart, MD

KEYWORDS

• Vulvar • Pruritus • Differential diagnosis
• Lichen simplex chronicus • Treatment

Vulvar pruritus can be caused by a wide spectrum of pathologies, the most common being candidiasis, contact dermatitis, lichen simplex chronicus (LSC), and lichen sclerosus. LSC begins with an inciting itch sensation for which scratching and rubbing yield pleasure and relief, which can trigger a chronic itch-scratch cycle. The tendency toward LSC cannot be cured, but the symptoms generally can be controlled. Prompt treatment with superpotent corticosteroids usually breaks the itch-scratch cycle. Careful attention to irritants and secondary infection prevents this from becoming a significant ongoing problem.

VULVAR PRURITUS

Vulvar pruritus is a common and distressing condition that affects nearly all women at some point in their lives. Vulvar pruritus describes an itch that feels good when scratched versus an itch that may be described as irritating, prickly, or burning. In the evaluation of vulvar pruritus, true itching is limited to a sensation that produces at least a desire to scratch or rub.

Patients with vulvar pruritus seek care from family practioners, gynecologists, internists, pediatricians, and dermatologists. When patients present themselves for care they are often frustrated by the effect that the pruritus has had on their daily living, and many have already failed multiple home or over-the-counter remedies.[1] Providers are often challenged to diagnose and treat this nonspecific symptom. This is because vulvar pruritus is physiologically complicated by its unique location, emotionally complicated by the impact it has on the patient, and diagnostically complicated and time consuming for the health care provider. This article provides a practical and clinical approach to the evaluation of vulvar pruritus and then focuses specifically on one common cause, LSC.

The location of the vulva at the junction of the urinary, genital, and gastrointestinal tracts, where cutaneous skin transitions to mucosal skin, creates a unique skin surface.[2] The vulva contains glabrous, nonglabrous, and mucosal skin. Local factors including warmth, moisture, and friction can complicate skin conditions by increasing the effect of irritants and prolonging irritant contact time. Moisture and warmth minimize and alter the characteristic presentation of scale, which is often used to differentiate common dermatoses.[1–4] In addition, the combination of warmth, moisture, and friction create the

There are no financial disclosures or conflicts of interest to report.
The views expressed here do not necessarily reflect the views of the United States Navy.
Department of Dermatology, Naval Health Clinic New England, 43 Smith Road, Newport, RI 02841, USA
E-mail address: kristen.stewart@med.navy.mil

Dermatol Clin 28 (2010) 669–680
doi:10.1016/j.det.2010.08.004
0733-8635/10/$ – see front matter. Published by Elsevier Inc.

equivalent of occlusion, which must be considered as a potential complicating factor of treatment with topical corticosteroids.

Skin symptoms of the vulva are often overlooked. Outside of gynecology and pediatrics, the vulva is infrequently examined during routine visits, and a patient is unlikely to have a vulvar examination unless she mentions her symptoms. In addition, the examination of the vulva is difficult, because even the normal appearance of the vulva varies with age and natural skin color. Finally, when examined, signs of vulvar skin disease are often subtle, difficult to distinguish from variations of normal, and atypical compared with classic cutaneous presentations.

Although the findings on physical examination may be subtle to the provider, the impact of vulvar pruritus is anything but subtle to the patient. Vulvar pruritus, or any form of vulvar irritation or discomfort, affects all aspects of a patient's life including simple activities of daily living, exercise, and sexual encounters, and the psychologic well-being of relationships and self-worth. Often there are underlying fears that the symptoms are caused by undiagnosed cancer, a sexually transmitted infection, poor hygiene, or that there will never be relief. The implications of these fears cannot be overstated.

To further complicate this medical condition, social cues, embarrassment, and the fears noted previously are often obstacles to the patient seeking care. Women often suppose that the cause of their vulvar itching is either a yeast infection or an allergic reaction.[3] Patients commonly invest an extraordinary amount of money in over-the-counter products, and time in hygiene routines that likely exacerbate the symptoms, complicate the history and physical examination, and delay presentation to a medical provider.

In addition to these complicating factors affecting the patient's presentation of vulvar pruritus, the provider further must overcome many obstacles. The time, equipment, and support required to perform an adequate history and examination can be cumbersome during a routine appointment. After interviewing, the patient must undress, be positioned for adequate exposure, and be examined with suitable lighting and ideally in the presence of a chaperoning assistant. To further confound the evaluation, both the recognition of normal findings and the subtle changes of vulvar disease require experience to appreciate.

In summary, vulvar pruritus is a common and distressing condition for patients, and its presentation is often delayed and complicated by home remedies. The true prevalence cannot be accurately estimated. Vulvar pruritus is a symptom, and an underlying cause must be sought and not assumed. This is best accomplished by obtaining a careful history of vulvar care regimens and treatments, performing a detailed physical examination, and considering a broad differential diagnosis.

Patient History

With any vulvar complaint it is imperative to gather a pertinent history. An efficient way to accomplish this uses a patient questionnaire that may be completed by the patient before seeing the provider. Tailoring such a form to one's own practice facilitates and expedites the patient encounter.

The interview should start with the patient defining her symptom. A patient may struggle to describe her complaint and should be offered a variety of descriptors, such as itch, burn, rawness, pain, tingling, and irritation. Itch, in its most basic form, is a sensation that causes a desire to scratch and for which scratching yields pleasure or relief. The patient who complains primarily of irritation, burning, rawness, soreness, or stinging generally exhibits problems that represent a different differential diagnostic than vulvar pruritus.[4] Some patients describe pain symptoms occurring as a result of rubbing or scratching.

Next, define the location of the pruritus as generalized, limited to a few areas, or localized to the vulva. Some patients hesitate to name or point to the area of involvement and may simply state, "it itches down there." In these cases, use the physical examination to teach the patient anatomic terms and encourage her to use her hand to show you where and how she scratches the affected skin.[3,4]

Ask the patient to identify triggers that make the pruritus better or worse, and seek to identify associations, such as vaginal discharge, relation to coitus and menses, contraception, lubrication, and sanitary products. Take time to ask the patient what she thinks the cause is and what may be her fears. Obtain a list of prescribed and over-the-counter treatments, the length of use, and the results of such treatments. Inquire about personal hygiene routines, including cleansers, douches, and use of washcloths, and determine how the products are used and how frequently.[4,5]

Gather pertinent historical information, including age, allergies, medications, and relevant surgeries, and conduct a directed review of systems. Identify preexisting conditions, such as abnormal Pap smears, genital warts, genital herpes simplex virus infection, herpes zoster, diabetes, allergic rhinitis, asthma, eczema, or psoriasis. Does she have a diagnosis of fibromyalgia, irritable bowel syndrome, interstitial cystitis, or chronic fatigue syndrome? When was her most recent pregnancy and menstrual cycle? Is she postmenopausal? Is there a family history of genitourinary disease?

Physical Examination

The physical examination should include a whole-body mucocutaneous examination, looking for stigmata of skin disease, such as eczema, psoriasis, and lichen planus, which may play a role in vulvar symptoms. A complete genital examination with positioning for adequate exposure and lighting should include examination of the entire anogenital area. Inspect the entire vulva for subtle erythema, swelling, lichenification, and hyperppigmentation or hypopigmentation and the presence of scarring. Have the patient point to her primary area of pruritus. Take a biopsy of any abnormal findings that cannot be defined or are suspicious for malignancy.

Because vaginal disease can have great affect on the vulva, the vaginal mucosa should be included in the examination. A sample of the vaginal secretions should be studied microscopically for the presence of clue cells, lactobacilli, hyphae, pseudohyphae, or budding yeast. As needed, bacterial and fungal cultures should be ordered.

Differential Diagnosis of Vulvar Pruritus

Vulvar pruritus is a symptom that can be caused by any vulvar irritation or inflammation. Because it can be the result of a variety of different conditions, the provider must search for the cause. Vulvar pruritus can be characterized as acute or chronic, or primary or secondary. Vulvar pruritus can be secondary to skin conditions, such as infections, irritants, hormonal changes, infestations, neoplasms, medications, or systemic disease (**Box 1**).

The most common causes of vulvar itching are infection and skin disease. Vulvar pruritus can be caused by infections, such as vulvovaginal candidiasis, trichomonas, gonorrhea, *Chlamydia*, and bacterial vaginosis. In addition to pruritus, these infections often are associated with abnormal vaginal discharge. When abnormal vaginal discharge accompanies vulvar pruritus a work-up including potassium hydroxide (KOH) and wet mount are required. Bacterial, fungal, and viral cultures also may be necessary.

Vulvovaginal candidiasis is the most common cause of acute-onset vulvar pruritus, and it is the most common cause of vulvar pruritus diagnosed by gynecologists (**Fig. 1**). Presumptive diagnosis and empiric treatment must be avoided in women with chronic vulvovaginal pruritus, however, because many genital skin problems are mistakenly attributed to candidiasis.

It is important to look for candidiasis in every itchy patient and confirm infection by microscopy or culture. Vulvovaginal candidiasis caused by *Candida albicans* commonly is associated with an itching and burning sensation and a thick, white, curd-like discharge that is worse premenstrually.[6] Non-albicans *Candidiasis* is usually asymptomatic, but can produce irritation, burning, and soreness.[4] Candidiasis is not just a primary problem, but also occurs as a superinfection when topical corticosteroids and oral antibiotics

Box 1
Differential diagnosis of vulvar pruritus

Dermatoses

*Irritant contact dermatitis

*Allergic contact dermatitis

*Lichen simplex chronicus

*Lichen sclerosus

*Lichen planus

*Psoriasis

Seborrheic dermatitis

Plasma cell vulvitis

Dermatographism

Papular acantholytic dyskeratosis

Infectious causes

Fungal: *candidiasis, tinea cruris

Bacterial: group A streptococcus, *Staphylococcus aureus, Trichomonas vaginalis, Neisseria gonorrhea, Chlamydia trachomatis*

Viral: herpes simplex virus, human papilloma virus, molluscum contagiosum

Infestations: scabies, lice, enterobiasis

Neoplasms

*Vulvar intraepithelial carcinoma

*Extramammary Paget disease

Syringomas

Mammary-like gland adenomas (hidradenoma papilliferum)

Langerhans cell histiocytosis

Basal cell carcinoma

*More common causes

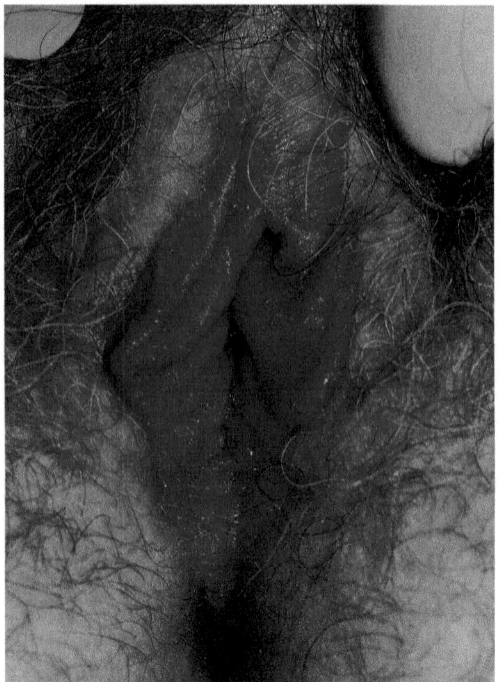

Fig. 1. Vulvovaginal candidiasis is the most common cause of sudden-onset itching; a fungal preparation showing yeast forms confirms the diagnosis of *Candida* suggested by red, puffy, modified mucous membranes with skin-fold fissures.

are used to treat underlying conditions.[4] Additionally, be aware that treatment with antifungal imidazole creams can cause a secondary irritant contact dermatitis (ICD), complicating the clinical picture.

Less commonly, such infections as herpes simplex virus, human papilloma virus, and molluscum contagiosum may provoke a sensation of itch. Note, however, that herpetic infections more commonly cause a burning pain, and human papilloma virus and molluscum are most likely to be asymptomatic. Consider perineal streptococcal disease secondary to group A streptococci, especially in pediatric patients.[6] Dermatophyte infections of anogenital skin are uncommon in women, and usually accompanied by involvement of the feet and toenails; a fungal preparation of scale from affected vulvar skin shows dermatophytosis.

The most likely skin diseases to present as vulvar pruritus include LSC; irritant and allergic contact dermatitis (ACD); lichen sclerosus; tinea cruris (much more common in men); lichen planus; psoriasis; and seborrheic dermatitis. As noted previously, characteristic scale seen on other parts of the body is commonly minimized or absent on the vulva because of moisture, which makes it difficult to distinguish these dermatoses by physical examination. Classic lesions identified elsewhere on a full-body skin examination can assist in narrowing the differential diagnosis. LSC is an important cause of primary vulvar pruritus and may complicate any of the other vulvar dermatoses. Therefore, it is discussed separately in detail later.

Contact dermatitis can be caused by irritants or allergens (**Fig. 2**). Vulvar skin is notably more sensitive to irritants and allergens than skin elsewhere on the body because of occlusion, hydration, and susceptibility to friction. Acute ICD occurs minutes to hours after exposure secondary to a strong irritant, such as urine or medications including trichloroacetic acid or podophylotoxin.[7] Much more common is the chronic form of ICD, where the cumulative effect of repeated, low-grade irritation causes damage to the skin barrier.[7,8] Overwashing, application of irritating hygiene products, lubricants, douches, and urinary and fecal incontinence (secondary to any variety of lower bowel disorders) can cause vulvar irritation and pruritus.[7–9] In response, some patients develop extensive hygiene routines secondary to fears of odor or infection, which further exacerbate the problem. Treatment of

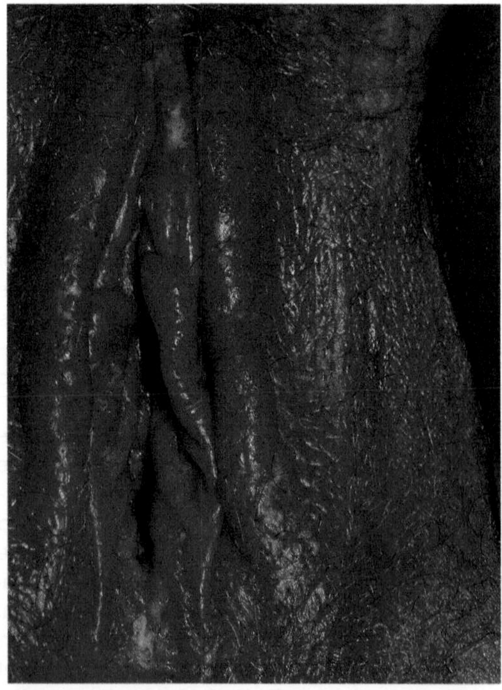

Fig. 2. This patient with irritant contact dermatitis from overwashing and allergic contact dermatitis from topical diphenhydramine exhibits edema of the labia minora, redness, and superficial erosions.

ICD consists of avoiding all irritants. It is important to inquire about incontinence, hygiene products, and cleansing habits and to give patients educational instructions on how to clean the vulvar area without causing irritation.

ACD occurs less frequently than ICD and is a delayed response that requires prior sensitization. Acute ACD is suspected on the basis of sudden onset of excruciating itching and vesiculation or erosion with exudation. The classic example of acute ACD is caused by poison ivy or poison oak. The diagnosis of chronic ACD, however, is more difficult, because both the history and clinical findings can be indistinguishable from, and overlap with, chronic ICD and LSC. Chronic ACD may accompany other skin problems and may occur as a result of treating preexisting symptoms. Potential sensitizers relevant to the vulva include topical anesthetics, particularly benzocaine, which is found in Vagisil; topical antibiotics; topical antifungal imidazole creams; topical corticosteroids; and preservatives.[7,10,11] The relevance of fragrances and nickel in vulvar ACD is unclear.[10–12] A diagnosis of ACD should be suspected in patients who apply multiple agents to their skin and whose pruritus does not respond to usual therapy.[8]

ACD should be ruled out by patch testing in any recalcitrant, chronic, or recurrent vulvar dermatosis. Testing to a standard patch series, and a medicament, cosmetic, and preservative series, plus "use testing" of all topical medicaments applied by the patient is recommended.[7,10–12] The therapy consists of avoidance of the chemical in the future and local skin care, which requires knowing all products that may contain this allergen, in addition to basic topical corticosteroid ointment use and nighttime sedation.

Lichen sclerosus is another skin disease in which pruritus is a main presenting symptom. Physical examination reveals atrophic, hypopigmented-to-white, crinkled, fragile plaques classically distributed in a figure-eight pattern around the vulva, perineal body, and perianal skin (**Fig. 3**). As the disease progresses, the main symptom shifts from pruritus to pain, which can be associated with a late physical finding of scarring with agglutination of normal genital structures.[4,8,13] The distinct presence of the labia minora may be lost and the clitoral hood may be scarred down.

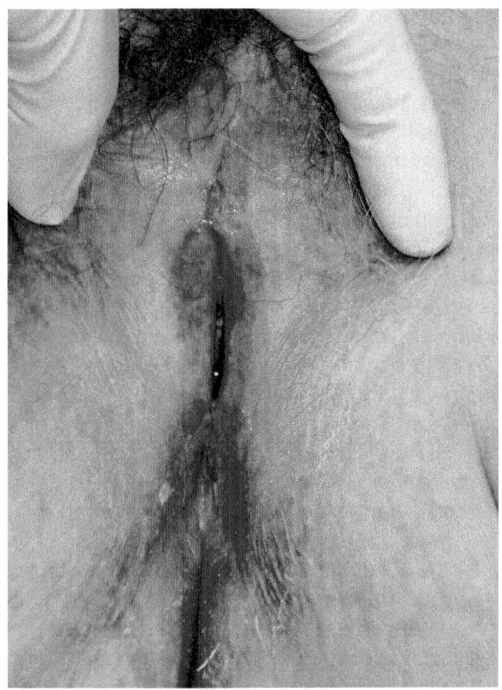

Fig. 3. Lichen sclerosus is manifested by white epithelium and a predisposition for resorption of the labia minora and scarring of the clitoral hood over the clitoris.

Lichen planus is another scarring vulvar dermatosis that has multiple morphologies including erosive, classic lacy, white, reticulate striae, and uniformly white plaques (**Fig. 4**).[8] The skin findings may be indistinguishable from lichen sclerosus and either asymptomatic, painful, or pruritic.

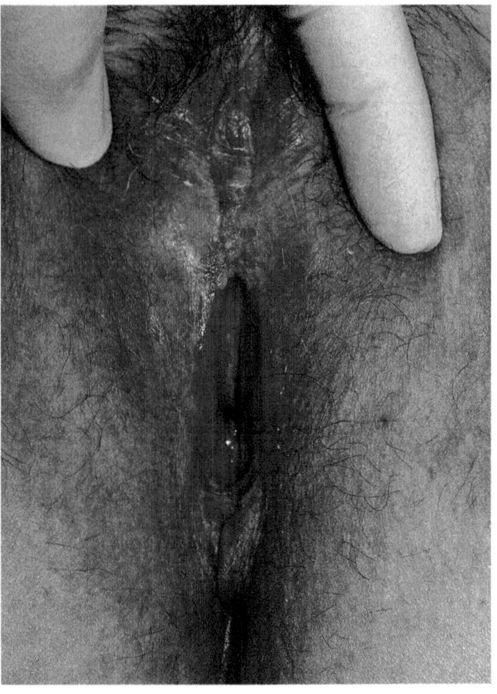

Fig. 4. Vulvar lichen planus is most often manifested by vestibular erosions, loss of vulvar architecture caused by scarring, and surrounding white epithethium; patients experience both itching and pain.

Commonly in lichen planus, there is associated disease in the vagina and oral mucosa. A biopsy can help to distinguish these two scarring diseases; however, obtaining a diagnostic biopsy can be difficult in subtle disease.

Classic psoriasis vulgaris, inverse psoriasis, and pustular psoriasis can all occur in the genital region. In skin folds, the classic silvery scale is replaced with a subtle, shiny texture (**Fig. 5**). A recent article correlates vulvar discomfort, manifested as pruritus or a burning sensation occurring in women with psoriasis, with depressive symptoms and encourages dermatologists to consider genital symptoms when evaluating psoriatic patients.[14] The erythematous plaques of vulvar psoriasis are considered to be well-demarcated compared with LSC, contact dermatitis, and seborrheic dermatitis. Seborrheic dermatitis is uncommon on the vulva and is usually associated with the simultaneous appearance of typical seborrhea on the scalp and central face.[8] The red, intertriginous plaques of psoriasis also can be difficult to distinguish clinically from tinea cruris and candidiasis. In-office KOH preparations and cultures are recommended.

Benign or malignant neoplasms are rare causes of vulvar pruritus. Physical examination should identify the presence of a focal neoplasm, and a prompt biopsy yields the diagnosis. Recent case reports in the literature describe syringomas,[15] mammary-like gland adenomas (also known as hidradenoma papilliferum),[16] Langerhans cell histiocytosis,[17] and basal cell carcinomas[18] presenting as vulvar pruritus. Vulvar intraepithelial neoplasm, previously known as Bowen disease or squamous cell carcinoma in situ, and extramammary Paget disease may clinically mimic the erythematous plaques of dermatitis.[8,19,20] Any condition unresponsive to corticosteroids requires biopsy to rule out vulvar intraepithelial neoplasm or extramammary Paget disease.

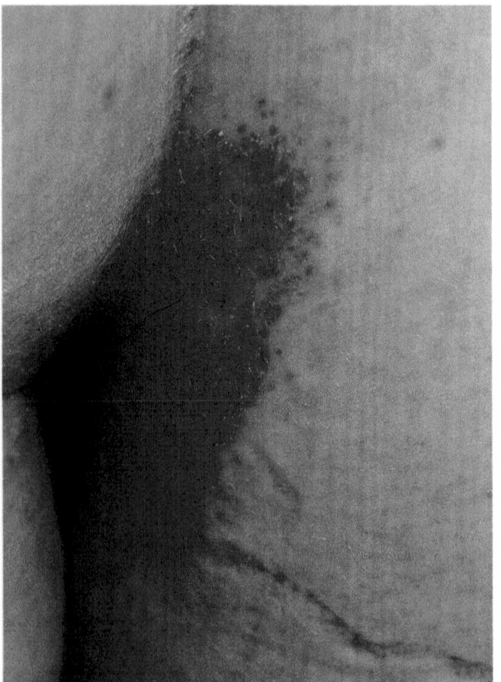

Fig. 5. Like most dermatoses that produce itching, psoriasis presents with red plaques; however, unlike extragenital psoriasis, anogenital psoriasis exhibits very subtle rather than heavy silvery scale.

Infestations, such as pediculosis pubis, scabies, and enterobiasis,[21] are in the differential diagnosis of pruritus vulvae patients, especially when the onset is acute and the pruritus is notably worse at night. A review of the literature reveals case reports of dermatographism,[22] papular acantholytic dyskeratosis,[23] and plasma cell vulvitis[24] as rare causes of vulvar pruritus.

Stress is common in patients who suffer from chronic itching. Depression and anxiety may be side effects of the chronic symptom or may be triggers that perpetuate the itching. To provide comprehensive care for the patient, the associated stress must be addressed, including, as appropriate, acknowledgment of her discomfort, committing to work with her until some amount of relief is found, prescribing antidepressants, and referral for professional counseling. In addition, the relevance of other treatable generalized conditions, such as diabetes, immunosuppression, and obesity, which may contribute to symptomatology, must be considered.

In cases where the cause of vulvar pruritus is secondary to a vulvar disorder, the pruritus usually resolves with treatment of the underlying disease. However, despite an adequate evaluation, often the cause of vulvar pruritus cannot be clearly identified. In these cases, treating the pruritus and reducing the inflammation with topical corticosteroids followed by reevaluation may uncover the underlying cause.

LICHEN SIMPLEX CHRONICUS

LSC of the vulva is one of the most common primary causes of vulvar pruritus and can be a secondary complication in any pruritic vulvar disease. LSC can be considered a localized, chronic variant of atopic dermatitis.[25] Dermatologists consider eczema, atopic dermatitis, neurodermatitis, and LSC essentially as a continuum of the same disease process.

Primary LSC arises in normal-appearing skin and when occurring in the anogenital area may be referred to as "pruritus vulvae," "pruritus scroti," or "pruritus ani." Primary LSC tends to occur in patients with an atopic diathesis. Atopy is defined as a personal or family history of allergic rhinitis, allergic conjunctivitis, hay fever, or asthma. Atopic patients are likely to experience itch secondary to irritation. The initial pruritus can be provoked by as little inciting event as touching, overcleaning, or tight clothing. Rubbing or scratching results in intense pleasure. The scratching and rubbing cause the skin to thicken and damages its protective barrier. This results in more scratching and increased susceptibility to irritants and infection. The continued irritation caused by the rubbing and scratching produces an itch-scratch cycle, which defines LSC.[4,8,25]

In secondary LSC, the itch-scratch cycle is instigated by any underlying vulvar condition, such as vulvovaginal candidiasis, lichen sclerosus, lichen planus, psoriasis, tinea cruris, and neoplasms. In both primary and secondary LSC, stress, heat, sweating, activity, and friction commonly aggravate the sensation of itch. Nighttime pruritus is common and the patient may not realize that they are scratching while they sleep.[4,8,25]

Patient History

Classically, patients with vulvar LSC present with a marked, relentless, intractable pruritus that has been present for weeks, months, or years. This is an itch that feels good when scratched verses an itch that may be described as irritating, prickly, or burning. In treating women with vulvovaginal pruritus, true itching produces a desire to scratch or rub: it is a "hands on" symptom.[4] Most patients are conscious of the itch-scratch cycle and can minimize rubbing or scratching by day; however, a few are completely unaware of their own behavior or may only scratch while asleep.

Many patients report that the pruritus started with a yeast infection or at a time of stress, but that the symptom persisted despite resolution of what was regarded as the inciting event. Any type of irritation, which may include heat and sweating and friction, worsens the itching. Further, irritation from bathing, topical medications, clothing, and sanitary pads also may exacerbate the pruritus.

Physical Examination

On careful examination, epidermal thickening or lichenified plaques with accentuated skin markings secondary to rubbing are present, either unilaterally or bilaterally (**Figs. 6–11**). If the patient uses her nails to scratch, the skin will be erythematous, likely with linear or angular excoriation and erosion. In the vulvar area this occurs most commonly overlying the labia majora, but also may involve labia minora, perineum, and vestibule and may extend to perianal skin. Depending on the patient's natural skin color, chronicity of symptoms, and the extent of the patient's scratching or rubbing, the skin changes may vary from normal to a very subtle erythema; to ruddy brown, secondary to hyperpigmentation; to whitish, secondary to the presence of scale in this moist area.[4,8,25]

Pubic hair in the area involved may be broken or lessened secondary to friction. Scratching, rubbing, topical treatments, and hygiene practices can lead to secondary changes, including erosions, ulcers, fissures, and crusting. Occasionally, the itch develops into a burning sensation or pain because of these secondary changes. This damage of the skin barrier leads to increased vulnerability to secondary infection and irritants. Mixed signs and symptoms can result when the LSC is secondary to another condition.

Full cutaneous examination may reveal eczematous changes on other skin surfaces or stigmata of atopy, such as keratosis pilaris, follicular

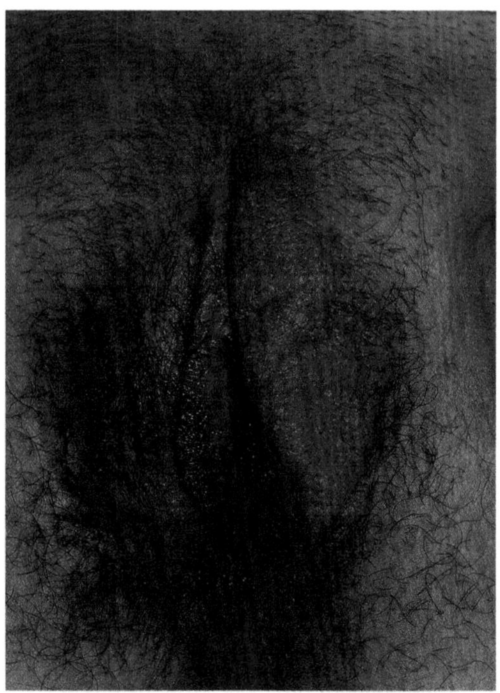

Fig. 6. Lichen simplex chronicus is characterized by thickening produced by rubbing and called lichenification. Rubbing also breaks hair.

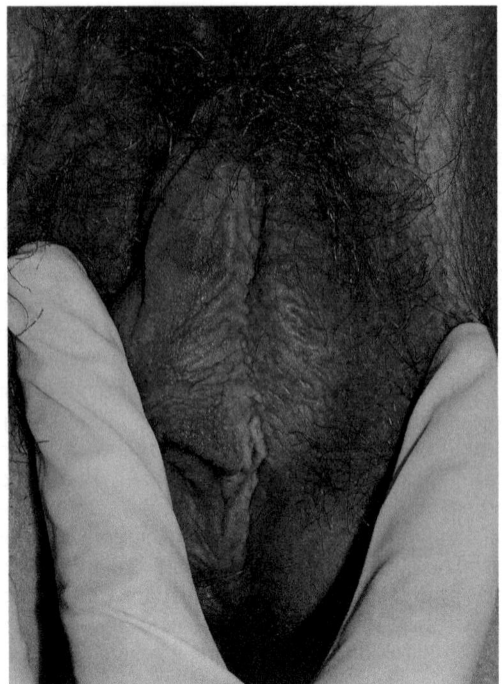

Fig. 7. Lichenification of the left interlabial sulcus is manifested by an accentuation of normal skin markings. Thick skin in moist areas often appears hypopigmented.

accentuation, xerosis, Dennie-Morgan lines, or hyperlinear palms.

Evaluation

LSC can usually be distinguished from other common pruritic vulvar conditions by a history of itching and pleasure with scratching accompanied by skin changes consistent with scratching or

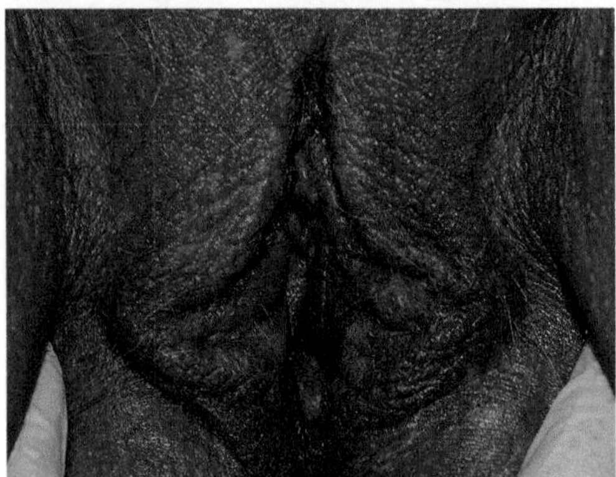

Fig. 8. Excoriations, irregular erosions produced by scratching, are common in patients with lichen simplex chronicus, as seen here in a setting of lichenification.

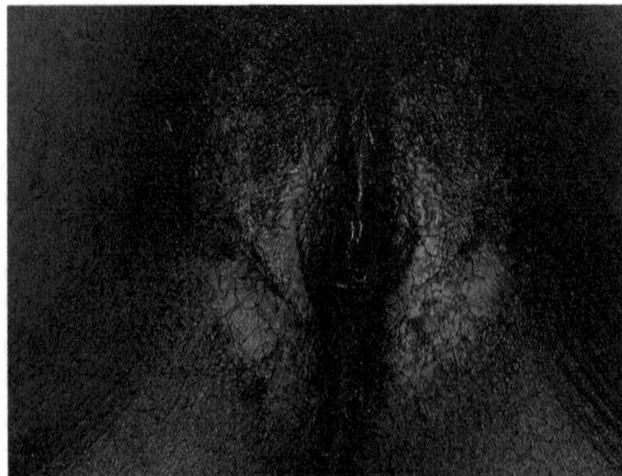

Fig. 9. White color with lichen simplex chronicus often occurs in patients of color; both postinflammatory hypopigmentation as seen on the perineum, and hypopigmentation from thickened, moist lichenification of the hairbearing surface of the labia majora occur.

rubbing. The differentiation of primary from secondary LSC is more difficult. Generally, this is done by a screen for infection and obvious skin disease, and treatment of LSC with subsequent reevaluation after clearing for persistent underlying disease. The most commonly found underlying conditions include candidiasis, contact dermatitis,

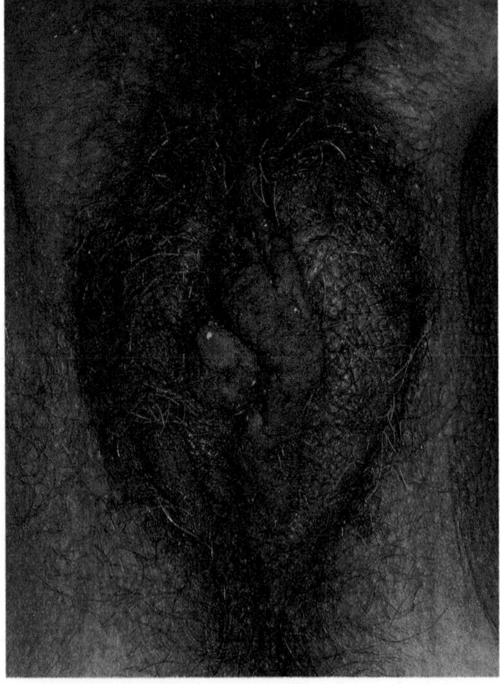

Fig. 10. Inflammation in patients with normally dark complexion generally appears hyperpigmented rather than red.

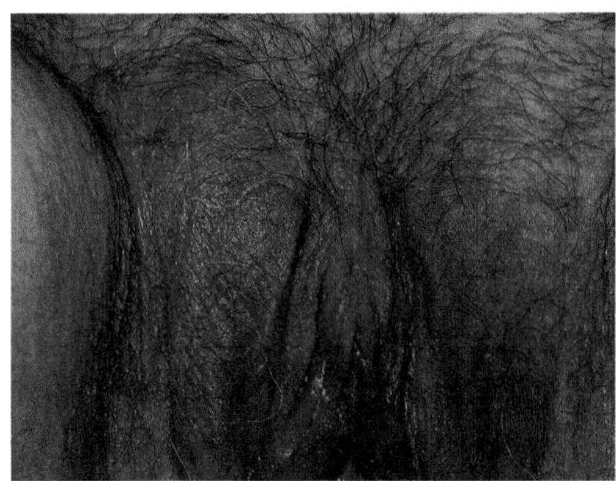

Fig. 11. The severity of pruritus of lichen simplex chronicus does not necessarily correlate with the degree of lichenification on examination; this woman with excruciating itching of the right anterior vulva shows only minor thickening compared with the left vulva.

psoriasis, and lichen sclerosus, but as discussed previously it is important to consider a broad differential. Bacterial and fungal cultures, and KOH preparations, are helpful in diagnosing secondary infections. If the diagnosis is in doubt, rule out an underlying condition with a skin biopsy. Histologically, LSC reveals hyperkeratosis, hypergranulosis, acanthosis, spongiosis, and a chronic inflammatory infiltrate.

Treatment

The key to successfully treating LSC is concomitant, combination therapy including a potent topical corticosteroid, nighttime sedation as needed, symptomatic antipruritic treatment with topical anesthetics, appropriate treatment of secondary bacterial and fungal infections, avoidance of all irritants, and identification and treatment of underlying conditions.

Topical corticosteroids decrease inflammation and break the itch-scratch cycle.[25,26] The modified mucous membranes of the vulva are relatively corticosteroid resistant, requiring potent corticosteroids. A superpotent corticosteroid, such as clobetsol diporpionate 0.05% ointment, applied very sparingly twice daily for 4 weeks, is usually sufficient. Hair-bearing skin, medial thighs, and perianal skin atrophy more easily than glabrous skin and are at risk for steroid dermatitis. Therefore, these areas should be followed very carefully. Patients should be examined monthly initially when on daily clobetasol. An in-office demonstration of how much ointment to apply, and to exactly what areas, can improve compliance and outcome and decrease risk of side effects.

The topical calcineurin inhibitors, tacrolimus ointment and pimecrolimus 1% cream, are nonsteroidal anti-inflammatory agents that have been approved as second-line treatments for eczema. They work as immunomodulators, blocking the release of inflammatory cytokines from T lymphocytes. Especially relative to the treatment of vulvar dermatoses, the draw to these medications stems from the lack of side effects, such as atrophy, striae, and steroid dermatitis associated with first-line topical corticosteroids. The recent literature contains multiple articles documenting the efficacy of topical calcineurin inhibitors in vulvar disease.[27–30] In September 2009, Goldstein and colleagues[30] summarized the case reports, case series, and open-label prospective studies regarding topical calcineurin inhibitors and vulvar dermatoses and concluded that, as with eczema elsewhere on the body, topical calcineurin inhibitors should remain second-line therapies in vulvar dermatoses for patients who are intolerant or resistant to topical corticosteroids. Of note, these medications often burn on application, although this is minimized when the medication is stored in a refrigerator. Also, these medications are black-boxed by the Food and Drug Administration for its risk for the production of squamous cell carcinoma and lymphoma.

Itching is often worse at night, when a significant amount of scratching or rubbing occurs. Nighttime sedation can help to eliminate nighttime scratching. Only a very little scratching and rubbing is necessary to perpetuate LSC. Hydroxyzine and diphenhydramine are sedating but produce REM sleep during which patients still rub. Tricyclic medications, such as amitriptyline and doxepin, induce deep sleep and sedate for a longer period (about 10 hours) and are more effective.[31] Because patients with chronic anogenital symptoms are often depressed and anxious, any antidepressant effects of such nighttime sedation may be beneficial.[32] Amitriptyline and doxepin at a dose of 10 to 100 mg 2 hours before bedtime are usually effective. The initial dosage should be low and increased as needed, because some patients become oversedated with higher initial doses and will not take the medication again. Warn the patient that dry eyes and mouth, constipation, and increased appetite may occur.

Because it takes time for the topical corticosteroid to have enough effect to noticeably decrease the vulvar pruritus, patients also require symptomatic relief. Lidocaine (Xylocaine) jelly 2% may be applied as often as needed as a cooling, nonirritating, and nonallergenic anesthetic. Avoid Vagisil and its generics that contain benzocaine and resourcinol, and topical diphenhydramine, all of which are sensitizers.

Screen and treat secondary infections with oral antibiotics and oral antifungal medications as needed to avoid the irritation of topical medications. Women with LSC who have thickened, lichenified skin and excoriations are at risk for candidiasis and bacterial superinfection. Cutaneous candidiasis is likely when there is a glazed texture of the skin, crural crease erythema, satellite collarettes or pustules, or skin-fold fissures. In the presence of classic physical findings, treatment can be empiric, but consider obtaining a culture first in the setting of chronic symptoms. Oral fluconazole, 150 mg once weekly, or nystatin ointment twice daily for 1 to 2 weeks is recommended. The imidazole creams are effective against most *Candida* species, but the cream vehicles tend to further irritate vulvar skin. For concerns about bacterial superinfection, cepalexin, 500 mg twice a day for a week, is an effective and inexpensive therapy.[33] When treating a patient with topical corticosteroids and oral antibiotics, anticipate the likelihood of a secondary yeast infection and add fluconazole, 150 mg once a week, preventively.

The patient should be instructed to wash with water only, using soft fingertips. Alert the patient to avoid inadvertent rubbing that commonly accompanies the use of washcloths. The vulvar skin can be hydrated by soaking in a tub of water at a comfortable temperature followed by application of a bland emollient, such as white petrolatum. All other treatments should be discontinued. Avoid soap; bubble baths; douches; lubricants; and exacerbating factors, such as excessive washing, heat, and friction. Fingernails are the worst irritants. Encourage the patient to cut her nails and, if possible, to wear gloves at nighttime.

A patient may be frustrated by previous ineffective treatments and by the effect the pruritus has had on her life and relationships. Some may argue and hesitate to try another topical corticosteroid, because previous treatments did not work. It is important to acknowledge the patient's concerns and to include her partner in discussions regarding diagnosis and treatment. Treatment failures often are caused by the use of a topical corticosteroid without the control of other factors (eg, secondary infection, irritants, and nighttime scratching) and by using too low potency a corticosteroid for too short a duration.[34] Patients need to understand that LSC can be controlled but not cured. The itch sensation in response to irritation is likely to recur. Written instructions listing the diagnosis, treatment instructions, reliable Internet resources, and a scheduled follow-up appoint in 4 weeks go a long way in securing a good patient-physician relationship (**Box 2**).

If a patient fails to improve, start by clarifying what the patient was actually doing for treatment. Reexamine the patient and consider underlying skin conditions, secondary infections, and a possible allergy to the treatment itself. Biopsy or rebiopsy and consider patch testing.[35] Pay attention to mood and affect in those who do not respond to usual therapy, because depression may be a persistent trigger of symptoms and warrant evaluation and treatment. Consider alternative treatments, such as antidepressants and hypnosis, to treat the associated distress and sleep interruption. A review of the literature reveals a case report in which long-standing, idiopathic, genital pruritus resolved after five sessions of self-hypnosis training. A trial of amitriptyline or

Box 2
Example of patient instructions

Diagnosis: Lichen simplex chronicus.

The treatment of lichen simplex chronicus is a lot of work. It is important to follow these instructions carefully.

1. Apply tiny amount of clobetasol ointment to affected area twice daily.
2. Minimize nighttime scratching; take amitriptyline, 10 mg, by mouth 1–2 hours before bedtime. Start by taking one tablet nightly and increase by one tablet (maximum 10) each night until sleep is restful and without scratching. If you feel too sedated in the morning, reduce dosage.
3. Apply a liberal amount of lidocaine 2% jelly as often as needed for discomfort.
4. To prevent a yeast infection while using a topical corticosteroid ointment, take fluconazole, 150 mg once weekly.
5. A very important part of the treatment is careful skin care to avoid irritation. Washing the skin is the most common irritation for skin. Washing dissolves the natural oils in the skin and allows tiny, invisible cracks that itch. Wash with warm water using only gentle fingertips rather than rough washcloths.

Avoid: hot water, harsh soaps, and washcloths.

Avoid: medications other than those prescribed as mentioned.

Avoid: rough fabric, tight clothes, and overheating.

Avoid: panty liners, douches, perfumes, and deodorants.

Schedule a follow-up appointment in 4 weeks.

gabapentin aimed at treating a neuropathy may be of benefit in recalcitrant cases.

SUMMARY

Vulvar pruritus can be caused by a wide spectrum of pathologies, the most common being candidiasis, contact dermatitis, LSC, and lichen sclerosus. LSC begins with an inciting itch sensation for which scratching and rubbing yield pleasure and relief, which can trigger a chronic itch-scratch cycle. The tendency toward LSC cannot be cured, but the symptoms generally can be controlled. Prompt treatment with superpotent corticosteroids usually breaks the itch-scratch cycle. Careful attention to irritants and secondary infection prevents this from becoming a significant ongoing problem.

REFERENCES

1. Farage MA, Miller KW, Ledger WJ. Determining the cause of vulvovaginal symptoms. Obstet Gynecol Surv 2008;63(7):445–64.
2. Turner MLC, Marinoff SC. General principles of diagnosis and treatment of vulvar disease. Dermatol Clin 1992;10(2):275–81.
3. Margesson LJ. Vulvar disease pearls. Dermatol Clin 2006;24:145–55.
4. Lynch PJ, Edwards L. Red plaques with eczematous features. In: Lynch PJ, Edwards L, editors. Genital dermatology. New York: WB Saunders; 1994. p. 27–34.
5. Pincus SJ. Vulvar dermatoses and pruritus vulvae. Dermatol Clin 1992;10(2):297–308.
6. Bohl TG. Overview of vulvar pruritus through the life cycle. Clin Obstet Gynecol 2005;48(4):786–807.
7. Bauer A, Rodiger C, Grief C, et al. Vulvar dermatoses – irritant and allergic contact dermatitis of the vulva. Dermatology 2005;210(2):143–9.
8. Lynch PJ. Vulvar pruritus and lichen simplex chronicus. In: Black M, editor. Obstetrical and gynecologic dermatology. St. Louis (MO): Mosby; 2002. p. 157–66.
9. Farage MA, Miller KW, Berardesca E, et al. Incontinence in the aged: contact dermatitis and other cutaneous consequences. Contact Dermatitis 2007;57(4):211–7.
10. Utaş S, Ferahbaş A, Yildiz S. Patients with vulval pruritus: patch test reports. Contact Dermatitis 2008;58(5):296–8.
11. Haverhoek E, Reid C, Gordon L, et al. Prospective study of patch testing in patients with vulval pruritus. Australas J Dermatol 2008;49(2):80–5.
12. Lucke TW, Fleming CJ, McHenry P, et al. Patch testing in vulval dermatoses: how relevant is nickel? Contact Dermatitis 1998;38(2):111–2.
13. Ball SB, Wojnarowski F. Vulvar dermatoses: lichen sclerosus, lichen planus, and vulval dermatitis/lichen simplex chronicus. Semin Cutan Med Surg 1998;17:182–8.
14. Zamirska A, Reich A, Berny-Moreno J, et al. Vulvar pruritus and burning sensation in woman with psoriasis. Acta Derm Venereol 2008;88(2):132–5.
15. Kavala M, Can B, Zindanci I, et al. Vulvar pruritus caused by syringoma of the vulva. Int J Dermatol 2008;47(8):831–2.
16. Scurry J, van der Putte SC, Pyman J, et al. Mammary-like gland adenoma of the vulva: review of 46 cases. Pathology 2009;41(4):372–8.
17. Elas D, Benda JA, Galask RP. Langerhans' cell histiocytosis of the vulva: the Iowa experience. J Reprod Med 2008;53(6):417–9.
18. Saini R, Sarnoff DS. Basal cell carcinoma of the vulva presenting as unilateral pruritus. J Drugs Dermatol 2008;7(3):288–90.
19. Pascual JC, Perez-Ramos M, Devesa JP, et al. Extramammary Paget's disease of the groin with underlying carcinoma and fatal outcome. Clin Exp Dermatol 2008;33(5):595–8.
20. Kehoe S, Luesley D. Pathology and management of vulval pain and pruritus. Curr Opin Obstet Gynecol 1995;7(1):16–9.
21. Day S. Threadworm: an infrequent clinical finding in a genitourinary medicine clinic attendee presenting with ano-genital irritation. Int J STD AIDS 2009;20(5):362–3.
22. Sherertz EF. Clinical pearl: symptomatic dermatographism as a cause of genital pruritus. J Am Acad Dermatol 1994;31:1040–1.
23. Wang L, Yang XC, Hao F, et al. Papular acantholytic dyskeratosis of the vulva. Eur J Dermatol 2009;19(4):402–3.
24. Goldstein AT, Christopher K, Burrows LJ. Plasma cell vulvitis: a rare cause of intractable vulvar pruritus. Arch Dermatol 2005;141(6):789–90.
25. Lynch PJ. Lichen simplex chronicus (atopic/neurodermatitis) for the anogenital region. Dermatol Ther 2004;17(1):8–19.
26. Virgili A, Bacilleri S, Corazza M. Managing vulvar lichen simplex chronicus. J Reprod Med 2001;46(4):343–6.
27. Reitamo S, Wollenberg A, Schopf E, et al. Safety and efficacy of 1 year of tacrolimus ointment for long-term treatment of atopic dermatitis. Arch Dermatol 2000;136:999–1006.
28. Weisshaar E. Successful treatment of genital pruritus using topical immunomodulators as a single therapy in multi-morbid patients. Acta Derm Venereol 2008;88(2):195–6.
29. Sarifakioglu E, Gumus II. Efficacy of topical pimecrolimus in the treatment of chronic vulvar pruritus: a prospective case series–a non-controlled, open labeled study. J Dermatolog Treat 2006;17(5):276–8.

30. Goldstein AT, Parneix-Spake A, McCormick CL, et al. Pimecroliums cream 1% for treatment of vulvar lichen simplex chronicus: an open-label, preliminary trial. Gynecol Obstet Invest 2007;64(4):180–6.
31. Aoki T, Kushimoto H, Hishikawa Y, et al. Nocturnal scratching and its relationship to the disturbed sleep of itchy subjects. Clin Exp Dermatol 1991;16: 268–72.
32. Bhatia MS, Gautam RK, Bedi GK. Psychiatric profile of patients with neurodermatitis. J Indian Med Assoc 1996;94:445–6.
33. Abeck D, Mempel M. *Staphylococcus aureus* colonization in atopic dermatitis and its therapeutic implications. Br J Dermatol 1998;139(Suppl. 53):13–6.
34. Lagro-Janssen, Sluis S. Effectiveness of treating nonspecific pruritus vulvae with topical steroids: a randomized controlled trial. Eur J Gen Pract 2009; 15(1):29–33.
35. Virgili A, Bacilieri S, Corazza M. Evaluation of contact sensitization in vulvar lichen simplex chronicus. A proposal for a battery of selected allergens. J Reprod Med 2003;48(1):33–6.

Vulvodynia: New Concepts and Review of the Literature

Vlada Groysman, MD

KEYWORDS

- Vulvodynia • Genital tract • Vulvar discomfort
- Multifactorial disorder

Vulvodynia is defined by the International Society for Study of Vulvovaginal Disease (ISSVD) as "vulvar discomfort, most often described as burning pain without relevant visible findings or a specific, clinically identifiable, neurologic disorder."[1] Patients with vulvodynia often describe it as chronic vulvar burning, stinging, irritation, rawness, and, rarely, pruritis.[2] It may be felt only during sexual intercourse, experienced continually, or triggered by nonsexual activities such as walking.[3–6] Although believed in the past to be an uncommon condition, vulvodynia is a major contributing cause for patient referral. Data from a population-based study funded by the National Institutes of Health found that 15.7% of women reported lower genital tract discomfort persisting 3 months or longer.[7] Recent population-based studies show estimates as high as 28%, with 1 study showing that 39% of women who suffer from chronic vulvar pain fail to seek treatment.[7] Frequency of vulvodynia is underestimated partially because of the belief of the medical community that this problem is psychological and thus is not in their realm, and also because affected women are reluctant to discuss their symptoms because of fear of neglect. Vulval pain has been highlighted as a highly prevalent condition that is associated with substantial disability.[8] Although vulvodynia is a multifactorial pain syndrome in which psychological, social, and sexual function interact, it is a diagnosis of exclusion, in which treatable causes such as dermatoses, infection, neoplasia, and neurologic disorder must be ruled out; patients must be properly classified and also appropriate education and psychological support/counseling must be administered. As vulvodynia receives increased attention by both the medical profession and the media, more women are seeking care, information, and guidance.

CAUSES

Infection and Vulvodynia

The causes of vulvodynia are unknown; however, several hypothesis have been proposed to identify causative factors. One of the most consistently reported clinical findings associated with the onset of vulvodynia is a history of frequent yeast infections. A chronic subclinical yeast infection was believed to play a role in the development of symptoms, but the use of antifungal medications has been shown to be inadequate for patients with undocumented yeast infection.[9–11] It is not clear whether the culprit is the yeast itself, the treatments undertaken that can sensitize the tissue, an underlying sensitivity present in the tissue, or simply the most common diagnosis made for unexplained symptoms. A recent study suggested that diverse urogenital infections such as yeast infection, urinary tract infection, trichomonas, and human papilloma virus (HPV) may precede the onset of vulvodynia, with multiple assaults significantly compounding risk.[12,13] However, this has not been a consistent finding within other studies, and prospective studies documenting

The author has financial relationships to disclose.
No funding support was provided for the purposes of this article.
Department of Dermatology, University of Alabama at Birmingham, EFH 414, 1530 3rd Avenue South, Birmingham, AL 35294-0009, USA
E-mail address: vlgroysman@yahoo.com

Dermatol Clin 28 (2010) 681–696
doi:10.1016/j.det.2010.07.002

urogenital infections in association with vulvodynia are warranted.

Although HPV was initially reported as a frequent cause of vulvodynia, testing for HPV has shown that this virus is absent in most women with vulvar pain.[14–17] One recent study observed that the low rate of observed infection in women with vulvodynia, and the diversity of HPV types detected in the patient population studied, suggest incidental virus carriage rather than direct cause and effect.[18,19]

Genetic Factors

Gerber and colleagues[20] conducted studies on genetic predisposition and the onset of vulvodynia. They found that more affected women were homozygous for allele 2 in the interleukin-1β receptor antagonist and for allele 2 interleukin-1β gene than nonaffected women. Each of these alleles has been associated with prolonged inflammatory response. Susceptibility to vulvodynia might be influenced by carriage of this polymorphism. They concluded that these findings strongly imply that women with vulvodynia may be at increased risk for a proinflammatory immune response to be triggered by a variety of stimuli and may have difficulty in terminating an inflammatory event that involves interleukin-1β production. A similar deficit in interleukin-1receptor antagonist production has been shown to contribute to chronic inflammation in individuals with inflammatory bowel disease. The investigators also stated that some women have a genetic predisposition to develop a chronic inflammatory response after an inciting event, such as a yeast infection. The prolonged inflammation could trigger other events such as increased sensitivity in both genital and nongenital areas of the body. It has been reported that affected women have more somatic pain disorders and show increases in sensitivity to nongenital touch, pain, and temperature.[21–23]

Vulvodynia as a Neuropathic Disorder

Vulvodynia has features that are characteristic of other chronic neuropathic pain conditions. These features include the persistent and burning quality of the pain, the allodynia and hyperpathia, the absence of physical findings on examination, lack of associated pathologic condition of the tissues, and strong association with depression, and are all reminiscent of other neuropathic syndromes such as regional pain syndrome (formerly reflex sympathetic dystrophy), and pudendal neuralgia.[8,24–29] The transition from the nociceptive to neuropathic pain is key in vulvodynia because it underlies the shift from a pain disorder in which sexual intercourse elicits pain to a pain disorder that is progressive and ongoing even with the avoidance of any further intercourse.[8,28] The role of neuropathic pain in vulvodynia is supported by a documented response to agents used to treat neuropathic pain. Immunohistochemistry has shown altered density of nerve endings such as the vanilloid receptor VR1 (TRPV1), which is expressed by nociceptors, and is triggered by capsaicin, noxious heat, protons, and chemicals produced during inflammation; as well as increased number of intraepithelial free nerve endings, calcitonin-related gene peptide (peptide found in nerve fibers), lowered tactile and pain thresholds, nociceptor sensitization, and overall peripheral nerve hyperplasia.[30–34] Several studies report successful treatment of localized vulvodynia with botulin toxin A.[35–38] Moreover, increased blood flow and erythema in the posterior vestibular mucosa have been shown in vulvodynia via laser Doppler perfusion imaging of the superficial blood flow in the vestibular mucosa. Researchers postulated that such observation is the result of both neovascularization and angiogenesis along with the release of neuropeptides from C fibers in the skin, which produces an axon reflex causing vasodilatation and increased blood flow.[39]

Pelvic Floor Abnormalities and Vulvodynia

Most women with vulvodynia exhibit pelvic floor abnormalities. Pelvic floor performance is significantly lower in affected patients in terms of contractile and resting ability and stability and efficiency of contraction.[40–44] Pelvic floor abnormality may serve as causative or aggravating factors in the development of vulvodynia. Rehabilitation of pelvic floor muscles via surface electromyography has been successful in reducing pain and increasing sexual interest, pleasure, and activity.[8]

Hormonal Influence

Hormones have a role in the genesis and continuance of many pain syndromes. Some clinic-based studies support an association between hormonal contraception and vulvodynia. The effect of oral contraceptives (OCs) on vulvar epithelium is largely unknown, however they may "alter the vaginal epithelium by promoting loss of a cyclic pattern, low karyopyknotic index and the appearance of navicular cells with marked curling and folding."[45,46] The presence of estrogen from OCs and the increased number of parabasal cells (a marker of atrophy), is unexpected. According to a recent study, women taking OCs have lower mechanical pain thresholds in the vestibular region compared with controls.[45] Other studies suggest that there is only a modest risk of OC use and vulvodynia, and that risk is confined to women whose exposure occurred before the age of 18 years. It is often difficult to assess whether OCs truly influence the risk of vulvodynia because OC preparations are variable.

However, hormone supplementation influences sensory discrimination and pain sensitivity. Estrogen is known to affect inflammatory neuropeptides involved in chronic pain, in which the lack of estrogen is associated with increased density of sympathetic, parasympathetic, and sensory nerve fibers in the vulva, whereas acute or chronic estrogen administration may result in a decrease in the total and sympathetic fiber numbers.[45,46] Moreover, estrogen regulates uterine sympathetic nerve remodeling through actions on myometrium, ganglion, and intermediary pituitary factors. Vaginal dysfunction during menopause is generally assumed to occur because of diminished estrogen-mediated trophic support of vaginal target cells. In addition, studies show that increased sympathetic innervation may change vasoconstriction and promote vaginal dryness, whereas sensory axon proliferation may contribute to symptoms of pain, burning, and itching associated with menopause and vulvodynia.[47,48] Estrogen can therefore both lower the pain threshold and be a potent mediator of peripheral nerve remodeling.

Vulvodynia is a multifactorial disease. Although most clinicians find that depression and anxiety are often associated with the disease and sometimes exacerbate it, studies do not support a psychosexual dysfunction as a primary cause of vulvodynia. Data show that vulvodynia results in a significant psychosocial effect and, compared with dermatologic disorders conventionally regarded as affecting well-being, patients with vulvodynia experienced a more severe effect on quality of life.[49] However, some experienced vulvologists are certain that psychosexual dysfunction is the major causal factor.[22] Also, conditions such as interstitial cystitis, headaches, fibromyalgia, and irritable bowel syndrome are overrepresented in women with vulvodynia, with depression compounding, and at times worsening, the condition. Although clinical management should begin with careful examination to rule out skin disease and infection, overall psychosocial effects should also be addressed during treatment.

Diagnosis

Getting the terminology

Assessment of a woman with possible vulvodynia includes both history and physical findings. A good assessment is essential to differentiate between vulvar pain caused by an objective abnormality, and vulvodynia, in which pain is unassociated with abnormal clinical findings; to differentiate between the different subsets of vulvodynia (localized, generalized, provoked, unprovoked, or overlapping) according to ISSVD terminology (**Box 1**).[1] A systematic assessment is essential in both early diagnosis and appropriate management of vulvodynia. Previous descriptions of vulvodynia have grouped patients according to whether pain is provoked by coitus (vulvar vestibulitis syndrome) or generalized and neuropathic pain (dysesthetic vulvodynia). Recent terminology debates have questioned whether the term vulvodynia should be replaced by dysesthesia, and the term vestibulitis avoided because there is no inflammation in vulvodynia. Definitions of pain provocation, quality, duration, and distribution vary. Terminology developed by the ISSVD recommends standardization of the definition of vulvar pain and the classification of vulvodynia into subtypes of generalized versus localized and provoked versus unprovoked.[3,50–52] Generalized specifies involvement of the whole vulva, and localized specifies involvement of a portion of

Box 1
ISSVD Terminology and Classification of Vulvar Pain (2003)

A) Vulvar Pain Related to a Specific Disorder[53]

- **1) Infectious** (eg, candidiasis, herpes, etc)
- **2) Inflammatory** (eg, lichen planus, immunobullous disorders, etc)
- **3) Neoplastic** (eg, Paget's disease, squamous cell carcinoma, etc)
- **4) Neurologic** (eg, herpes neuralgia, spinal nerve compression, etc)

B) Vulvodynia

- **1) Generalized**
  - **a) Provoked** (sexual, nonsexual, or both)
  - **b) Unprovoked**
  - **c) Mixed** (provoked and unprovoked)
- **2) Localized** (vestibulodynia, clitorodynia, hemivulvodynia, etc)
  - **a) Provoked** (sexual, nonsexual, or both)
  - **b) Unprovoked**
  - **c) Mixed** (provoked and unprovoked)

Data from Moyal-Barracco M, Lynch PJ. 2003 ISSVD terminology and classification of vulvodynia: a historical perspective. J Reprod Med 2004;49:772–7.

vulva, such as vestibule (vestivulodynia), clitoris (clitorodynia), hemivulva (hemivulvodynia).[53] Unprovoked implies discomfort that occurs spontaneously, without a trigger, provoked asserts that the discomfort is caused by physical contact, such as intercourse, clothing pressure, tampon use, cotton-tipped pressure or fingertip pressure.[53] The ISSVD has recommended elimination of the term dysesthesia because it is an "unnecessary modification of previous terminology."[53]

Moreover, vulvodynia is a diagnosis of exclusion; it occurs in the absence of clinically identifiable findings such as active or chronic infection of the vulva, inflammation, neoplasia, spasmodic pelvic musculature, trauma, or a neurologic disorder as evident in peripheral neuropathy, pudendal neuralgia, herpes neuralgia, spinal nerve compression, and so forth.[54–56] These can often be ruled out on examination. Sphincter dysfunction, weakness in the lower limbs, sensory changes such as anesthesia of the affected area, allodynia, and symmetric sensation of bilateral limbs should be assessed.

Examination

A complete genitourinary physical examination is recommended in assessing a patient with vulvodynia. The examination should include visual inspection of the external genitalia and labia for erythema, erosions, crusting, pallor, dryness and ulceration, and hypopigmentation, and it should include a speculum.[57,58] A pediatric-sized speculum, and single-digit internal examination to evaluate pelvic floor muscle strength and tenderness is advised for patient comfort.[8] A wet mount is often helpful in evaluation of vaginal secretions for yeast, pH, and white blood cells.[2]

Candida is usually the first working diagnosis that needs to be ruled out. Itching is a predominant symptom in *Candida albicans* infection with secondary pain and rawness. Some organisms, such as *Candida glabrata*, *Candida parapsilosis*, *Candida krusei*, and *Saccharomyces cerevisae*, can cause symptoms similar to vulvodynia such as burning, soreness, rawness, and irritation. These organisms are difficult to detect and treat, and they are often not responsive to initial antifungal therapy. A fungal culture is imperative in diagnosis, because it is easy to miss these organisms on microscopic analysis. In contrast with *C albicans*, the organisms listed earlier do not produce pseudohyphae or hyphae in the vagina, but form small, budding yeast. Isolation of a fungal organism does not ensure that the cause of the symptoms has been identified, but the treatment could help in case the symptoms are related. On physical examination, creamy white curds are visible on the vaginal walls, and there is vulvar erythema, rarely with pustules.[8,53,54]

A routine vaginal culture is indicated for a patient with vulvar pain, because some patients exhibit a heavy growth of group B *Streptococcus*. Although group B *Streptococcus* is usually an asymptomatic colonizer of vagina, many clinicians believe that it occasionally produces vulvar burning or irritation. These patients may benefit from penicillin administration.[59]

Skin diseases of the vulva or vagina can also cause pain. Such conditions as lichen planus are a common cause of vulvar pain. Approximately 50% of women with cutaneous lichen planus have genital involvement. Erosive lichen planus is a distinct subtype of the disease, which manifests as vestibular, introitus, and vaginal erosions, resulting in inflammatory vaginal discharge even in the absence of vulvar involvement. There is also contact bleeding and marked erythema of vaginal mucosa. Erosive lichen planus is a scarring disease, therefore loss of the normal architecture of the vulva is common, and, in severe cases, results in obliteration of the vaginal canal. Inflammatory vaginitis may occasionally be caused by other erosive skin diseases, such as cicatricial pemphigoid, pemphigus vulgaris, bullous pemphigoid, erythema multiforme, and fixed drug eruption.[12,54,60–62] More common noninfectious causes of vaginal inflammation include atrophic vaginitis and a clinical syndrome seen in premenopausal women consisting of diffuse vaginal erythema and vaginal secretions that are microscopically purulent and exhibit increase in immature epithelial cells. Sobel[63,64] named this syndrome desquamative inflammatory vaginitis. Lichen sclerosis is another chronic inflammatory disease with a predilection for the anogenital region. It often presents with pruritis as the most frequent symptom, and clinical signs such as pallor, atrophy, fissures, and foci of hyperkeratosis. Dyspareunia is a common complaint.

Vulvar dermatitis may also present with symptoms of dyspareunia; however, the main symptom is again pruritis. It has traditionally been classified into endogenous dermatitis, such as seborrheic dermatitis, atopic dermatitis, and lichen simplex chronicus, and exogenous dermatitis from irritants and allergic contact dermatitis. However, there is often an overlap. Lichenification, excoriations, and, at times, fissures are evident on examination. Biopsy of a specific skin finding is necessary. Recent study reported that 61% of women who presented with chronic vulvar pain had identifiable disease on biopsy. The remaining 39 % had nonspecific findings. The investigators recommended performing biopsies in patients who present with vulvodynia symptoms even in the absence of skin or mucosal changes. This recommendation has been debated in the literature.[65] However, biopsy of a specific skin finding is often best to avoid false positives, and evaluation by a trained dermatopathologist is essential.[25,66,67]

Evaluation of Psychosocial Effects

Vulvodynia often significantly affects a woman's psychological health. Reports of psychosocial stress are common in the literature and include depression, altered body image, impaired social relationships, altered sexual function, and difficulty in physical activities and daily activities of life. An overall decrease in quality of life is seen in women with vulvodynia.[8,68]

As with other areas, conflicting studies exist regarding the psychosocial effect of vulvar discomfort. The only consistent psychological effect in women with vulvodynia was difficulty with sexual functioning. Although studies find that affected women's physiologic sexual arousal is not impaired, because of fear of sexual intimacy from previous experiences with pain with intercourse, patients become fearful and thus sexual arousal is decreased. It is often necessary to perform a psychosexual assessment or to send patient and partner to be properly evaluated.[69,70]

Treatment

The management of vulvodynia includes nonspecific supportive measures (**Box 2**) as well as specific therapies directed toward the treatment of neuropathic pain, pelvic floor muscle dysfunction, and the psychosexual factors and sequelae (**Box 3**).

Education

Patients who have vulvodynia often endure multiple therapeutic modalities. First, it is essential to properly diagnose and identify the pain pattern of vulvodynia. It is important to fully educate the patient and the partner and to fully explain both the condition and treatment options. Always introduce the concept early in the treatment process and warn that initial treatment is a trial of therapy.[53,57,71–74] Validation of the patient's symptoms is invaluable in treatment. Many women are convinced that their symptoms result from a yeast infection or are fearful that their symptoms signify a serious underlying medical illness or future infertility. Patients need reassurance regarding these concerns and that their symptoms are not caused by a sexually transmitted or life-threatening disease. The self-management program that the Robert Wood Johnson Medical School-University of Medicine and Dentistry of New Jersey used during a vulvodynia clinical trial introduces empowerment through individual self-management. It consists of 3 components, including a psychoeducation component that involves understanding of exacerbating and alleviating factors, mental preparation and generalized awareness of their condition, and the ability to control factors affecting the condition. Learning to manage factors was empowering to patients. The second component involved physically training the pelvic floor through understanding the physiology of pelvic pain and learning exercises to decrease the painful sensations. The third component of self-management is sexual preparation of both patient and partner, which consists of learning other forms of sexual pleasure. The study found these techniques to be highly effective because the woman empowers herself through taking control of the condition and her response to the condition.[8]

There are almost no scientific data on the efficacy of therapies for vulvodynia. Clinical trials are primarily limited to small, open series of patients, and placebo-controlled studies are too small to yield useful data. However, because vulvodynia

Box 2
Nonspecific activities for managing vulvodynia

Validate symptoms, be supportive

Treat any objective abnormalities

Topical estrogens (estradiol vaginal cream [Estrace] can be used intravaginally or topically) (conjugated equine estrogen [Premarin])

Discontinue irritants (eg, excessive washing, irritating lubricants, tight clothing, douching, nonessential medications, sanitary pads, hair dryers)

Apply lubrication during sexual activity (eg, vegetable oil, Astroglide)

Apply lylocaine 2% jelly or 5% ointment for pain 20 minutes before sexual activity

Apply cold compresses (eg, crushed ice, frozen peas, gel pack)

Address and manage depression

Offer education (including written material) for both patient and partner

Refer patient for membership in National Vulvodynia Association

Refer both patient and partner for sex therapy and counseling to help cope with symptoms

Box 3
Standard therapy for vulvodynia

Treat abnormal visible conditions such as infections, dermatoses, and both malignant and premalignant conditions

Vulvar care measures; avoidance of irritants

Topical medications

- Lidocaine 5% jelly at introitus at bedtime
- Nitroglycerine
- Amitriptyline 2%, baclofen 2% (±ketofen 2%)
- Capsaicin

Oral medications:

- Antidepressant class
  - Tricyclic medications (≤150 mg/d)
  - Venlafaxine extended release (150 mg/d)
  - Duloxetine (60 mg twice a day)
- Anticonvulsant class
  - Gabapentin (≤3600 mg/d)
  - Pregabalin (≤300 twice a day)

Injections

- Triamcinolone 10 mg/mL, 0.2–0.4 mL into trigger point
- Botulinum toxin A injections
- Intralesional interferon (IFN)-α (no longer used)

Pelvic floor physical therapy

Pelvic floor surface electromyography and biofeedback

Low-oxalate diet with calcium citrate supplementation (controversial)

Cognitive-behavioral therapy (CBT), sexual counseling

Surgery (for vestibulodynia only) localized excision/vestibulectomy/perineoplasty

has gained recognition as a common and treatable entity, more studies are ongoing. A broad range of possible management strategies exists, but the trial and error approach is necessary to find the most effective treatment of a patient. The concern is that few of the treatment strategies have been confirmed in randomized controlled trials.[75–77] However, therapies should not be disregarded because of lack of randomized controlled clinical trials, because this is a complicated and difficult-to-treat condition.

Vulvar Care and Topical Preparations

A variety of general nonspecific measures are available to increase the comfort level of women with vulvodynia (see **Box 2**). All potential irritants should be eliminated, including the frequent application of medications, particularly creams that contain alcohols and other irritating substances. Excessive washing of the vulvar region by patients is common, and many commercial lubricants (eg, K-Y lubricating jelly [Ortho McNeil, Raritan, NJ, USA]) may cause irritation. Astroglide (BioFilm, Vista, CA, USA) and vegetable oil are good alternatives. Xylocaine (AstraZeneca, Wilmington, DE, USA) 2% jelly (does not burn on application) and 5% ointment (brief burning sensation on application but is more potent) can help relieve the symptoms of burning in many women and, when applied liberally 20 minutes before sexual activity, may facilitate intercourse. Zolnoun and colleagues[79] trialed 5% lidocaine ointment in 61 patients with vulvodynia, and a significant increase in patients' ability to have intercourse was noted (76% of women reported ability to have intercourse, compared with 36% before treatment).[78–81] In this study, patients applied the ointment on the cotton ball and placed it in the vestibule overnight. Patients continued to apply the preparation for 7 weeks, although some applied it for a longer period of time. Danielsson and colleagues[66] compared application of topical lidocaine gel with biofeedback in 46 women and found improved sexual function in both groups at 12 months. Lidocaine application does have side effects, so it is important to instruct patients that transient penile numbness may occur for sexual partners and that a remote chance of lidocaine toxicity exists.[57] A condom may decrease such side effects. Application of topical anesthetics may result in significant increase in the degree of comfort during intercourse.[72,78]

The application of cold compresses or ice to the vulva may help relieve symptoms. Rinsing and patting dry the vulva after urination may be helpful. Use of hair dryers should be discouraged. Benzocaine is the anesthetic in Vagicaine (Clay-Park Laboratories Inc, Bronx, NY, USA) and Vagisil (Combe Inc, White Plains, NY, USA), but this may cause allergic contact dermatitis and should be avoided. Diphenhydramine (Benadryl; Warner Wellcome, Morris Plains, NJ, USA), present in many topical anesthetics and anti-itch preparations, is also is a common sensitizer that should be avoided.[54]

The topical immune response modifier imiquimod (Aldara, 3M Pharmaceuticals) has been suggested as a potential therapy because of its stimulation of the cellular immune system and induction of cytokines such as IFN-α. However, this medication is a potential irritant and no clinical studies on its use in vulvodynia have been published. Topical and oral corticosteroids are not useful for vulvar pain, except in the case of accompanying inflammatory skin disease such as lichen planus.

Some clinicians anecdotally describe improvement in premenopausal and non–estrogen-deficient women by avoidance of all painful stimuli, including intercourse, for 1 to 2 months, along with the application of estrogen creams to the affected area. A study by Eva and colleagues[82] showed decreased estrogen receptor expression in women with vulvar dysfunction; thus introduction of estrogen, both vaginally and topically, may improve both vulvar and vaginal atrophy and associated pain.

Steinberg and colleagues[83] retrospectively evaluated the effects of capsaicin 0.025% applied daily for 12 weeks with preventative application of lidocaine. Although results showed a significant improvement of vulvar pain, the investigators did not indicate a specific number of patients in whom the therapy was effective. Moreover, given the prior application of lidocaine, it is impossible to isolate the effect of capsaicin. Murina and colleagues[84] also studied the application of capsaicin cream preceded by an application of lidocaine, but did so with a prospective design, a higher dosage, and a longer treatment duration. Results indicated that 59% of participants reported an improvement of their vestibular pain, but the symptoms recurred 2 weeks after capsaicin discontinuation. Despite the preventive application of lidocaine, all participants indicated an intense burning sensation after capsaicin use. Care should be taken with the application of capsaicin because of its potential as a strong irritant.[78] Topical nitroglycerin has been reported to improve symptoms associated with vulvodynia, but headache was a significant side effect of treatment.[85]

Oral Medications

Pharmacologic therapies, both oral and topical, are a mainstay of vulvodynia management. Specific first-line therapy for most patients with either form of vulvodynia is standard therapy for neuropathic pain. A survey of 167 providers who treat vulvar pain was conducted in 2005. The most commonly used treatment of vulvodynia was tricyclic antidepressants (TCAs). There was no difference in the use of physical therapy, estrogens, injected or topical steroids, IFN, or laser therapy to treat generalized and localized vulvodynia. Respondents were more likely to use TCAs, gabapentin, and psychiatric care, and less likely to use local anesthesia and vestibulectomy.[86]

Antidepressants

Although most antidepressants do not confer specific relief from neuropathic pain, several are useful in this regard: tricyclic medications, venlafaxine, and duloxetine. Tricyclic medications, particularly amitriptyline (Elavil, AstraZeneca) and desipramine (Norpramin, Aventis Pharmaceuticals, Bridgewater, NJ, USA), improve pain substantially in most patients who can tolerate doses of 100 to 150 mg.[8,54,87] Patients must be counseled that, although these medications are known primarily for their antidepressant effects, they are also being used for their beneficial effects on neuropathic pain. Many information sheets provided by pharmacies currently list these medications as commonly indicated for pain (although the pain indications are not approved by the US Food and Drug Administration). Patients who believe they are receiving the medication to treat depression are likely to feel deceived and therefore may not take their medication. With amitriptyline, patients should be started on half of a 10-mg tablet and the dose should be gradually increased to minimize potential adverse reactions until the total dose is 150 mg or until symptoms are controlled, whichever occurs first. Other side effects include constipation, weight gain, urinary retention, tachycardia, blurred vision, and confusion. Serious side effects include seizures, stroke, infarctions, agranulocytosis, and thrombocytopenia.[8] If unacceptable drowsiness or fatigue occurs, the dose can be decreased slightly and the patient given a week to acclimate before trying again to increase the dose. If the patient continues to experience drowsiness, desipramine, which is less sedating, can be substituted using the same dosing schedule (ie, target dose of 125–150 mg/d).[2] However, desipramine is more likely to produce anxiety and tremulousness compared with amitriptyline, so, occasionally, patients might benefit from combination therapy with these 2 drugs to minimize these side effects while maintaining the beneficial effects. Other side effects of tricyclic medications include dryness of the mouth and eyes, constipation, increased appetite, and, rarely, urinary retention. Reed and colleagues[88] showed that of 83 women taking a TCA at the first follow-up, 49 improved by more than 50%, compared with 30 of 79 not taking a TCA at follow-up. They concluded that women prescribed TCAs in general were more likely to have pain improvement compared with those women not taking these medications.[54,88]

Other antidepressants have been used for pain control. These selective serotonin and norepinephrine reuptake inhibitors, such as venlafaxine and duloxetine, have been used for women with vulvodynia. These medications are often used when a patient does not respond readily to the common tricyclics, and are often used in conjunction with anticonvulsants. Venlafaxine is started at 37.5 mg daily in the morning with an increase to 75 mg daily after 1 to 2 weeks. Medication can be increased gradually to 150 mg daily. When stopping the medication, it is important to wean slowly. Duloxetine is begun at 20 to 30 mg each day and titrated to as much as 60 mg twice a day. Because most selective serotonin reuptake inhibitors can theoretically inhibit the metabolism of tricyclics, monitoring tricyclic levels in these patients is prudent.[54,58,89–91]

Anticonvulsants

For women who cannot tolerate adequate doses of tricyclic medications or who fail to improve, gabapentin (Neurontin, Parke-Davis, Morris Plains, NJ, USA) may be considered. This medication is effective in diabetic neuropathy and postherpetic neuralgia at doses of 3600 mg/d or less.[92,93] Anecdotally, many clinicians have reported beneficial effects of gabapentin in treating vulvodynia.[94,95] Overall, this anticonvulsant is better tolerated and than tricyclic medications. However, it should be administered in divided doses 3 to 4 times a day, it is more expensive than amitriptyline, and it also has several side effects, including drowsiness, fatigue, dizziness, and ataxia. Serious reactions include leucopenia. Similar to tricyclic medications, this drug can be administered at low doses initially and gradually increased. Gabapentin comes in 100-, 300-, 400-, 600-, and 800-mg tablets. It is started at 300 mg by mouth daily for 3 days, then 300 mg by mouth twice daily for 3 days, and then 300 mg by mouth 3 times daily. It can be increased gradually to 3600 mg. Do not exceed 1200 mg in a dose and, for elderly patients, do not exceed 2700 mg/d. If there is a partial response to tricyclics, they may be continued at lower doses, such as 10 to 20 mg, in combination with gabapentin, and the combination of the 2 drugs may be better than either alone.[96]

A similar medication, pregabalin (Lyrica), can be used, titrating to as much as 150 mg twice a day. Side effects are similar to those of gabapentin. Carbamazepine (Tegretol; Novartis Corporation Pharmaceuticals) and Topiramate (Topamax, Ortho Pharmaceutical Corporation, Raritan, NJ, USA) have also been used to treat vulvodynia.[8,93,94,97]

Some women remain refractory to most commonly used oral therapy. Recent study evaluated the efficacy of a central nervous system agent, lamotrigine, which is an anticonvulsant with demonstrated benefits in both mood and pain syndromes. Lamotrigine (Lamictal, GlaxoSmithKline Pharmaceuticals, Durham, NC, USA) is an anticonvulsant and mood stabilizing agent that works by stabilizing the slow, inactivated conformation for the type IIA neuronal sodium channels, which prevents ongoing firing of action potentials in conditions of sustained neuronal depolarization. A study of 31 patients who completed the trial showed a clinically significant response to treatment with lamotrigine as shown by decreased pain scores and improved mood and anxiety symptoms. Subjects from the vulvodynia group had especially robust reductions on all measures of pain at both the 8- and 12-week visits.[98]

Pelvic Floor Physical Therapy and Biofeedback

Although it was once a second-line treatment of vulvodynia, pelvic floor therapy has become a major therapy in the treatment of vulvodynia.[99–101] Physical therapy has been shown to be efficacious in the treatment of vulvodynia and, in this author's opinion, is essential in successful management of vulvodynia. Pelvic floor physical therapy is widely available and effective. It involves the assessment of the patient history and pelvic musculature, joints, and muscle tension. The function of related structures, such as bowel and bladder, is assessed as well. Most therapists use a weekly session focused on exercise for the pelvic girdle and floor, soft tissue mobilization, and joint manipulation.[89,99–101]

Physical therapy has the advantage of treating the associated abnormalities that may worsen the symptoms of vulvodynia, such as joint pain, fibromyalgia, and interstitial cystitis. A study performed by Hartman and colleagues[72] sought to identify current practice trends of physical therapists in the United States. treating women with localized, provoked vulvodynia. Assessment modalities used by more than 70% included detailed history; assessment of posture, tension in the pelvic floor, pelvic girdle, associated pelvic structures, and bowel/bladder function; strength testing of abdominals and lower extremities; and voiding diaries. Nearly 70% used exercise for the pelvic girdle and pelvic floor; soft tissue mobilization/myofascial release of the pelvic girdle, pelvic floor, and associated structures; joint mobilization/manipulation; bowel/bladder retraining and help with contact irritants, dietary changes; and sexual function.[72] An evaluation by a physical therapist may identify and help alleviate dysfunctional aspects of the musculoskeletal system, such as the obturator internus and coccygeus muscles, and the sacrospinous and sacrotuberous ligaments.[67,100,101] Other areas that can be targeted by physical therapy include fascial attachment and tissue tension levels of the bladder and urethra, uterine mobility, and sacrococcygeal mobility and positioning.[101] Physical therapy treatment techniques include both internal and external soft tissue mobilization and myofascial release.[40,45,66,100]

A recent retrospective study reported the response rate of 24 patients with either vulvar vestibulitis syndrome or dysesthetic vulvodynia who were treated with pelvic floor rehabilitation by the Glazer method and concomitant physical therapy.[99,101] Patients with vulvodynia are more likely than asymptomatic women to exhibit increased resting pelvic floor muscle tension with fasciculation, but overall weakness.[102] This profile probably predates symptoms and may predispose these women to the development of vulvodynia. These abnormalities are too subtle to be identified during physical examination, but they can be identified by surface electromyography (Glazer method). Biofeedback training helps patients learn exercises to strengthen weakened pelvic floor muscles and to relax these muscles, with a resultant reduction in pain. The Glazer method uses a small vaginal probe (about the size of a tampon) with electrical sensors connected to a computer. If pelvic floor abnormalities are identified by surface electromyography, then retraining the pelvic floor muscles with twice-daily exercises can be extremely beneficial. A home training device can be attached to the vaginal probe so the patient can monitor the effectiveness of her exercise regimen as a biofeedback procedure.[35] The exercises must be performed regularly, and improvement is generally observed after several months. After 8 to 12 months, the exercises can be discontinued and patients generally retain the improvement in symptoms, although the profile of high resting tension of pelvic floor muscles, fasciculation, and weakness usually returns.[99,102] A retrospective study in Italy assessed a total of 145 women diagnosed with vulvodynia who were treated with weekly biofeedback and transcutaneous electroanalgesia (TENS), in association with functional electrical stimulation and home therapy with stretching exercises for the pelvic floor. An improvement of vulvar pain was seen in 75.8% of subjects. The study concluded that pelvic floor relaxation with biofeedback and electroanalgesia is safe and effective in improving vulvar pain and dyspareunia in women with vulvodynia.[98] Another study in Italy assessed 40 women with vulvodynia who underwent transcutaneous electrical nerve stimulation. Twice-weekly active TENS or sham treatments were delivered through a vaginal probe via a calibrated dual channel YSY-EST device. Women of both groups underwent 20 treatment sessions. The study concluded that marked improvement was shown in most women compared with placebo.[103] Moreover, recent literature on vulvodynia also mentions a novel therapeutic approach to treatment of the disease with noninvasive cortical stimulation. This may be effective in very resistant cases.[104,105]

Intralesional Injections

Clinically, botulinum toxin A blocks the cholinergic innervation of the target tissue. Recently, it has been shown to be effective in women with vulvodynia.[106] Several studies have concluded that conditions and symptoms that are caused by pelvic floor spasms, daily pelvic pain, and dyspareunia are most likely to be improved by botulinum toxin A. Limited data regarding use for provoked vestibulodynia indicate an improvement in pain scores. A recent study in Korea examined 7 women with pain on genitalia that could not be controlled with conventional pain managements. Between 20 and 40 U of botulinum toxin A were used in each injection. Injection sites were the vestibule, levator ani muscle, or the perineal body. Repeat injections were administered every 2 weeks if the patient's symptoms had not fully subsided. In all patients, pain disappeared with botulinum toxin A injections. Five patients needed to be injected twice; the other 2 patients needed only 1 injection. The study did not observe complications related to botulinum toxin A injections, such as pain, hemorrhage, infection, or muscle paralysis, but potential problems with botulinum toxin A injection include toxin reactions, urinary and fecal incontinence, urinary retention, and secondary treatment failure caused by antibody production.[21,107–109] In a case study by Romito and colleagues,[110] the 2 participants reported complete pain relief within 2 to 7 days after the injections, lasting for 5 to 6 months.[111] Dykstra and Presthus[106] conducted a study with 12 patients who reported a significant reduction of their pain for 8 to 14 weeks after the injection, with a higher dosage leading to a longer-lasting effect. Nevertheless, only 25% of patients reported a significant improvement of their quality of life on follow-up. The optimum dose and injection technique of botulinum toxin has not been determined, which probably explains the different conclusions of these studies.

IFN-α has been reported to be beneficial, primarily when injected locally.[112–115] It was initially advocated in vulvar vestibulitis, because there was an association with HPV and vulvar pain. Recent studies have disputed that notion. However, a report of a focal depression in natural killer lymph cell activity in patients with vulvodynia supports the use of IFN.[115] The most common regimen consists of IFN-α 1 million units injected 3 times per week for 4 weeks circumferentially at the periphery of the vestibule. In this procedure, the vestibule is divided into 12 areas as in a clock face; for example, a first injection could be given at the 6:00 position, the second injection at the 7:00 position, and so on until the entire periphery has been injected once. Patients may experience flu-like symptoms such as fever, malaise, and myalgias; pretreatment with acetaminophen or ibuprofen may minimize these symptoms.[112–114] In addition, patients may experience significant injection-site pain, which may be relieved by pretreatment of 20 to 30 minutes with a topical anesthetic. Improvement 1 year after IFN-α therapy is variable.[112–114]

Although topical steroids do not help patients with vulvodynia, trigger point injections are useful, especially when a patient occasionally reports pain that is localized in origin. When one of these trigger points is identified, 0.2 to 0.3 mL of 3 mg/mL triamcinolone acetonide injected into the affected area may substantially improve pain within 1 to 2 weeks.[2,116] An additional injection 4 to 6 months later occasionally resolves the pain permanently. Some investigators combine triamcinolone acetonide 0.1% injections with bupivacaine, with injections into a specific area or as a pudendal block. Segal and colleagues[117] examined the effects of subcutaneous injections of betamethasone plus lidocaine administered at 1-week intervals in the vestibule. At follow-up, the participant indicated a complete relief of her pain and improvement in sexual intercourse. The efficacy of methylprednisolone injections plus lidocaine were studied prospectively by Murina and colleagues.[84] Results revealed that 32% of participants had a complete remission of their pain symptoms, and 36% of the patients showed improvement.

Surgical Therapy

Another treatment option for patients with vulvar vestibulitis syndrome is surgical excision of the vestibule.[18,31,118–124] It is commonly the last treatment option for patients with vestibulodynia because most experts believe that surgery should be reserved for long-standing cases of severe vulvar pain and after all other managements have yielded unsatisfactory results.[55,118,125,126]

Three approaches are often used in the surgical treatment of vulvodynia, including a local excision (clinical identification and removal of extreme painful areas), total vestibulectomy (skin, mucous membrane, hymen, and adjacent tissue are removed, along with vestibular glands and transaction of Bartholin ducts), and perineoplasty (tissues of perineum removed ending just above the anal orifice), in which denervation of the vestibule (vestibuloplasty) has been shown to be ineffective.[55,118,125–129] Many surgeons remove all areas of the vestibule, including areas that do not exhibit pain, because vestibulectomy failures result in recurrences in remaining vestibule tissue. About 85% of patients experience a cure or remarkable improvement in their symptoms after surgery.[55,118,125–129] However, dehiscence, recurrence of symptoms, or worsening of pain occasionally occurs after vestibulectomy. Although vestibulectomy was once the treatment of choice for vulvar vestibulitis syndrome, the scarcity of experienced surgeons, the discomfort of the procedure, the cost, and the success of less-aggressive therapies have relegated this procedure to second- or third-line therapy.

Laser Therapy

Early reports of some forms of laser ablation described improvement in vulvodynia.[130–135] However, worsening pain and recurrence are common,[24] and laser treatment is now contraindicated in women with vulvar pain. Laser ablation of the vulvar epithelium is an alternative to the vestibulectomy, but laser therapy for vulvodynia remains a controversial issue. Reid and colleagues[130] advocated the use of flashlamp-excited dye laser to selectively photocoagulate symptomatic subepithelial blood vessels in 168 women and the removal of painful Bartholin glands in 52 women not responsive or not suited to flashlamp-excited dye laser photothermolysis. The study showed statistically significant clinical improvement. Results of laser therapy for vulvodynia compare similarly with vestibulectomy. Complete response occurs in 62% versus improvement in 92%.[130] Ketoprofen-neodymium:yyttrium-aluminum-garnet (KTP-Nd:YAG) laser treatment has been used in the treatment of vulvodynia, with a study examining patient response after 2 years. Sixty-eight percent reported less pain with sexual intercourse and 29% reported no change. The KTP-Nd:YAG laser and pulsed-dye laser offer the benefit of being absorbed by vasculature and thus encouraging collagen remodeling.[136] Because angiogenesis and increased nerve density are characteristics of vulvodynia, the laser is used to disrupt this phenomenon and to advance collagen remodeling without changing the innate structure.[136] CO_2 laser therapy for vulvodynia was not recommended in a study of 3 cases of vulvodynia after CO_2 laser treatment of condylomata acuminata or bowenoid papulosis of the female genital mucosa. Laser treatment was associated with a delay in healing and chronic pain.

Dietary Modifications

The theory that high urinary and tissue oxalate levels cause pain in some patients has led to the use of a low-oxalate diet and mealtime calcium citrate supplementation. The addition of oral calcium citrate (Citracal), 2 tablets (200 mg and 950 mg) orally 3 times a day, is used to neutralize oxalates in the urine.[137] One theory is that oxalate may irritate the vestibulum and may be a contributing cause to vulvodynia pain over a long period.[57,58] Other studies have indicated that patients with vulvodynia do not have increased oxalate levels, and that there is no correlation between oxalate levels and symptom improvement, so most vulvologists do not find dietary modification useful for vulvodynia.[138–141]

Counseling

Vulvodynia is often devastating, affecting a patient's personal relationships and quality of life. Depression is a common symptom and should be addressed.[28] Sargeant and O'Callaghan[116] reported that women with vulvar pain reported significantly worse mental health-related quality of live than women without vulvar pain. In their study, illness perceptions played an important role in the women's mental health-related quality of life. The clinician should make it clear that counseling and antidepressant therapy are recommended not to treat their pain, but because they can minimize the depression and disruption of personal relationships.[68,69,142] A referral to couples counseling is ideal and can help the patient and her partner cope with vulvodynia. Patients need to understand that referral to therapy does not meant that a patient's condition is imagined; therapy is just another tool in the treatment of vulvodynia. Sex therapy, couples counseling, and psychotherapy can be important in proper management of patient.[108,137,143,144] A therapist with expertise in sex therapy is preferred to help the couple to discover alternative types of painless sexual activity.

Behavioral interventions for chronic pain emphasize a self-management approach, deemed more effective than more conventional medical and rehabilitation therapies.[145] CBT for vulvodynia can help to decrease pain, reduce fear and anxiety associated with pain, and reestablish satisfying sexual functioning.[23,42,146,147] Kuile and colleagues[148] evaluated the efficacy of therapy in a group format; the investigators reported that participants had a significant reduction of vulvar pain, in addition to a significant improvement of sexual satisfaction and perceived pain control.[149] Masheb and colleagues[150] tested the efficacy of CBT and supportive psychotherapy (SPT) in women with vulvodynia. Participants had statistically significant decreases in pain severity, with 42% achieving clinical improvement; participants in CBT reported greater treatment improvement and satisfaction than participants in SPT. Bergeron and colleagues[151] conducted the only randomized study that examined CBT. More specifically, participants were randomized either to CBT, biofeedback, or vestibulectomy. The participants of the 3 treatment groups reported noteworthy improvements of their pain.[83,151] The average pain reduction was 47% to 70% for vestibulectomy, 19% to 35% for biofeedback, and 21% to 38% for CBT. Although vestibulectomy was shown to be appreciably more successful than the 2 other treatments in terms of pain decline, the 3 treatments resulted in equal levels of improvement. Moreover, the CBT group presented a significantly lower dropout rate than the vestibulectomy group, and participants were more content with their treatment than those who took part in biofeedback.

SUMMARY

Vulvodynia is a multifactorial chronic pain disorder that is distressing to the patient and exigent to the physician. Although the condition is common, it remains little understood, so patients remain undiagnosed and untreated or undertreated for many years. Although multiple therapies exist in the treatment of vulvodynia, few randomized controlled clinical trials have been performed. Thus, treatment should be individualized and tailored to a patient's diagnosis, symptoms, and psychosexual functioning. Patient education is also important and is facilitated by patient brochures providing assurance that vulvodynia is a real disease. In addition, joining the National Vulvodynia Association (www.nva.org), a clearinghouse for information and updates on vulvar

pain, helps to inform patients and to alleviate the sense of isolation that patients may experience.

REFERENCES

1. Moyal-Barracco M, Lynch PJ. 2003 ISSVD terminology and classification of vulvodynia. A historical perspective. J Reprod Med 2004;49:772–7.
2. Edwards L. New concepts in vulvodynia. Am J Obstet Gynecol 2003;189(3):S24–30.
3. Petersen C, Lundvall L, Kristensen E, et al. Vulvodynia. Definition, diagnosis and treatment. Acta Obstet Gynecol Scand 2008;87(9):893–901.
4. McKay M. Vulvodynia: diagnostic patterns [abstract]. Dermatol Clin 1992;10:423–33.
5. Turner ML, Marinoff SC. Association of human papillomavirus with vulvodynia and the vulvar vestibulitis syndrome [abstract]. J Reprod Med 1988; 33:533–7.
6. Byrne MA, Walker MM, Leonard J, et al. Recognizing covert disease in women with chronic vulval symptoms attending an STD clinic: value of detailed examination including colposcopy [abstract]. Genitourin Med 1989;65:46–9.
7. Harlow BL, Stewart EG. A population-based assessment of chronic unexplained vulvar pain: have we underestimated the prevalence of vulvodynia [abstract]? J Am Med Womens Assoc 2003;58:82–8.
8. Bachmann GA, Rosen R, Pinn VW, et al. Vulvodynia: a state of-the-art consensus on definitions, diagnosis and management. J Reprod Med 2006; 51:447–56.
9. Bornstein J, Livnat G, Stolar Z, et al. Pure versus complicated vulvar vestibulitis: a randomized trial of fluconazole treatment. Gynecol Obstet Invest 2000;50:194–7.
10. Munday PE. Response to treatment in dysaesthetic vulvodynia. J Obstet Gynaecol 2001;21:610–3.
11. Schmidt S, Bauer A, Greif C, et al. Vulvar pain. Psychological profiles and treatment responses. J Reprod Med 2001;46:377–84.
12. Bergeron S, Binik YM, Khalife S, et al. Vulvar vestibulitis syndrome: reliability of diagnosis and evaluation of current diagnostic criteria. Obstet Gynecol 2001;98:45–51.
13. Nguyen RH, Sanson D, Harlow BL. Urogenital infections in relation to the occurrence of vulvodynia. J Reprod Med 2009;54(6):385–92.
14. Marks TA, Shroyer KR, Markham NE, et al. A clinical, histologic, and DNA study of vulvodynia and its association with human papillomavirus [abstract]. J Soc Gynecol Investig 1995;2:57–63.
15. Morin C, Bouchard C, Brisson J, et al. Human papillomaviruses and vulvar vestibulitis [abstract]. Obstet Gynecol 2000;95:683–7.
16. Shafik A. Pudendal canal syndrome as a cause of vulvodynia and its treatment by pudendal nerve decompression [abstract]. Eur J Obstet Gynecol Reprod Biol 1998;80:215–20.
17. Cox JT. Deconstructing vulval pain. Lancet 1995; 345:53.
18. Gaunt G, Good A, Stanhope CR. Vestibulectomy for vulvar vestibulitis. J Reprod Med 2003;48: 591–5.
19. Traas MA, Bekkers RL, Dony JM, et al. Surgical treatment for the vulvar vestibulitis syndrome. Obstet Gynecol 2006;107:256–62.
20. Gerber S, Bongiovanni A, Ledger W, et al. Interleukin-1β gene polymorphism in women with vulvar vestibulitis syndrome. Eur J Obstet Gynecol Reprod Biol 2003;107(1):74.
21. Pukall CF, Binik YM, Khalife S, et al. Vestibular tactile and pain thresholds in women with vulvar vestibulitis syndrome [abstract]. Pain 2002;96: 163–75.
22. Mascherpa F, Bogliatto F, Lynch P, et al. Vulvodynia as a possible somatization disorder: more than just an opinion. J Reprod Med 2007;52(2):107–10.
23. Brauer M, ter Kuile MM, Janssen SA, et al. The effect of pain-related fear on sexual arousal in women with superficial dyspareunia. Eur J Pain 2007;11(7):788–98.
24. Graziottin A, Castoldi E, Montorsi F, et al. Vulvodynia: the challenge of "unexplained" genital pain [abstract]. J Sex Marital Ther 2001;27:503–12.
25. Tschanz C, Salomon D, Skaria A, et al. Vulvodynia after CO_2 laser treatment of the female genital mucosa [abstract]. Dermatology 2001;202:371–2.
26. McKay M. Vulvodynia: a multifactorial clinical problem [abstract]. Arch Dermatol 1989;125: 256–62.
27. Edwards L, Mason M, Phillips M, et al. Childhood sexual and physical abuse: incidence in patients with vulvodynia [abstract]. J Reprod Med 1997; 42:135–9.
28. Bodden-Heidrich R, Kuppers V, Beckmann MW, et al. Psychosomatic aspects of vulvodynia: comparison with the chronic pelvic pain syndrome [abstract]. J Reprod Med 1999;44:411–6.
29. Granot M, Zimmer EZ, Friedman M, et al. Association between quantitative sensory testing, treatment choice, and subsequent pain reduction in vulvar vestibulitis syndrome. J Pain 2004;5:226–32.
30. Bohm-Starke N, Hilliges M, Falconer C, et al. Neurochemical characterization of the vestibular nerves in women with vulvar vestibulitis syndrome [abstract]. Gynecol Obstet Invest 1999;48:270–5.
31. Chaim W, Meriwether C, Gonik B, et al. Vulvar vestibulitis subjects undergoing surgical intervention: a descriptive analysis and histopathological correlates. Eur J Obstet Gynecol Reprod Biol 1996;68: 165–8.

32. Slone S, Reynolds L, Gall S, et al. Localization of chromogranin, synaptophysin, serotonin, and CXCR2 in neuroendocrine cells of the minor vestibular glands: an immunohistochemical study [abstract]. Int J Gynecol Pathol 1999;18:360–5.
33. Chadha S, Gianotten WL, Drogendijk AC, et al. Histopathologic features of vulvar vestibulitis [abstract]. Int J Gynecol Pathol 1998;17:7–11.
34. Tympanidis P, Casula M, Yiangou Y, et al. Increased vanilloid receptor VR1 innervation in vulvodynia. Eur J Pain 2004;8(2):129–33.
35. Gunter J. Vulvodynia: new thoughts on a devastating condition. Obstet Gynecol Surv 2007;62(12):812–9.
36. Woodruff JD, Parmley TH. Infection of the minor vestibular gland. Obstet Gynecol 1983;62:609–12.
37. Melzack R. The McGill Pain Questionnaire: major properties and scoring methods. Pain 1975;1: 277–99.
38. Ashton AK. The new sexual pharmacology: a guide for the clinicians. In: Leiblum SR, editor. Principles and practice of sex therapy. 4th edition. New York: Guilford Press; 2007. p. 509–41.
39. Bohm-Starke N, Hilliges M, Blomgren B, et al. Increased blood flow and erythema in the posterior vestibular mucosa in vulvar vestibulitis. Obstet Gynecol 2001;98(6):1067–74.
40. Glazer HI, Marinoff SC, Sleight IJ. Web-enabled Glazer surface electromyographic protocol for the remote, real-time assessment and rehabilitation of pelvic floor dysfunction in vulvar vestibulitis syndrome. A case report. J Reprod Med 2002;47:728–30.
41. Bergeron S, Brown C, Lord MJ, et al. Physical therapy for vulvar vestibulitis syndrome: a retrospective study. J Sex Marital Ther 2002;28:183–92.
42. Bergeron S, Lord MJ. The integration of pelvi-perineal re-education and cognitive-behavioral therapy in the multidisciplinary treatment of the sexual pain disorders. Sex Marital Ther 2003;18: 135–41.
43. Meana M, Binik I, Khalife S, et al. Affect and marital adjustment in women's rating of dyspareunic pain. Can J Psychiatry 1998;43:381–5.
44. Payne KA, Binik YM, Amsel R, et al. When sex hurts, anxiety and fear orient attention towards pain. Eur J Pain 2004;9:427–36.
45. Harlow BL, Vitonis AF, Stewart EG. Influence of oral contraceptive use on the risk of adult-onset vulvodynia. J Reprod Med 2008;53(2):102–10.
46. Bohm-Stark N, Johannesson U, Hilliges M, et al. Decreased mechanical pain threshold in the vestibular mucosa of women using contraceptives. J Reprod Med 2004;49:888–92.
47. Straub R. The complex role of estrogens in inflammation. Endocr Rev 2007;28(5):521–74.
48. Ting AY, Blacklock AD, Smith PG. Estrogen regulates vaginal sensory and autonomic nerve density in the rat. Biol Reprod 2004;71(4):1397–404.
49. Ponte M, Klemperer E, Sahay A, et al. Effects of vulvodynia on quality of life. J Am Acad Dermatol 2009;60(1):70–6.
50. O'Hare PM, Sherertz EF. Vulvodynia: a dermatologist's perspective with emphasis on an irritant contact dermatitis component [abstract]. J Womens Health Gend Based Med 2000;9:565–9.
51. Masheb RM, Lozano C, Richman S, et al. On the reliability and validity of physician ratings for vulvodynia and the discriminant validity of its subtypes. Pain Med 2004;5:349–58.
52. American College of Obstetricians and Gynecologists. Vulvar nonneoplastic epithelial disorders. Int J Gynaecol Obstet 1998;60:181–8.
53. Lynch PJ. Vulvodynia: a syndrome of unexplained vulvar pain, psychologic disability and sexual dysfunction. J Reprod Med 1986;31:773–80.
54. Haefner H, Collins S, Davis GD, et al. The vulvodynia guideline. J Low Genit Tract Dis 2005;9:40–51.
55. Goldstein AT, Klingman D, Christopher K, et al. Surgical treatment of vulvar vestibulitis syndrome: outcome assessment derived from a postoperative questionnaire. J Sex Med 2006;3:923–31.
56. Landry T, Bergeron S, Dupuis M-J, et al. The treatment of provoked vestibulodynia: a critical review. Clin J Pain 2008;24(2):155–71.
57. Goldstein AT, Burrows L. Vulvodynia. J Sex Med 2008;5:5–15.
58. Goldstein AT, Marinoff SC, Haefner HK. Vulvodynia: strategies for treatment. Clin Obstet Gynecol 2005; 48(4):769–85.
59. Zhu YZ, Yang YH, Zhang XL. [Vaginal colonization of group B *Streptococcus*: a study in 267 cases of factory women] [abstract]. Zhonghua Liu Xing Bing Xue Za Zhi 1996;17:17–9 [in Chinese].
60. Bergeron S, Binik YM, Khalife S, et al. The treatment of vulvar vestibulitis syndrome: towards a multimodal approach. Sex Marital Ther 1997;12: 305–11.
61. Bergeron S, Binik YM, Khalife S. In favor of an integrated pain-relief treatment approach for vulvar vestibulitis syndrome. J Psychosom Obstet Gynaecol 2002;23:7–9.
62. O'Connell TX, Nathan LS, Satmary WA, et al. Non-neoplastic epithelial disorders of the vulva. Am Fam Physician 2008;77(3):321–6.
63. Edwards L, Friedrich EG Jr. Desquamative vaginitis: lichen planus in disguise [abstract]. Obstet Gynecol 1988;71:832–6.
64. Edwards L. Desquamative vulvitis [abstract]. Dermatol Clin 1992;10:325–37.
65. Bowen AR, Vester A, Marsden L, et al. The role of vulvar skin biopsy in the evaluation of chronic vulvar pain. Am J Obstet Gynecol 2008;199(5): 467,e1–6.
66. Danielsson I, Torstensson T, Brodda-Jansen G, et al. EMG biofeedback versus topical lidocaine

gel: a randomized study for the treatment of women with vulvar vestibulitis. Acta Obstet Gynecol Scand 2006;85:1360–7.
67. Zolnoun D, Hartmann K, Lamvu G, et al. A conceptual model for the pathophysiology of vulvar vestibulitis syndrome. Obstet Gynecol Surv 2006;61(6):395–401.
68. Turk DC, Okifuji A. Psychological factors in chronic pain: evolution and revolution. J Consult Clin Psychol 2002;70:678–90.
69. Bergeron S, Khalife S, Glazer HI, et al. Surgical and behavioral treatments for vestibulodynia: two-and-one-half year follow-up and predictors of outcome. Obstet Gynecol 2008;111(1):159–66.
70. Ayling K, Ussher JM. "If sex hurts, am I still a woman?" The subjective experience of vulvodynia in hetero-sexual women. Arch Sex Behav 2008;37:294–304.
71. Haefner HK. Report of the International Society for the study of Vulvovaginal disease: terminology and classification of vulvodynia. J Low Genit Tract Dis 2007;11(1):48–9.
72. Hartmann D, Strauhal MJ, Nelson CA. Treatment of women in the United States with localized, provoked vulvodynia: practice survey of women's health physical therapists. J Reprod Med 2007;52(1): 48–52.
73. Kamdar N, Fisher L, MacNeill C. Improvement in vulvar vestibulitis with montelukast. J Reprod Med 2007;52(10):912–6.
74. Yoon H, Chung WS, Shim BS. Botulinum toxin A for the management of vulvodynia. Int J Impot Res 2007;19(1):84–7.
75. Reed BD, Haefner HK, Punch MR, et al. Psychosocial and sexual functioning in women with vulvodynia and chronic pelvic pain: a comparative evaluation [abstract]. J Reprod Med 2000;45:624–32.
76. Honig E, Mouton JW, van der Meijden WI. Can group B streptococci cause symptomatic vaginitis [abstract]? Infect Dis Obstet Gynecol 1999;7: 206–9.
77. Reed BD, Sen A, Gracely RH. Effect of test order on sensitivity in vulvodynia. Clin J Pain. J Reprod Med 2007;24(2). February 2008.
78. Murina F, Radici G, Bianco V. Capsaicin and the treatment of vulvar vestibulitis syndrome: a valuable alternative? MedGenMed 2004;6:48.
79. Zolnoun DA, Hartmann KE, Steege JF. Overnight 5% lidocaine ointment for treatment of vulvar vestibulitis. Obstet Gynecol 2003;102:84–7.
80. Morrison GD, Adams SJ, Curnow JS, et al. A preliminary study of topical ketoconazole in vulvar vestibulitis syndrome. J Dermatolog Treat 1996;7(4):219–21.
81. Pagano R. Vulvar vestibulitis syndrome: an often unrecognized cause of dyspareunia. Aust N Z J Obstet Gynaecol 1999;39:79–83.
82. Eva LJ, MacLean AB, Reid WM, et al. Estrogen receptor expression in vulvar vestibulitis syndrome. Am J Obstet Gynecol 2003;189(2):458–61.
83. Steinberg AC, Oyama IA, Rejba AE, et al. Capsaicin for the treatment of vulvar vestibulitis. Am J Obstet Gynecol 2005;192:1549–53.
84. Murina F, Tassan P, Roberti P, et al. Treatment of vulvar vestibulitis with submucous infiltrations of methylprednisolone and lidocaine. An alternative approach. J Reprod Med 2001;46:713–6.
85. Walsh KE, Berman JR, Berman LA, et al. Safety and efficacy of topical nitroglycerin for treatment of vulvar pain in women with vulvodynia: a pilot study. J Gend Specif Med 2002;5(4):21–7.
86. Updike GM, Wiesenfeld HC. Insight into the treatment of vulvar pain: a survey of clinicians. Am J Obstet Gynecol 2005;193(4):1404–9.
87. McKay M. Dysesthetic ("essential") vulvodynia: treatment with amitriptyline [abstract]. J Reprod Med 1993;38:9–13.
88. Reed BD, Caron AM, Gorenflo DW, et al. Treatment of vulvodynia with tricyclic antidepressants: efficacy and associated factors. J Low Genit Tract Dis 2006;10(4):245–51.
89. Munday P, Buchan A, Ravenhill G, et al. A qualitative study of women with vulvodynia II. Response to a multidisciplinary approach to management. J Reprod Med 2007;52(1):19–22.
90. Murina F, Bernorio R, Palmiotto R. The use of Amielle vaginal trainers as adjuvant in the treatment of vestibulodynia: an observational multicentric study. Medscape J Med 2008;10:23.
91. Plante AF, Kamm MA. Life events in patients with vulvodynia. BJOG 2008;115:509–14.
92. Backonja M, Beydoun A, Edwards KR, et al. Gabapentin for the symptomatic treatment of painful neuropathy in patients with diabetes mellitus: a randomized controlled trial [abstract]. JAMA 1998;280:1831–6.
93. Rose MA, Kam PC. Gabapentin: pharmacology and its use in pain management. Anaesthesia 2002;57:451–62.
94. Sasaki K, Smith CP, Chuang YC, et al. Oral gabapentin (neurontin) treatment of refractory genitourinary tract pain [abstract]. Tech Urol 2001;7:47–9.
95. Ben-David B, Friedman M. Gabapentin therapy for vulvodynia. Anesth Analg 1999;89:1459–60 Citation.
96. Fisher RS, Sachdeo RC, Pellock J, et al. Rapid initiation of gabapentin: a randomized, controlled trial. Neurology 2001;56(6):743–8.
97. Harris G, Horowitz B, Borgida A. Evaluation of gabapentin in the treatment of generalized vulvodynia, unprovoked. J Reprod Med 2007;52(2): 103–5.
98. Dionisi B, Anglana F, Inghirami P, et al. Use of transcutaneous electrical stimulation and

biofeedback for the treatment of vulvodynia (vulvar vestibular syndrome): result of 3 years of experience. Minerva Ginecol 2008;60(6):485–91.
99. Glazer HI. Dysesthetic vulvodynia: long-term follow-up after treatment with surface electromyography-assisted pelvic floor muscle rehabilitation [abstract]. J Reprod Med 2000;45:798–802.
100. McKay E, Kaufman RH, Doctor U, et al. Treating vulvar vestibulitis with electromyographic biofeedback of pelvic floor musculature [abstract]. J Reprod Med 2001;46:337–42.
101. Hartmann EH, Nelson C. The perceived effectiveness of physical therapy treatment on women complaining of chronic vulvar pain and diagnosed with either vulvar vestibulitis syndrome or dysesthetic vulvodynia. Journal of Women's Health 2001;25:13–8.
102. Glazer HI, Jantos M, Hartmann EH, et al. Electromyographic comparisons of the pelvic floor in women with dysesthetic vulvodynia and asymptomatic women [abstract]. J Reprod Med 1998; 43:959–62.
103. Murina F, Bianco V, Radici G, et al. Transcutaneous electrical nerve stimulation to treat vestibulodynia: a randomised controlled trial. BJOG 2008;115(9): 1165–70.
104. Cecilio SB, Zaghi S, Cecilio LB, et al. Exploring a novel therapeutic approach with noninvasive cortical stimulation for vulvodynia. Am J Obstet Gynecol 2008;199(6):e6–7.
105. Nair AR, Klapper A, Kushnerik V, et al. Spinal cord stimulator for the treatment of a woman with vulvovaginal burning and deep pelvic pain. Obstet Gynecol 2008;111(2 Pt 2):545–7.
106. Dykstra DD, Presthus J. Botulinum toxin type A for the treatment of provoked vestibulodynia: an open-label, pilot study. J Reprod Med 2006;51:467–70.
107. Sobel JD. Desquamative inflammatory vaginitis: a new subgroup of purulent vaginitis responsive to topical 2% clindamycin therapy [abstract]. Am J Obstet Gynecol 1994;171:1215–20.
108. Marinoff SC, Turner ML. Vulvar vestibulitis syndrome: an overview [abstract]. Am J Obstet Gynecol 1991;165:1228–33.
109. Rao A, Abbott J. Using botulinum toxin for pelvic indications in women. Aust N Z J Obstet Gynaecol 2009;49(4):352–7.
110. Romito S, Bottanelli M, Pellegrini M, et al. Botulinum toxin for the treatment of genital pain syndromes. Gynecol Obstet Invest 2004;58:164–7.
111. Brown CS, Glazer HI, Vogt V, et al. Subjective and objective outcomes of botulinum toxin type A treatment in vestibulodynia: pilot data. J Reprod Med 2006;51:635–41.
112. Horowitz BJ. Interferon therapy for condylomatous vulvitis [abstract]. Obstet Gynecol 1989;73:446–8.
113. Marinoff SC, Turner ML, Hirsch RP, et al. Intralesional alpha interferon: cost-effective therapy for vulvar vestibulitis syndrome [abstract]. J Reprod Med 1993;38:19–24.
114. Gerber S, Bongiovanni AM, Ledger WJ, et al. A deficiency in interferon-alpha production in women with vulvar vestibulitis. Am J Obstet Gynecol 2002;186:361–4.
115. Masterson BJ, Galask RP, Ballas ZK. Natural killer cell function in women with vestibulitis. J Reprod Med 1996;41(8):562–8.
116. Sargeant HA, O'Callaghan FV. The impact of chronic vulval pain on quality of life and psychosocial well-being. Aust N Z J Obstet Gynaecol 2007; 47(3):235–9.
117. Segal D, Tifheret H, Lazer S. Submucous infiltration of betamethasone and lidocaine in the treatment of vulvar vestibulitis. Eur J Obstet Gynecol Reprod Biol 2003;107:105–6.
118. McCormack WM, Spence MR. Evaluation of the surgical treatment of vulvar vestibulitis [abstract]. Eur J Obstet Gynecol Reprod Biol 1999;86:135–8.
119. Schneider D, Yaron M, Bukovsky I, et al. Outcome of surgical treatment for superficial dyspareunia from vulvar vestibulitis [abstract]. J Reprod Med 2001;46:227–31.
120. Bornstein J, Zarfati D, Goldik Z, et al. Vulvar vestibulitis: physical or psychosexual problem [abstract]? Obstet Gynecol 1999;93:876–80.
121. Solomons CC, Melmed MH, Heitler SM. Calcium citrate for vulvar vestibulitis: a case report [abstract]. J Reprod Med 1991;36:879–82.
122. Bergeron S, Bouchard C, Fortier M, et al. The surgical treatment of vulvar vestibulitis syndrome: a follow-up study. J Sex Marital Ther 1997;23:317–25.
123. Meana M, Binik YM, Khalife S, et al. Biopsychosocial profile of women with dyspareunia. Obstet Gynecol 1997;90:583–9.
124. Arnold LD, Bachmann GA, Rosen R, et al. Vulvodynia:characteristics and associations with comorbidities and quality of life. Obstet Gynecol 2006; 107:617–24.
125. Goetsch MF. Simplified surgical revision of the vulvar vestibule for vulvar vestibulitis. Am J Obstet Gynecol 1996;174:1701–5.
126. Bornstein J, Goldik Z, Stolar Z, et al. Predicting the outcome of surgical treatment of vulvar vestibulitis. Obstet Gynecol Surv 1997;52:618–9.
127. Kehoe S, Luesley D. Vulvar vestibulitis treated by modified vestibulectomy. Int J Gynaecol Obstet 1999;64:147–52.
128. Lavy Y, Lev-Sagie A, Hamani Y, et al. Modified vulvar vestibulectomy: simple and effective surgery for the treatment of vulvar vestibulitis. Eur J Obstet Gynecol Reprod Biol 2005;120:91–5.
129. Bornstein J, Abramovici H. Combination of subtotal perineoplasty and interferon for the treatment of vulvar vestibulitis. Gynecol Obstet Invest 1997;44:53–6.

130. Reid R, Omoto KH, Precop SL, et al. Flashlamp-excited dye laser therapy of idiopathic vulvodynia is safe and efficacious. Am J Obstet Gynecol 1995;172:1684–96 [discussion: 1696–701].
131. Adanu RMK, Haefner HK, Reed BD. Vulvar pain in women attending a general medical clinic in Accra, Ghana. J Reprod Med 2005;50(2):130–4.
132. Arnold LD, Bachmann GA, Rosen R, et al. Assessment of vulvodynia symptoms in a sample of US women: a prevalence survey with a nested case control study. Am J Obstet Gynecol 2007; 196(2):e1–6.
133. Friedrich EG Jr. Vulvar vestibulitis syndrome. J Reprod Med 1987;32:110–4.
134. Goetsch MF. Vulvar vestibulitis: prevalence and historic features in a general gynecologic practice population. Am J Obstet Gynecol 1991;164: 1609–14.
135. Harlow BL, Wise LA, Stewart EG. Prevalence and predictors of chronic lower genital tract discomfort. Am J Obstet Gynecol 2001;185: 545–50.
136. Leclair CM, Goetsch MF, Lee KK, et al. KTP-Nd:YAG laser therapy for the treatment of vestibulodynia, a follow-up study. J Reprod Med 2007;52:53–8.
137. Greenstein A, Militscher I, Chen J, et al. Hyperoxaluria in women with vulvar vestibulitis syndrome. J Reprod Med 2006;51:500–2.
138. Baggish MS, Sze EH, Johnson R. Urinary oxalate excretion and its role in vulvar pain syndrome. Am J Obstet Gynecol 1997;177:507–11.
139. Metts JF. Vulvodynia and vulvar vestibulitis: challenges in diagnosis and management. Am Fam Physician 1999;59:1547–56, 1561–2.
140. Danielsson I, Sjoberg I, Ostman C. Acupuncture for the treatment of vulvar vestibulitis: a pilot study [abstract]. Acta Obstet Gynecol Scand 2001;80: 437–41.
141. Powell J, Wojnarowska F. Acupuncture for vulvodynia [abstract]. J R Soc Med 1999;92:579–81.
142. Bachmann GA, Rosen R, Arnold LD, et al. Chronic vulvar and other gynaecologic pain: prevalence and characteristics in a self-reported survey. J Reprod Med 2006;51(1):3–9.
143. Kandyba K, Binik YM. Hypnotherapy as a treatment for vulvar vestibulitis syndrome: a case report. J Sex Marital Ther 2003;29:237–42.
144. Pukall CF, Kandyba K, Amsel R, et al. Efficacy of hypnosis for the treatment of vulvar vestibulitis syndrome: a preliminary investigation. J Sex Med 2007;4:417–25.
145. Reissing ED, Binik YM, Khalife S, et al. Vaginal spasm, pain, and behavior: an empirical investigation of the diagnosis of vaginismus. Arch Sex Behav 2004;33:5–17.
146. Davis HJ, Reissing ED. Relationship adjustment and dyadic interaction in couples with sexual pain disorders: a critical review of the literature. Sexual and Relationship Therapy 2007;22(2):245–54.
147. Masheb RM, Brondolo E, Kerns RD. A multidimensional, case-control study of women with self-identified chronic vulvar pain. Pain Med 2002;3(3):253–9.
148. Kuile MM, Weijenborg PT. A cognitive-behavioral group program for women with vulvar vestibulitis syndrome (VVS): factors associated with treatment success. J Sex Marital Ther 2006;32:199–213.
149. Fowler RS. Vulvar vestibulitis: response to hypocontactant vulvar therapy. J Low Genit Tract Dis 2000;4:200–3.
150. Masheb RM, Kerns RD, Lozano C, et al. A randomized clinical trial for women with vulvodynia: cognitive-behavioral therapy vs. supportive psychotherapy. Pain 2009;141(1-2):31–40.
151. Bergeron S, Binik YM, Khalifé S, et al. A randomized comparison of group cognitive-behavioral therapy, surface electromyographic biofeedback, and vestibulectomy in the treatment of dyspareunia resulting from vulvar vestibulitis. Pain 2001;91:297–306.

ADDITIONAL RESOURCES FOR CLINICIANS AND PATIENTS: WEB SITES

American College of Obstetricians and Gynecologists. Available at: http://www.acog.org/publications/patient_education/bp127.cfm

International Society for the Study of Vulvovaginal Disease (ISSVD). Available at: http://www.issvd.org

National Vulvodynia Association. Available at: http://www.nva.org

Vulval Pain Society. Available at: http://www.vulvalpainsociety.org

Vulvar Pain Foundation. Available at: http://www.vulvarpainfoundation.org

Contact Dermatitis of the Vulva

Bethanee J. Schlosser, MD, PhD

KEYWORDS

- Vulva • Female genitalia • Allergic contact dermatitis
- Irritant contact dermatitis • Contact dermatitis

Inflammatory dermatoses and cutaneous infections commonly affect the vulva. Cultural taboos, embarrassment, and fear may prevent women from reporting vulvar pruritus, pain, and cutaneous eruptions to their health care providers. As a result, women often self-medicate using a myriad of over-the-counter and/or herbal remedies. Vulvar disease is often multifactorial. Diagnosis of vulvar diseases can be challenging because of the effect of local factors (moisture, friction), clinical manifestations, which differ from nongenital cutaneous sites, and the frequent concomitant presence of multiple diagnoses. Lack of knowledge by practitioners causes underrecognition and misdiagnosis of vulvar disorders, which leads to repeated failure to improve despite use of multiple medications.

Whether self-induced or iatrogenic, contact dermatitis frequently complicates vulvar disorders. Contact dermatitis results from exposure to exogenous agents, either irritants or allergens. Irritant contact dermatitis (ICD) affects the vulva more often than allergic contact dermatitis (ACD).[1] Acute, subacute, and chronic forms exist. Subacute and chronic contact dermatitis, either allergic or irritant, typically present with eczematous changes ranging from mild erythema to lichenified, thick erythematous plaques with excoriation, fissures, and weeping. Severe, acute contact dermatitis may be bullous, erosive, and extremely painful.

The vulva is particularly susceptible to ICD and ACD.[2,3] Vulvar skin has been shown to react more intensely to some irritants (eg, benzalkonium chloride, maleic acid) than forearm skin; however, vulvar skin may not be more susceptible than other skin areas to all irritants.[2,4] The barrier function of vulvar skin is compromised by moisture (urine, vaginal discharge), enzymes (stool residua), friction, and heat, all of which constitute the normal vulvar environment.[5] Estrogen is integral in maintaining the strength and integrity of vulvar tissues. Estrogen deficiency, as occurs during premenarche, oral contraceptive use, postpartum, lactation, and menopause, decreases the barrier function of the vulvar epithelium.[5,6] Persistent contact with urine can alone cause irritant dermatitis, widely recognized as diaper dermatitis in infants. Urinary incontinence, secondary to pelvic floor muscle weakness and laxity, severely affects up to 20% of women aged 80 years and older.[7] Obesity and limitations in physical mobility, which reduce the ability to touch and visually inspect the vulva, can significantly impede a patient's ability to keep the vulva clean and dry. Additional risk factors for vulvar contact dermatitis include preexisting dermatosis, occlusion (from natural skin folds, sanitary napkins), poor nutritional status, overzealous hygiene practices, and concomitant microbial infections (ie, candidiasis, infectious diarrhea).

ICD of the vulva is more common than ACD.[1] Both types of contact reactions may occur simultaneously and have overlapping features clinically and histologically. Contact dermatitis should be considered early in the evaluation of patients with chronic vulvar symptoms (pruritus, irritation) with or without abnormal findings on examination. In patients with other vulvar dermatoses, contact reactions should be suspected in patients who do not respond appropriately to therapy.[8] Vulvar contact dermatitis may result from direct application, inadvertent transfer from other body sites, local exposure to

Funding sources: None.
Department of Dermatology, Northwestern University, 676 North Saint Clair Street, Suite 1600, Chicago, IL 60611, USA
E-mail address: bschloss@nmff.org

Dermatol Clin 28 (2010) 697–706
doi:10.1016/j.det.2010.08.006
0733-8635/10/$ – see front matter

products excreted in the urine and/or feces after oral consumption, and systematized contact reactions. This article addresses the most common causes of ICD and ACD affecting the vulva and provides practical recommendations for evaluation and management.

IRRITANT CONTACT DERMATITIS

ICD is common, although the exact prevalence remains unclear. ICD results from cutaneous exposure to substances that cause direct cytotoxicity to keratinocytes without prior sensitization. Irritants can remove surface lipids and water-holding substances, damage cell membranes, and denature keratins and other proteins.[9–11]

Severe, acute ICD is equivalent to a caustic burn and manifests as erythema, edema, and vesicles, which evolve quickly into erosions and superficial ulcerations (**Fig. 1**). Subacute and chronic irritant reactions present with poorly demarcated erythematous patches and plaques with variable scale and excoriations. Patients may complain of burning, rawness, stinging pain, and/or itching. Severe irritant dermatitis can progress to punched-out ulcers with elevated, indurated borders (erosive diaper dermatitis of Jacquet) or erythematous to violaceous pseudoverrucous papules and nodules (granuloma gluteale infantum). These clinical presentations are well recognized in infants with chronic diaper dermatitis but may also occur in adults.[12] Significant pain and dysuria may occur in the context of vulvar erosions. Irritant reactions may also manifest as stinging and burning in the absence of identifiable skin changes.[13]

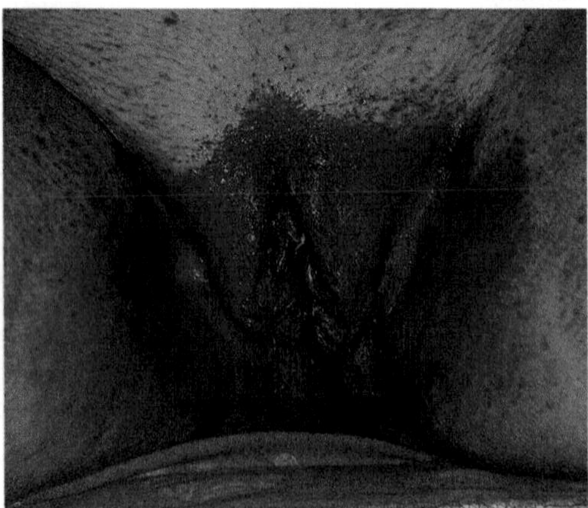

Fig. 1. Severe, erosive ICD of the vulva to witch hazel. Note the relative sparing of the inferior genitoinguinal creases in which natural occlusion of skin folds minimized irritant contact. (*Courtesy* of Dr Lynette J. Margesson, Manchester, NH.)

Greater concentrations of a given irritant are more likely to cause dermatitis. Common classes of irritants include acids, alkalis, surfactants, solvents, oxidants, and enzymes.[14] More specifically, urine, feces, sweat, topical medications, overzealous cleansing practices, and feminine hygiene products cause irritant contact reactions (**Box 1**).[6] Strong irritants usually cause immediate symptoms, which facilitate correlation between the culprit product and disease. Weaker irritants cause more subtle changes and are therefore less often suspected.

Douches contain both irritants and sensitizers. Douches that contain acids or alkalis can become irritants if not diluted properly by the patient during preparation. The main irritants in douches are alum, citric acid, and lactic acid. Sodium bicarbonate and sodium borate are alkalis that cause irritant contact reactions.[15]

Box 1
Common vulvar irritants

Body Fluids

- Abnormal vaginal discharge
- Feces (enzymes)
- Semen
- Sweat
- Urine (ammonia)

Excessive bathing

Feminine hygiene products

- Depilatories
- Douches
- Feminine hygiene wipes
- Lubricants
- Panty liners
- Sanitary napkins/pads

Heat

- Heating pads
- Hair dryer

Medications

- Alcohol-based creams and gels
- Bichloroacetic acid, trichloroacetic acid
- Cantharidin
- Fluorouracil
- Imiquimod
- Phenol
- Podophyllin
- Propylene glycol
- Spermicides (foaming agents, emulsifiers)

Soaps and detergents (including bubble baths)

ALLERGIC CONTACT DERMATITIS

ACD represents a delayed (type IV) hypersensitivity reaction that occurs in a genetically predisposed individual after sensitization to an allergen. This type of immunologic reaction involves antigen presentation by Langerhans cells, antigen recognition in the context of MHC class II molecules by T cells, and subsequent T-cell activation and proliferation. Allergens are typically low molecular weight, lipid-soluble molecules.[14] Because there is a delay between exposure to the allergen and onset of symptoms or physical abnormalities (typically 48–72 hours), allergens may not be readily recognized. Acute ACD results from exposure to a strong allergen to which the patient was previously sensitized and presents as an acute, vesiculobullous eruption with severe pruritus and/or pain; patients typically seek care immediately. Significant erythema, edema, coalescing vesicles, and ulcerations occur (**Figs. 2** and **3**). Vesicles may assume linear or geometric configurations reflecting areas of allergen contact when transferred by fingers or when touched by plant leaves. Robust allergic reactions may become generalized, especially affecting sites of previous contact dermatitis to the same allergen (recall phenomenon). Chronic ACD may result from intermittent or prolonged exposure to a relatively weak allergen and presents as subacute inflammation with variable degrees of pruritus; there is often a pattern of exacerbation and remission, which parallels allergen exposure.[16] Chronic ACD manifests as erythematous to hyperpigmented, lichenified plaques with variable scale and excoriation (**Fig. 4**). In dark-skinned patients, hyperpigmentation may be prominent and can mask erythema.

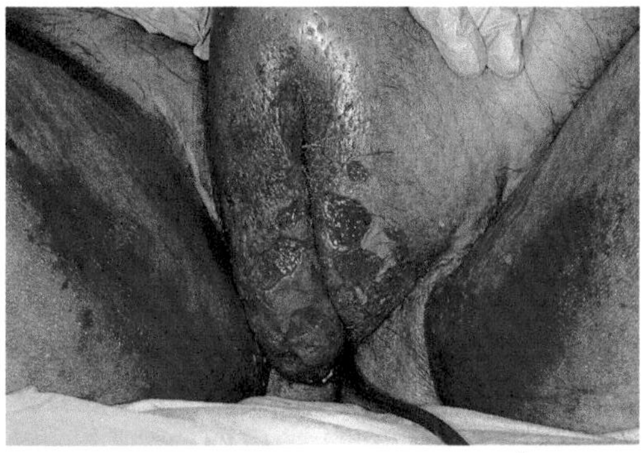

Fig. 3. Severe ulcerative ACD to benzocaine. Note severe ulceration of the labia majora with urinary catheter in place. The proximal medial thighs are frequently affected because of inadvertent contact and spreading of vulvar allergens. (*Courtesy* of Dr Lynette J. Margesson, Manchester, NH.)

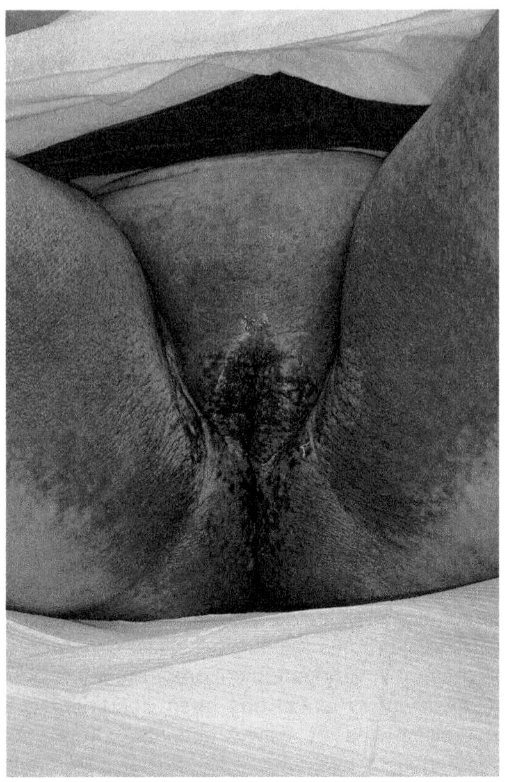

Fig. 2. Acute erosive ACD to benzocaine. Note the background of erythema and lichenification involving the mons and medial thighs. (*Courtesy* of Dr Lynette J. Margesson, Manchester, NH.)

Vulvar ACD was first reported in the literature in 1990.[17] ACD has been assessed in numerous studies of patients with pruritus vulvae or other vulvar dermatoses, and numerous allergens have been identified (**Box 2**).[8,12,18–20] Patients with pruritus vulvae and pruritic vulvar dermatoses are at higher risk for developing contact dermatitis because of their frequent, and potentially excessive, use of topical anesthetics (eg, benzocaine) and other products in the quest for symptom relief.[19] The most frequently identified allergens in large studies include neomycin,[8,17,19] "caine" anesthetics (benzocaine, dibucaine hydrochloride),[19,21] fragrance,[19,21] balsam of Peru,[8] and nickel.[8,20,21]

Medicaments are agents used to treat, prevent, or alleviate the symptoms of disease. Culprit allergens in medicaments reflect local prescribing practices and vary geographically.[22] Frequently cited medicaments in vulvar ACD include topical anesthetics, antibiotics, corticosteroids, antiseptics, and preservatives.[20,22] Of 135 patients with chronic vulvar pruritus and discomfort who underwent patch testing, 63 (47%) had at least 1 positive patch reaction, and 39 (29%) were considered

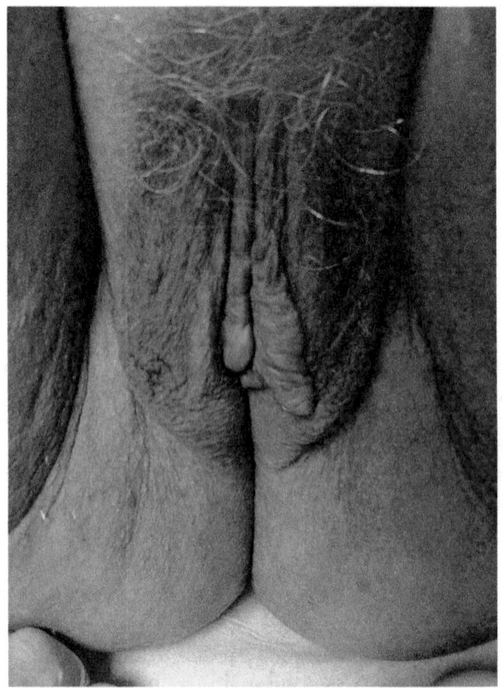

Fig. 4. Chronic ACD with mild erythema, scaling, lichenification, and areas of hyperpigmentation. (*Courtesy of* Dr Bethanee J. Schlosser, Chicago, IL.)

relevant to the patient's clinical condition. Medicaments and their components accounted for most of the positive reactions.[8] Lewis and colleagues[19] showed similar results when 121 women with pruritus vulvae underwent patch testing; 57 (47%) had at least 1 relevant positive patch reaction, of which medicaments or their components were the most common allergens. Utas and colleagues[23] performed patch testing on 50 women with pruritus vulvae including women treated for primary vulvar dermatoses; 26 (52%) of the women had at least 1 positive patch reaction, and 8 (16%) were deemed relevant. The most frequent relevant allergens were fragrance, preservatives, and medicaments. Brenan and colleagues[21] obtained positive patch test results in 42% of 50 patients with chronic vulvar symptoms; medicaments (including "caine" mix and ethylenediamine) and fragrance were common allergens identified.

Neomycin is the most common allergen among topical antibiotic preparations. Positive patch test reactions are observed in 11.6% of adults and 8% of children.[24] Drugs that cross-react with neomycin include bacitracin, streptomycin, kanamycin, gentamicin, and tobramycin.[25]

The "caine" anesthetics are widely recognized causes of ACD. Ester anesthetics (benzocaine, procaine, tetracaine) are the best-known allergens and cross-react with para-aminobenzoic acid, paraphenylenediamine, sulfa drugs, thiazide diuretics, and azo and aniline dyes.[25] Unfortunately, benzocaine continues to be widely available in over-the-counter topical anti-itch preparations (ie, Vagisil). A history of sulfa allergy or adverse reaction to hair dye can provide diagnostic clues to the culprit allergen. Amide anesthetics (bupivacaine, lidocaine, dibucaine, mepivacaine, and prilocaine) are less potent and less common sensitizers. Patients may have simultaneous ACD to both classes of topical anesthetics.[26]

Topical corticosteroids may be sensitizers, due to the steroid molecule itself or its vehicle components. Patch testing to tixocortol pivalate (Class A), budesonide (Class B and D), and hydrocortisone-17-butyrate (Class D2) detects most cases of topical corticosteroid-induced ACD.[15]

More than 5000 fragrance materials are used at present.[15] In general, fragrance allergy is common; the North American Contact Dermatitis Group has demonstrated sensitivity to fragrance mix I or balsam of Peru in 9.1% and 10.6% of patients, respectively.[27] Balsam of Peru (*Myroxylon pereirae*) and fragrance mix I (a mix of 8 fragrances) have conventionally been used to screen patients for fragrance allergy. Fragrance mix II, which contains lyral, citral, farnesol, citronellol, hexyl cinnamic aldehyde, and coumarin, began to be used in 2007. Balsam of Peru is a naturally occurring compound of benzyl acetate, benzyl alcohol, cinnamic acid, cinnamic alcohol, cinnamic aldehyde, eugenol, and isoeugenol, derived from Central and South American fir trees. Balsam of Peru is a useful marker for fragrance allergy, with a positive patch reaction in more than 50% of fragrance-allergic patients.[15] Sensitivity to balsam of Peru and/or fragrance has been implicated in pruritus vulvae and chronic vulvar dermatoses.[8,19–21,28]

Ethylenediamine hydrochloride is a stabilizer that became notorious for ACD to the original formulation of Mycolog cream.[15] Ethylenediamine hydrochloride is also the parent compound for the class of antihistamines that includes hydroxyzine and is a component of the asthma medication, aminophylline. Although the present formulation of Mycolog does not contain ethylenediamine hydrochloride, this sensitizer continues to be present in various topical preparations.

Sensitivity to nickel has been documented in several studies of vulvar patients. Crone and colleagues[29] evaluated 35 vulvar dermatitis patients with patch testing; positive reactions were documented in 26% with nickel being the most common. Similarly, Lucke and colleagues[28] demonstrated nickel sensitivity in 31% of 55

Box 2
Common vulvar allergens

Anesthetics

- Amides (dibucaine, lidocaine)
- Crotamiton
- Diphenhydramine
- Esters (benzocaine, tetracaine)

Antibiotics

- Bacitracin
- Neomycin
- Polymyxin
- Sulfonamides

Antifungals

- Imidazoles (clotrimazole, miconazole)
- Nystatin

Antiseptics

- Chlorhexidine
- Gentian violet
- Mercuric chloride
- Phenylmercuric salts
- Povidone iodine
- Thimerosal

Corticosteroids

Douches

- Benzethonium chloride
- Fragrance/perfumes
- Methyl salicylate
- Oil of eucalyptus
- Oxyquinoline
- Phenylmercuric acetate
- Thymol

Emollients

- Glycerin
- Jojoba oil
- Lanolin
- Propylene glycol

Fragrance

- Balsam of Peru
- Cinnamic alcohol, cinnamic aldehyde
- Eugenol
- Isoeugenol
- Hydroxycitronellal

Nail Polish

- Toluene-sulfonamide formaldehyde resin

Nickel

Preservatives

- Bronopol
- Diazolidinyl urea
- Formaldehyde
- Imidazolidinyl urea
- Kathon
- Quaternium 15

Rubber

- Latex
- Mercaptobenzothiazole
- Thiurams

Sanitary Napkins

- Acetyl acetone
- Formaldehyde
- Fragrance
- Methacrylates

Spermicides

- Hexylresorcinol
- Nonoxynol
- Oxyquinoline sulfate
- Phenylmercuric acetate and butyrate
- Quinine hydrochloride

patients with vulvar dermatoses, and approximately half of the patients experienced reduction in symptoms with avoidance of direct contact with nickel and/or adherence to a nickel-free diet. In the absence of direct nickel contact with the vulva, the role of nickel sensitivity in vulvar pruritus and dermatitis requires further evaluation.

Various spices and flavorings have also been linked to vulvar pruritus and dermatitis.[30,31] Fifty-three patients with chronic anogenital dermatitis underwent patch testing, and 35 (66%) showed at least 1 positive reaction.[30] In addition to noting sensitivity to nickel (18 patients), fragrance (9 patients), and preservatives (6 patients), positive reactions to spices, including curry mix, nutmeg, coriander, peppermint oil, and onion powder, were noted in 15 patients. These reactions were deemed relevant in 4 patients, with symptomatic and clinical improvement noted with avoidance of the allergens.

CLINICAL DIFFERENTIAL DIAGNOSIS

Acute vesiculo-erosive forms of contact dermatitis can mimic other bullous and ulcerative disorders (**Box 3**). The differential diagnosis of acute contact dermatitis includes herpes simplex virus infection, candidiasis, fixed-drug eruption, immunobullous disorders (pemphigus vulgaris, mucous membrane pemphigoid, bullous pemphigoid), and erosive lichen planus. The acute onset of the eruption favors contact dermatitis; immunobullous

Box 3
Clinical differential diagnosis of ICD and ACD

Acute vesiculoerosive contact dermatitis

- Bullous pemphigoid
- Candidiasis
- Erythema multiforme
- Fixed drug eruption
- Hailey-Hailey disease (benign familial pemphigus)
- Herpes simplex virus infection
- Lichen planus (erosive, bullous)
- Mucous membrane pemphigoid
- Pemphigus vulgaris

Chronic eczematous contact dermatitis

- Atopic dermatitis
- Candidiasis
- Erythrasma
- Extramammary Paget disease
- Lichen simplex chronicus
- Psoriasis
- Seborrheic dermatitis
- Squamous cell carcinoma in situ
- Tinea cruris

disorders and erosive lichen planus typically are more gradual in onset.

Subacute and chronic forms of ICD and ACD can be similar clinically to several eczematous and papulosquamous dermatoses (see **Box 3**). Atopic dermatitis, lichen simplex chronicus, seborrheic dermatitis, inverse psoriasis, and tinea cruris should be considered in the differential diagnosis. The less common but more serious diagnoses of squamous cell carcinoma in situ and extramammary Paget disease should also be considered for localized lesions.

EVALUATION

Contact dermatitis, both irritant and allergic, should be considered early in the evaluation of women with vulvar complaints and compatible clinical findings. In addition, contact dermatitis often complicates the management of other vulvar dermatoses. Patients with vulvar diseases that do not respond to appropriate treatment should be interviewed and evaluated for possible contact reactions.

Accurate diagnosis of ICD or ACD requires a high degree of suspicion and thorough investigation to correlate symptoms and clinical findings with the patient's exposure history. A thorough history of all vulvar products, medications (prescription, over-the-counter, and complementary), contraceptives, sexual products, and hygiene practices must be obtained to identify potential contactants. Questioning may reveal extreme hygiene practices including the use of bleach, lye, and antiseptic mouthwashes to cleanse the vulva, minimize odor, and/or prevent infection. In addition, cosmetics and products used elsewhere on the body may be culprits after inadvertent transfer to the genitalia from the hands (ie, toluene sulfonamide formaldehyde resin in nail polish as a cause of vulvar ACD). Products used by intimate partners may play a role, as close contact (via sexual activity, ie, connubial transfer, and shared living spaces) can result in irritant and allergen transfer. The interview should also address potential occupational and hobby exposures; a floral worker with vulvar dermatitis had a relevant positive patch reaction to primin.[30] The temporal relationship between the onset of recurrent episodes of dermatitis and food consumption should also be investigated; oral products may cause sensitization and dermatitis after excretion in the urine and/or feces.[31] There are myriad types of products about which patients should be questioned (see **Boxes 1** and **2**). Additional areas of cutaneous involvement should be investigated; concomitant eyelid dermatitis in patients with vulvar contact dermatitis is not uncommon and reinforces the importance of considering allergen transfer by touching.

The clinical features of ACD and ICD may be indistinguishable from each other as well as other vulvar dermatoses. Irritant and allergic contact reactions may occur simultaneously, further complicating the diagnosis. Histopathologic features may be nonspecific, with overlapping features noted between ICD and ACD. Histopathologic changes of ICD can vary according to the specific irritant and its concentration.[11] Low irritant concentrations typically cause epidermal spongiosis, mild superficial dermal edema, and a superficial perivascular lymphocytic inflammatory infiltrate.[32] High concentrations of irritant can result in ballooning of keratinocytes in the upper epidermis with variable degrees of cell necrosis and neutrophilic inflammation.[33] ACD demonstrates epidermal spongiosis, intraepidermal spongiotic vesicles, and a superficial dermal inflammatory infiltrate composed of lymphocytes, macrophages, and Langerhans cells. Eosinophils are present in variable numbers. Spongiosis becomes less prominent as lesions become more chronic.[34] Psoriasiform hyperplasia, typified by acanthosis, hyperkeratosis, and parakeratosis, may occur in chronic forms of both ACD and ICD.[34] Biopsy, for both routine histopathology and direct immunofluorescence, may be most useful in the setting of erosive lesions to exclude immunobullous disorders, erosive lichen planus, and other entities.

Patch testing is essential for accurate identification of allergens. For patch testing evaluation of vulvar dermatitis, the North American Contact Dermatitis Group standard and corticosteroid series are recommended. Additional series for medications, perfumes, preservatives, and other allergens may be performed, if indicated.[35] Patch tests are best interpreted at 48 and 72 hours with an additional reading obtained between 72 and 120 hours.[15] The relevance of positive patch reactions, either as a primary cause or an aggravating factor, must be considered. If a positive patch test reaction is identified, correlation with the clinical examination and history of exposures should be made.[36] Patients may be able to tolerate a medication containing a preservative to which they have a positive patch reaction because the concentration of the preservative in the preparation used is often less than the threshold needed to produce a clinical reaction.[37] Patch testing has not been shown to be helpful in patients who presented with vulvodynia (vulvar pain in the absence of any clinical abnormality).[28]

Patients should be provided with detailed written instructions regarding allergens to avoid and a list of safe alternatives. The Contact Allergen Replacement Database, available from the American Contact Dermatitis Society, is an invaluable tool (www.contactderm.org). Of note, fragrance-allergic patients should be educated that "unscented" products may actually contain low concentrations of masking fragrance (used to mask unpleasant chemical or fatty odors but not intended to convey their own scent). Patients should avoid such unscented products and instead seek "fragrance-free" products that possess no fragrance chemicals including masking fragrance.[15] When the safety of a product is unclear, sensitized patients may be advised to perform repeated open application testing (ROAT, twice-daily application to nondermatitic skin of the antecubital fossa). Because vulvar skin reacts differently to irritants and allergens than nongenital skin, and by definition the vulva is not an open area, ROAT has limited applicability in vulvar contact dermatitis.

The patient's estrogen status should be assessed. Normal saline wet mount preparations of vaginal discharge and pH measurement are essential. Signs of estrogen insufficiency include pH greater than 4.5, reduced or absent lactobacilli, and increased numbers of immature, parabasal keratinocytes, which appear as rounded cells with relatively high nuclear to cytoplasmic ratio.

Patients should be evaluated clinically for secondary infection by bacteria, fungi, and viruses. Clinical clues include fissuring, crusting, and pustules. Bacterial exudate cultures can be obtained from crusted erosions or unroofed pustules. Potassium hydroxide microscopy and fungal culture of pustule contents can assist in the diagnosis of vulvovaginal candidiasis. Herpes simplex virus cultures, Tzanck smears, and/or direct fluorescent antigen preparations should ideally be obtained from unroofed, intact pustules or vesicles. Clinical examination findings in conjunction with the results of laboratory testing should direct antimicrobial therapy.

TREATMENT

All potential irritants and allergens must be discontinued. Patients should be advised to cleanse the vulva no more than twice daily using only lukewarm (not hot) water without soap, cleanser, or detergent. Sitz baths, in which the patient fills the tub with only lukewarm water to cover the hips and buttocks, may be used for cleansing the vulva and for relief of pain or itching. For those patients that are not able to maneuver into a tub, a handheld shower spray can be used on a gentle setting for directed vulvar hygiene. Patients should be instructed to use only their hands to clean the vulva and to discontinue the use of all washcloths, loofahs and sponges. Patients should pat the vulva dry, avoiding rubbing and additional friction. Plain white petrolatum should be applied as an emollient and barrier and is especially important for fissured or eroded areas.

Erosions cause severe dysuria. Patients should be advised to apply a copious layer of plain white petrolatum to all eroded areas before and after each bathroom use. Patients may reduce dysuria further, either by urinating while seated in a shallow tube of lukewarm water or by pouring lukewarm water over the vulva during micturition.

Vesicles and weeping erosions produce additional moisture that can macerate vulvar tissues and cause further irritation. Sitz baths (5–10 minutes twice daily) or compresses are helpful in removing serous crusts and providing symptomatic relief. Dilute aluminum acetate solutions can be applied for short periods as compresses to facilitate desiccation.

Depending on the severity and chronicity of the vulvar dermatitis, a low- (hydrocortisone 2.5%), medium- (triamcinolone acetonide 0.1%), or high-potency (clobetasol propionate 0.05%, halobetasol 0.05%) topical corticosteroid ointment should initially be applied twice daily until lesions have healed completely (**Fig. 5**). Corticosteroid potency and frequency of dosing can be tapered as the dermatitis improves. For severe cases of contact dermatitis, including those that present with vesicular and/or erosive disease, systemic corticosteroids are indicated. Prednisone (40–60 mg daily in the morning or alternatively 0.5–1.0mg/kg/d based on ideal body weight) with gradual tapering over 14 to 21 days quickly provides dramatic relief of symptoms and clinical improvement, more so potentially for allergic rather than irritant reactions. Systemic corticosteroids may be given through intramuscular injection (triamcinolone acetonide, 1 mg/kg as a single dose); however, intramuscular injection precludes individualized tapering of medication dose and does not allow discontinuation of medication if a patient experiences adverse effects (ie, steroid psychosis). As symptoms improve, patients should be transitioned to the use of a topical corticosteroid ointment as noted above. Systemic prophylaxis for candidiasis (fluconazole 150 mg by mouth once weekly) should be considered in all patients treated with topical or systemic corticosteroids.[5]

Pruritus and associated scratching can perpetuate and promote inflammation, the so-called scratch-itch cycle. A combination of nonsedating and sedating antihistamines can be used for maximal symptom relief. Loratadine (10 mg), fexofenadine (60 mg), or cetirizine (10 mg) can be administered in the morning for relief of daytime pruritus; dosing may be increased to twice daily as needed. Hydroxyzine (25–100 mg) and doxepin (10–75mg) are the preferred sedating antihistamines for bedtime use daily to minimize scratching during sleep. Topical antipruritic medications (eg, diphenhydramine, lidocaine) should be avoided. Patients should be advised to avoid heat, which may increase histamine release and worsen pruritus. Instead, cool compresses, cool gel packs, or frozen vegetables wrapped in thin fabric can provide significant relief of pruritus; frozen products and ice should not be applied directly to the skin.

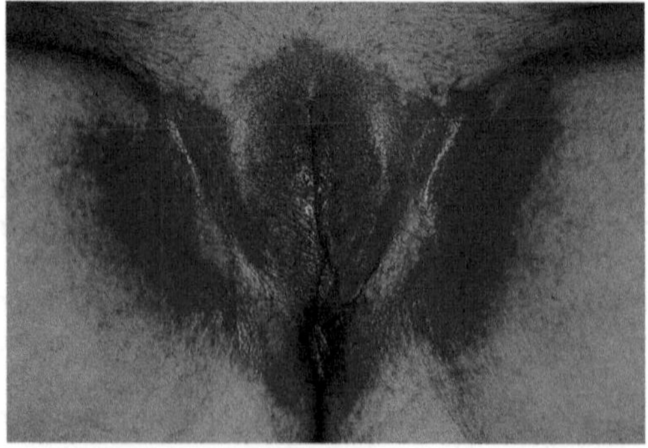

Fig. 5. Dramatic improvement in severe ICD to witch hazel (see **Fig. 1**) after discontinuation of product and treatment with topical corticosteroids. Sparing of the inferior genitoinguinal creases is more easily appreciated after resolution of acute edema and erosions. (*Courtesy* of Dr Lynette J. Margesson, Manchester, NH.)

If secondary infection by bacteria, fungi, or viruses is suspected, appropriate diagnostic testing should be performed, as discussed earlier. Clinical examination findings in conjunction with the results of laboratory testing should direct antimicrobial therapy. Systemic antimicrobial therapy should be used, when possible, rather than topical medications to avoid further irritant or allergic reactions and to minimize physical manipulation of the affected areas. In patients treated with systemic antibiotics, prophylaxis for secondary vulvovaginal candidiasis using fluconazole 150 mg by mouth once weekly should be considered.

Estrogen deficiency should also be corrected. Although estrogen deficiency may not be an issue of acute importance during the initial evaluation, failure to address estrogen deficiency may predispose the patient to recurrent contact dermatitis or other vulvar dystrophy in the future. Consideration should be given to the risks, benefits, and modes of administration in the context of the individual patient.

Comprehensive patient education, both verbal and written, is essential for successful resolution of the dermatitis and, more importantly, to prevent future irritant or allergic contact reactions. Patients should be followed closely during the initial phase of treatment to ensure patient adherence and to monitor for complications of therapy (ie, corticosteroid atrophy, secondary infection, and development of ACD or ICD to prescribed medications).

SUMMARY

Contact dermatitis, both irritant and allergic, should be considered early in the evaluation of women with vulvar complaints and compatible clinical findings. Such considerations are especially important with increased chronicity of symptoms and for those women who have seen multiple providers, as both scenarios increase the number of medicaments and other remedies used by patients. Vulvar contact dermatitis is more often caused by irritants than allergens. The most frequently noted allergens in patients with vulvar pruritus and/or dermatitis include medicaments, preservatives, fragrance, and nickel. Contact dermatitis may be the primary or secondary problem in patients with vulvar symptoms, and vulvar disease is often multifactorial.

An organized, stepwise approach to the evaluation and treatment of patients with vulvar complaints is required to successfully address each abnormality identified toward the end goal of a healthy vulva and happy patient.

REFERENCES

1. Mathias CG, Maibach HI. Dermatotoxicology monographs I. Cutaneous irritation: factors influencing the response to irritants. Clin Toxicol 1978;13(3): 333–46.
2. Britz MB, Maibach HI. Human cutaneous vulvar reactivity to irritants. Contact Dermatitis 1979;5(6): 375–7.
3. Farage M, Maibach HI. The vulvar epithelium differs from the skin: implications for cutaneous testing to address topical vulvar exposures. Contact Dermatitis 2004;51(4):201–9.
4. Elsner P, Wilhelm D, Maibach HI. Sodium lauryl sulfate-induced irritant contact dermatitis in vulvar and forearm skin of premenopausal and postmenopausal women. J Am Acad Dermatol 1990;23(4 Pt 1):648–52.
5. Margesson LJ. Contact dermatitis of the vulva. Dermatol Ther 2004;17(1):20–7.
6. Margesson LJ. Vulvar disease pearls. Dermatol Clin 2006;24(2):145–55, v.
7. Hannestad YS, Rortveit G, Sandvik H, et al. A community-based epidemiological survey of female urinary incontinence: the Norwegian EPINCONT study. Epidemiology of Incontinence in the County of Nord-Trondelag. J Clin Epidemiol 2000; 53(11):1150–7.
8. Marren P, Wojnarowska F, Powell S. Allergic contact dermatitis and vulvar dermatoses. Br J Dermatol 1992;126(1):52–6.
9. Effendy I, Maibach HI. Surfactants and experimental irritant contact dermatitis. Contact Dermatitis 1995; 33(4):217–25.
10. Pierard GE, Goffin V, Hermanns-Le T, et al. Surfactant-induced dermatitis: comparison of corneosurfametry with predictive testing on human and reconstructed skin. J Am Acad Dermatol 1995;33 (3):462–9.
11. Willis CM, Stephens CJ, Wilkinson JD. Epidermal damage induced by irritants in man: a light and electron microscopic study. J Invest Dermatol 1989;93(5):695–9.
12. Virgili A, Corazza M, Califano A. Diaper dermatitis in an adult. A case of erythema papuloerosive of Sevestre and Jacquet. J Reprod Med 1998;43(11): 949–51.
13. Kamarashev JA, Vassileva SG. Dermatologic diseases of the vulva. Clin Dermatol 1997;15(1): 53–65.
14. Marks JG, Elsner P, DeLeo VA. Contact & occupational dermatology. 3rd edition. St. Louis (MO): Mosby; 2002.
15. Fisher AA, Rietschel RL, Fowler JF. Fisher's contact dermatitis. 6th edition. Hamilton (ON): B C Decker; 2008.
16. Pincus SH. Vulvar dermatoses and pruritus vulvae. Dermatol Clin 1992;10(2):297–308.
17. Doherty VR, Forsyth A, MacKie RM. Pruritus vulvae: a manifestations of contact hypersensitivity? Br J Dermatol 1990;123(Suppl 37):26–7.
18. Goldsmith PC, Rycroft RJ, White IR, et al. Contact sensitivity in women with anogenital dermatoses. Contact Dermatitis 1997;36(3):174–5.
19. Lewis FM, Shah M, Gawkrodger DJ. Contact sensitivity in pruritus vulvae: patch test results and clinical outcome. Am J Contact Dermat 1997;8(3):137–40.
20. Nardelli A, Degreef H, Goossens A. Contact allergic reactions of the vulva: a 14-year review. Dermatitis 2004;15(3):131–6.
21. Brenan JA, Dennerstein GJ, Sfameni SF, et al. Evaluation of patch testing in patients with chronic vulvar symptoms. Australas J Dermatol 1996;37(1):40–3.
22. Bauer A, Rodiger C, Greif C, et al. Vulvar dermatoses—irritant and allergic contact dermatitis of the vulva. Dermatology 2005;210(2):143–9.
23. Utas S, Ferahbas A, Yildiz S. Patients with vulval pruritus: patch test results. Contact Dermatitis 2008;58:296–8.
24. Zug KA, McGinley-Smith D, Warshaw EM, et al. Contact allergy in children referred for patch testing: North American contact dermatitis group data, 2001–2004. Arch Dermatol 2008;144(10):1329–36.
25. Davis MD. Unusual patterns in contact dermatitis: medicaments. Dermatol Clin 2009;27(3):289–97, vi.
26. Gunson TH, Greig DE. Allergic contact dermatitis to all three classes of local anaesthetic. Contact Dermatitis 2008;59(2):126–7.
27. Warshaw EM, Belsito DV, DeLeo VA, et al. North American contact dermatitis group patch-test results, 2003-2004 study period. Dermatitis 2008; 19(3):129–36.
28. Lucke TW, Fleming CJ, McHenry P, et al. Patch testing in vulval dermatoses: how relevant is nickel? Contact Dermatitis 1998;38(2):111–2.
29. Crone AM, Stewart EJ, Wojnarowska F, et al. Aetiological factors in vulvar dermatitis. J Eur Acad Dermatol Venereol 2000;14(3):181–6.
30. Vermaat H, Smienk F, Rustemeyer T, et al. Anogenital allergic contact dermatitis, the role of spices and flavour allergy. Contact Dermatitis 2008;59(4):233–7.
31. Vermaat H, van Meurs T, Rustemeyer T, et al. Vulval allergic contact dermatitis due to peppermint oil in herbal tea. Contact Dermatitis 2008;58(6):364–5.
32. Willis CM, Young E, Brandon DR, et al. Immunopathological and ultrastructural findings in human allergic and irritant contact dermatitis. Br J Dermatol 1986;115(3):305–16.

33. Taylor RM. Histopathology of contact dermatitis. Clin Dermatol 1986;4(2):18–22.
34. White CR Jr. Histopathology of exogenous and systemic contact eczema. Semin Dermatol 1990; 9(3):226–9.
35. Virgili A, Bacilieri S, Corazza M. Evaluation of contact sensitization in vulvar lichen simplex chronicus. A proposal for a battery of selected allergens. J Reprod Med 2003;48(1):33–6.
36. Bruze M. What is a relevant contact allergy? Contact Dermatitis 1990;23(4):224–5.
37. Skinner SL, Marks JG. Allergic contact dermatitis to preservatives in topical medicaments. Am J Contact Dermat 1998;9(4):199–201.

Lichen Sclerosus

Ruth Murphy, PhD, MBChB, FRCP

KEYWORDS

• Lichen sclerosus • Childhood lichen sclerosus • Vulva
• Differentiated vulvar intraepithelial neoplasia

DISEASE PATHOGENESIS

Lichen sclerosus (LS) is a complex chronic inflammatory skin disease, with genetic, physiologic, and environmental factors that influence the clinical phenotype and disease outcome. It is generally accepted as an autoimmune disorder with a predilection for genital skin, but the exact target antigen and disease pathogenesis remain controversial. Hallopeau and Darier first described lichen sclerosus at the end of the nineteenth century as a variant of lichen planus (LP).[1–3] Now LP and LS are generally accepted as different entities on the basis of distinguishing clinical and histologic features, although the diseases overlap. Early stages of LS and LP can sometimes be difficult to differentiate clinically, and established cases of vulvar LS may develop introital LP. This crossover subgroup can be more refractory to treatment.[4,5]

The exact pathogenesis of LS remains unclear, although clinical observations are leading to a translational medical approach to unraveling disease pathogenesis. LS is considered to be an autoimmune disorder and, in common with other autoimmune diseases, is found more commonly in females. The condition has been associated clinically and immunologically with autoimmune thyroiditis, pernicious anemia, vitiligo, and alopecia areata.[6–10] These disorders should be considered in the evaluation of patients suspected of having LS and are useful both clinically in the diagnosis of LS and in the detection of other early subclinical autoimmune conditions. From clinical experience, patients with undiagnosed autoimmune thyroiditis may present with LS, which is more difficult to control until they return to a clinically euthyroid state.

The genetic contribution to the development of lichen sclerosus is also complex. Familial cases have been described in identical and nonidentical twins and siblings, although the inheritance pattern is not clearly established.[11] Genes that regulate the human leukocyte antigens (HLA) have been investigated to see if associations between HLA antigens and LS exist.[12,13] No associations have been found between HLA class 1 antigens, which occur on the surface of all nucleated cells and platelets. LS has been shown to be associated with type 2 antigens particularly DQ7, -8 or -9.[12,13] HLA type 2 antigens are expressed on immunocompetent cells that normally recognize foreign particles.

Established areas of lichen sclerosus show a T-lymphocyte dominant inflammatory infiltrate, sometimes with an associated lymphocytic vasculitis. When T-cell receptor gene rearrangement studies from affected penile and vulvar skin are performed, a monoclonal population of rearranged γ-chain gene of the T-cell receptor have been identified, which could explain the increased risk of malignant transformation in affected individuals.[14–17]

Because the inflammation in LS initially targets the basement membrane, resulting in apoptosis of basal cells, it has been postulated that the target antigen may lie in this region. Evidence for this comes from work showing circulating autoantibodies to the endothelial cell adhesion molecule, ECAM-1, in 67% of patients with LS.[18]

Antibodies targeting the basement membrane zone, (chiefly BP 180 and BP 230), have been identified in 30% of sera of affected patients.[18,19] The mechanism leading to the synthesis of these autoantibodies is not fully understood. Current theories postulate that oxidative stress as a result of DNA damage induced by reactive oxygen species, as a result of chronic inflammation, may lead to the disease and possibly any associated malignancy.[20]

There are no conflicts of interest.

Department of Dermatology, Queens Medical Centre, Nottingham University Teaching Hospitals, Nottingham NG7 2UH, UK
E-mail address: Ruthmurphy1@aol.com

Dermatol Clin 28 (2010) 707–715
doi:10.1016/j.det.2010.07.006
0733-8635/10/$ – see front matter

Debate continues with respect to the pathogenic role played by *Borrelia burgdorferi* infection in triggering LS. In Europe there is some supporting evidence for Borrelia infection and LS from polymerase chain reaction amplification of Borrelia-type genetic material in the patches of LS. This finding has not been replicated in studies from the United States.[21,22]

It is possible that Borrelia infection may act as one of several environmental triggers that can trigger LS in genetically susceptible individuals. Extragenital LS, occurring as patches that clinically resemble scleroderma, is reported to occur in approximately 6% of patients with vulvar lichen sclerosus.[4] It is known that lesional LS skin has altered extracellular matrix proteins similar to scleroderma, a condition that, in localized cutaneous disease, may coexist and show clinical similarities to LS.[23,24] Acrodermatitis chronica atrophicans, a sclerodermatous skin reaction to Borrelia, has clinical and histologic features of localized scleroderma, but the lesions are usually acral in distribution rather than genital.[25]

Finally, because the 2 peaks in incidence for vulvar LS occur during times of low estrogen, before puberty and after menopause, there is some debate as to the exact role played by hormones in disease pathogenesis.[26] In normal female genitals, the transition from vagina to vulva is marked by an increase in androgen receptors and a decrease in estrogen and progesterone receptors. Vulvar androgen receptor expression seems to be decreased in a subgroup of individuals with LS.[27,28] Work has been recently published that suggests that disturbance of androgen-dependent growth of the vulvar skin by oral contraceptive pills (OCPs), and especially OCP with antiandrogenic properties, might trigger the early onset of LS in a subgroup of susceptible young women.[29]

Therefore, lichen sclerosus is a complex disease expressed in individuals who are at increased risk of autoimmune disease. External triggers that may influence the exact timing of disease onset might include oxidative stress from chronic inflammation, hormonal manipulation from the use of oral contraceptive agents, and possibly even infection. The clinical features of the disease, treatment options, failures, and disease complications are discussed next.

CLINICAL FEATURES

LS preferentially affects women in the fifth or sixth decade of life as well as children.[30] The incidence of LS is lower in men than in women, but there is also a bimodal onset in the male population, with peaks of disease onset in young boys and then again in older men.[31] In children and adults, the presentation differs slightly. Vulval irritation, worsening at night, is the most frequent symptom reported in adults.[4] With disease progression, scratching and sclerotic changes lead to pain from erosions and fissures.[4,30] Progressive scarring and tissue adhesion results in narrowing of the introitus, which, caused by loss of elasticity, easily tears at the base of the posterior fourchette. This tearing makes sexual activity difficult or impossible and leads to significant psychosexual distress.[32,33]

Girls often present with irritation and soreness,[34] but not infrequently with constipation or urinary symptoms.[35] In the author's experience, children may also present with behavioral problems, particularly night fears and pain caused by their unexplained nocturnal discomfort and the reward of attention from a concerned parent.

The characteristic clinical appearance of lichen sclerosus is as plaques of ivory white, atrophic or thickened skin with ecchymoses and hemorrhage from repeated scratching of the sclerotic and thinned labia minora (**Figs. 1** and **2**). Although there are many skin diseases that exhibit white color, the crinkled texture change is classic and, generally, pathognomonic (**Fig. 3**); although shiny, smooth texture also occurs (see **Fig. 1; Fig. 4**). With time, the scratching leads to hyperkeratosis and superficial erosions (**Fig. 5**). Sometimes these changes can be difficult to differentiate from vulvar intraepithelial neoplasia (VIN), especially in asymptomatic individuals. With disease progression, the labia minora adhere to adjacent structures and often fissure (**Fig. 6**). These fissures are painful and can become infected secondarily with bacteria or yeast. The inflammation causes pigmentary disturbance, and symmetric hypermelanosis in the region of the labia minora frequently occurs and can cause concern and diagnostic uncertainty with respect to a vulval malignant melanoma (**Fig. 7**). As the disease progresses, there is scarring with labial resorption, burying of the clitoris, and narrowing of the introitus (see **Fig. 6**) and urethral strictures in males.

In children, the clinical findings are similar, but to an untrained clinician may resemble sexual abuse (see **Fig. 4**). Because lichen sclerosus exhibits the Koebner phenomenon at sites of trauma, some cases of LS may actually be aggravated by sexual abuse.[36,37] This topic is a contentious area, and if there is any diagnostic doubt, these children should be evaluated jointly with health care clinicians who are appropriately trained in safeguarding issues.

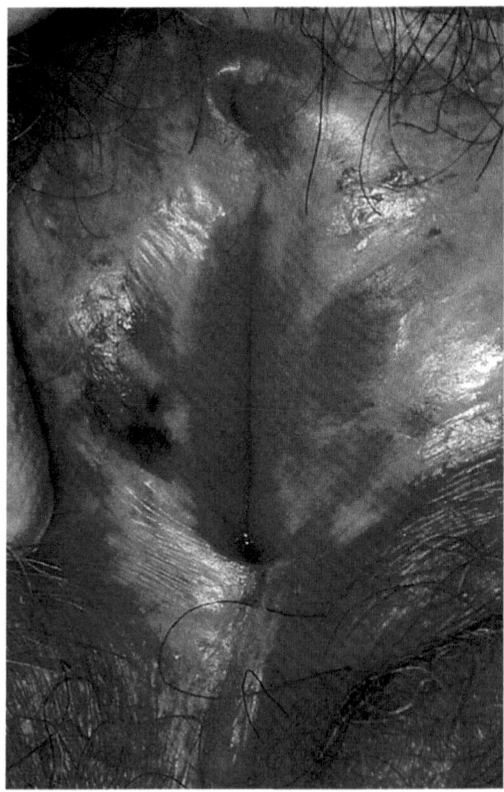

Fig. 1. Lichen sclerosus showing pallor, shiny texture, and resorption of the labia minora and agglutination of the clitoral hood; there is classic hemorrhage/purpura on the right labium majus and at the posterior fourchette. (*Courtesy of* Ruth Murphy, PhD, MBChB, FRCP, Nottingham, UK.)

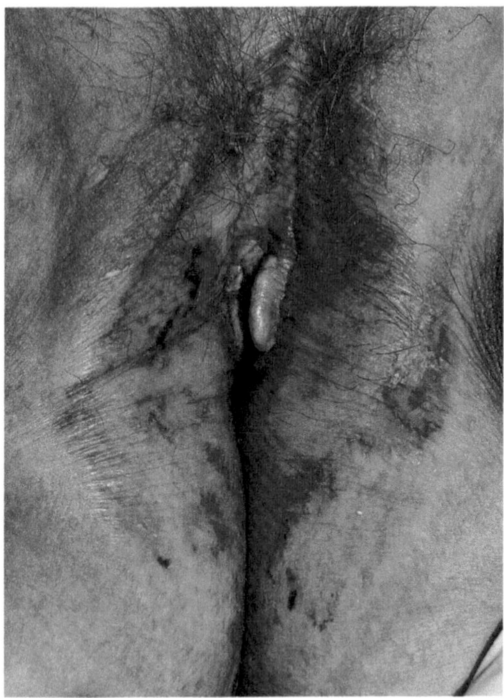

Fig. 2. White, crinkled plaques of lichen sclerosus, showing excoriations and purpura caused by scratching as well as partial resorption of the labia minora and clitoral hood. (*Courtesy of* Libby Edwards, MD, Charlotte, NC.)

Vulvar LS is usually a clinical diagnosis. In the early stages of the disease the diagnosis can sometimes be difficult. The main differential diagnoses are psoriasis, lichen planus, lichen simplex chronicus, and benign mucous membrane pemphigoid.[4] In the early stages, differentiation can be particularly challenging, and currently debate exists as to whether there is an increased prevalence of LS in patients with psoriasis and whether the 2 conditions more commonly coexist in the vulval region than we generally recognize.[38,39]

However, if there is diagnostic doubt, a vulval biopsy is recommended.[4] In children, the threshold for vulval biopsy is generally higher, and in most cases a trial of potent topical steroids is initially recommended.[4] Because vulval LS is usually responsive to high-potency topical steroids, any area resistant to therapy would be an absolute indication for biopsy to confirm the diagnosis or exclude malignancy in any age group.[4]

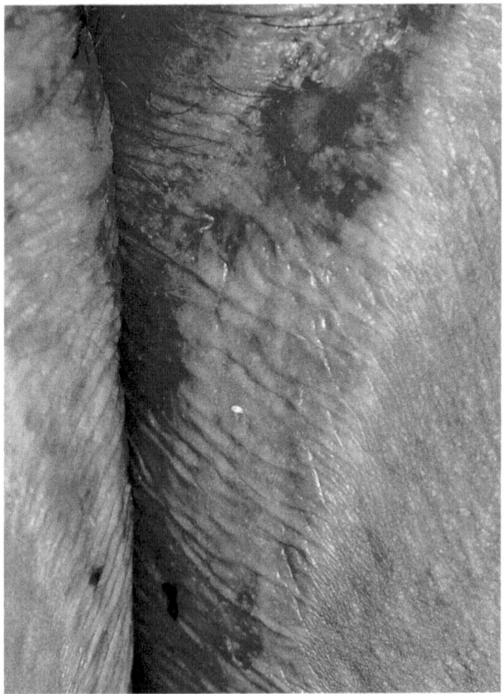

Fig. 3. Rubbing has resulted in erosions in this crinkled, fragile plaque of lichen sclerosus. (*Courtesy of* Libby Edwards, MD, Charlotte, NC.)

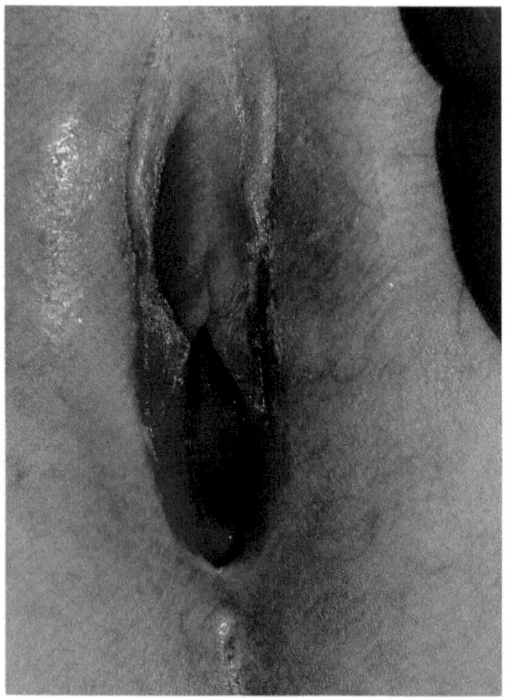

Fig. 4. Lichen sclerosus sometimes exhibits shiny or waxy skin, as in the prepubertal girl. Lichen sclerosus in girls can be difficult to diagnosis; the hypopigmentation is often more subtle, because of the naturally pale background of young genital skin. Also, the purpura and fissures are often mistaken for childhood sexual abuse. (*Courtesy of* Libby Edwards, MD, Charlotte, NC.)

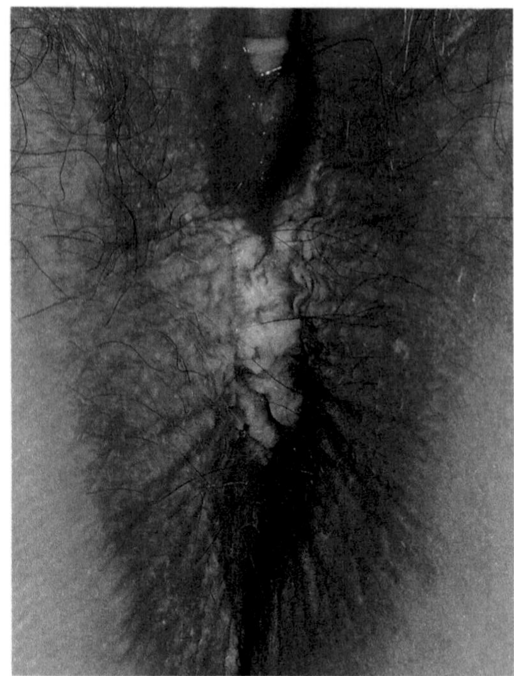

Fig. 5. Rubbing and scratching produce both excoriations and, as on the perineal body of this woman with lichen sclerosus, hyperkeratotic lesions and fissuring. Hyperkeratotic lichen sclerosus in postmenopausal women is the highest risk morphology for squamous cell carcinoma, and persistent lesions should be biopsied. (*Courtesy of* Libby Edwards, MD, Charlotte, NC.)

HISTOLOGY

The pathology for LS is often difficult to interpret, and a final diagnosis must always be made in the context of a true clinicopathologic correlation. There is no overall correlation between the histologic appearance and the length of time the disease has been present.[40] The classic features of uncomplicated LS are a thinned epidermis with hyperkeratosis, a wide band of homogenized collagen beneath the dermo-epidermal junction, and a lymphocytic infiltrate beneath the homogenized area.[41]

In the early stages of LS, not only is the clinical appearance sometimes hard to interpret but so is the histologic picture.[42] The features may be similar to psoriasis or lichen planus with irregular acanthosis, mild hyperkeratosis, hypergranulosis, mild lichenoid lymphocytic infiltrate with lymphocyte tagging and dilated blood vessels immediately under the basement membrane, focal basement membrane thickening, luminal hyperkeratosis of adnexal structures, submucosal edema and homogenization, lichenoid lymphocytic infiltrate, and lymphocyte exocytosis.[42]

The most important management point here is that the diagnosis of LS is usually clinical. A biopsy may be helpful but should not be interpreted in isolation. In early disease, the clinicopathological correlation may be difficult and such individuals may need follow-up and a repeat biopsy if the clinical findings significantly change and diagnostic uncertainty persists. A nonspecific biopsy does not rule out lichen sclerosus, although classic histologic findings confirm the diagnosis.

DISEASE COMPLICATIONS

The true morbidity associated with poorly controlled and undertreated vulvar LS is not known, although without doubt these patients often suffer for many years from genital discomfort and, sometimes, fear that the disorder is sexually transmitted and untreatable.[32] If untreated, lichen sclerosus leads to destruction and scarring of the normal genital architecture. Not infrequently, therefore, affected individuals report loss of sexual function from scarring and sometimes vulval

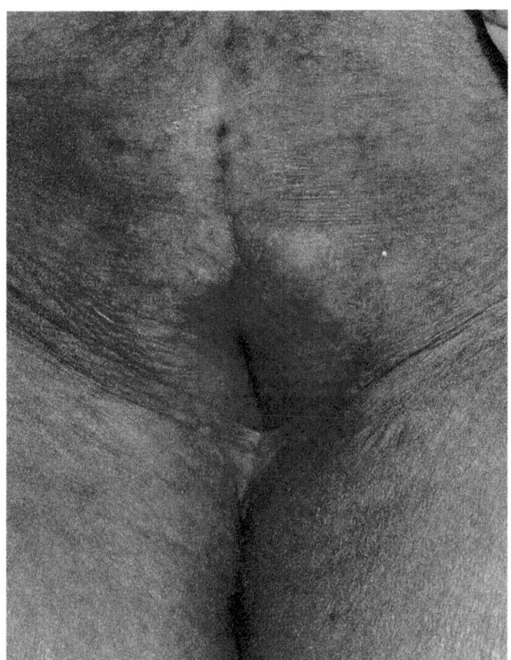

Fig. 6. Lichen sclerosus demonstrating anatomic changes as a result of scarring with adhesions over the clitoris, resorption of the labia minora, and reduction in the size of the introitus. (*Courtesy of* Libby Edwards, MD, Charlotte, NC.)

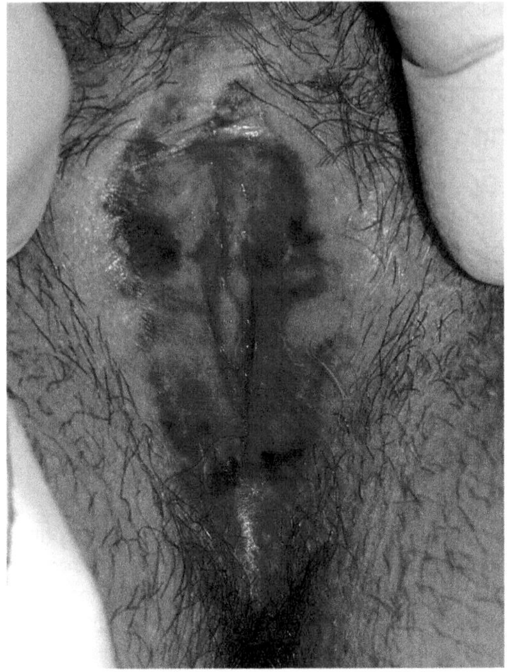

Fig. 7. Patchy hyperpigmentation of the modified mucous membranes can be a confusing occurrence, and often occurs late, when other signs and symptoms are abating. (*Courtesy of* Libby Edwards, MD, Charlotte, NC.)

dysesthesias following burned out LS.[32] This reported vulval discomfort can be misinterpreted by the unwary physician and patients as poorly controlled LS. It is an important distinction because the treatment is similar to that for other vulval pain disorders, and symptoms may even worsen with the continued use of ultrapotent topical steroids. Scarring can result in the development of a clitoral pseudocyst as adhesions form over the clitoral hood completely sealing the area and reducing sensation at this site, which may lead to anorgasmia. Keratin debris may then continue to accumulate below the clitoral hood, which leads to the development of a painful cyst. Surgical correction with circumcision is then necessary.[43]

With ongoing inflammation, lichen sclerosus can result in adhesion and resorption of the labia minora and a reduced introitus, which in sexually active patients, leads to dyspareunia. In the early stages, this may be corrected with the regular use of dilators, but with more established disease, surgical correction may be helpful followed by the use of dilators and ultrapotent topical steroids to prevent readhesion.[43] Because lichen sclerosus demonstrates koebnerization with trigger/recurrence at sites of injury and trauma, surgery, where possible, is best avoided.[42] When LS affects the penis, scarring can result in phimosis, as well as difficulty with micturition. It is not in the scope of an article about vulval disease to go into this in detail.

Perhaps the most controversial complication of LS is the estimated risk of malignancy confirmed in association with the disorder. Squamous cell carcinoma (SCC) is the most common malignancy described in association with anogenital LS (**Fig. 8**).[44] Although verrucous carcinoma, basal cell carcinoma, and malignant melanoma have all been reported on a background of LS.[45–47]

Vulval squamous cell carcinoma has an incidence of 1.5 per 100,000 women in Western communities, about one-eighth that of cervical cancer.[48] When cases of vulval SCC have been reviewed, about 60% appear to arise on a background of LS.[49–51] Two studies have shown that there is a definite risk in individuals with LS developing anogenital SCC.[26,52] Overall, the lifelong risk of developing LS in patients with diagnosed genital LS appears to be 5%.[26,44,45] From a clinical management point of view, it would be helpful to identify which individuals with LS are at particular risk of developing malignancy.

Evidence so far suggests that vulval SCC occurs in 2 patterns, the first is found predominantly in younger women and is multifocal, related to oncogenic human papillomavirus (HPV), and originates from undifferentiated VIN.[51] There is no

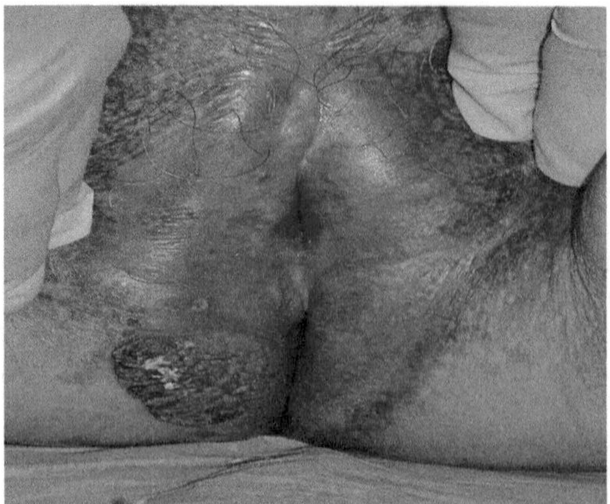

Fig. 8. Typical changes of longstanding lichen sclerosus showing pallor in a figure-of-eight distribution with adhesions over the clitoris, reduction in the size of the introitus, and an area of squamous cell carcinoma arising in differentiated VIN on the right perineum. (*Courtesy of* Ruth Murphy, PhD, MBChB, FRCP, Nottingham, UK.)

association with LS in this group. The second is found in older women, is unifocal, is not related to HPV, and can originate from VIN. In this group, LS is considered a predisposing factor. It is possible that HPV and LS are not mutually exclusive, but may act as cofactors in the pathogenesis of vulval SCC.[52,53]

The typical lesions of SCC are hyperkeratotic or ulcerated plaques, but any persistent vulval lesion should be biopsied. Individuals with persistent hyperkeratotic LS or a past history of SCC of the vulva should be followed up because these individuals appear to be at particular risk of developing well-differentiated VIN and then SCC.[4,52,53]

TREATMENT AND INVESTIGATIONS

As with many inflammatory conditions affecting the genital region, there is a lack of published, randomized, controlled trials for the treatment of lichen sclerosus. To address this, a Cochrane Systematic Review for Therapeutic Interventions for the Treatment of LS is currently ongoing. Treatment evidence so far is thus determined from the author's clinical practice and the British Association of Dermatologists-published guidelines for the diagnosis and management of LS.[4] Evaluation of the trials reported at that stage led to the recommendation that an ultrapotent topical steroid should be the first-line treatment in LS for either sex and for any age.[4] No data existed comparing steroid potency, frequency of application, and duration of steroid treatment.[4]

There are several versions of how these ultrapotent steroids should be used. A common treatment regimen is to prescribe clobetasol propionate ointment (less irritating than cream) for use once daily for 1 month, followed by alternate day usage for 1 month, and thereafter usage once or twice weekly to prevent disease flares. Other regimens exist and some advocate more intense clobetasol propionate treatment initially, followed by a discontinuation of therapy once the disease is under control. In the author's experience, the disease usually flares up again when the topical steroid is discontinued, which may result in delayed treatment and scarring. The author is also aware that not all patients with LS report symptoms.

It is recommended that individuals showing signs of disease activity, such as ecchymosis, hyperkeratosis, fissures, and adhesions, should be treated even if they are reported as asymptomatic.[4] It is not known whether treatment of LS will reduce the malignant potential of LS.

Published data are emerging suggesting that calcineurin inhibitors, such as tacrolimus and pimecrolimus, might be safe and effective first-line treatment options in the management of LS.[54] The Cochrane review will address these reports, but their biggest flaw to date is that the long-term follow-up data is missing with respect to malignancy, of particular importance for an at-risk patient group treated with immunosuppressive therapies.

TREATMENT FAILURE

LS is generally a steroid-responsive condition, which makes it satisfying to treat. Disease failures occur but are rare and may be caused by several factors. The most important point to establish is whether the diagnosis is correct, and if in doubt, a biopsy is essential. If the diagnosis is certain, then it is important to establish exactly what is meant by treatment failure.

If patients' symptoms of vulval itch and soreness persist and the physician observes hemorrhage, hyperkeratosis, and fissures, then the disease is poorly controlled. Usually this is caused by lack of compliance from fear of applying ultrapotent topical steroids to the anogenital region.[4] This fear is largely caused by instructions found on the package insert recommending that ultrapotent topical steroids should not be applied to the anogenital region. It is, therefore, well worth spending time at the point of diagnosis discussing these issues. Sometimes elderly or infirm individuals are not physically able to apply the topical steroids to the affected region and the involvement of a visiting nurse or caregiver to assist with application, if possible, can be helpful.

Treatment failure in children commonly occurs and may be associated with night pain. In the individuals that the author has treated, this is nearly always caused by under treatment of the LS because of parental anxiety or behavioral problems in the affected child. Consultations in this age group take longer and a greater level of reassurance is needed.

If patients with LS are describing pain and altered sensation, and the physical examination shows an improvement in the physical signs and evidence of controlled LS, then it is possible that the symptoms are caused by vulval dysesthesia, a secondary vulval pain syndrome, which needs reassurance; appropriate treatment, such as amityptiline or gabapentin; and not an increased use of topical steroids.

Sometimes individuals with vulval LS develop a secondary problem, such as allergic contact dermatitis or a bacterial and yeast infection. These problems can be investigated further by patch tests or culture and sensitivity. Risk factors for the development of allergic contact dermatitis are individuals with a history of reacting to creams or cosmetics elsewhere on the skin. Secondary bacterial or Candida infection often complicates the labial and vulval fissures in patients with LS and should be considered in unresponsive patients.

FOLLOW-UP AND PROGNOSIS

Patients should be followed up according to need. Initially a follow-up is helpful to ensure that there is adequate disease response and appropriate compliance with therapy. This initial follow-up is suggested at 3 months following the initiation of high-potency topical steroids, with a second follow-up at 6 months to check that the disease remains well controlled. If the disease is uncomplicated and well controlled, then patients can be discharged with an annual review in primary care.[4] If a primary care annual review is not possible, patients may be reviewed annually by a specialist. In reality, the risk of malignancy in this group is likely to be low and patients should be alerted to the development of VIN or an SCC by an area of skin thickening or persistent rawness that is resistant to therapy.

Patients who are poorly controlled, and those with ongoing hyperkeratosis, should be continuously followed up. A biopsy of the thickened skin in this group will usually show squamous hyperplasia, which can be difficult to differentiate from well-differentiated VIN. This group is at particular risk of developing SCC and needs careful observation. Individuals with LS who develop SCC affecting the vulva require lifelong follow-up.[4]

The prognosis in children with lichen sclerosus remains unclear. Earlier reports in children with LS reported complete resolution of the condition at puberty in a large proportion of the study population.[55] These findings have been refuted by another study in which, despite resolution of symptoms, some clinical signs remained, leading to the argument that LS persists into adulthood in most cases.[56] This finding is supported by the case of a young adult woman with documented LS resolving at puberty, who presented and died of vulvar squamous cell carcinoma.[57]

This case implies that, ideally, appropriate long-term follow-up is required in cases of childhood lichen sclerosus. As with adults, children require follow-up initially until disease control is established, and then until they are responsible enough to understand their condition and are aware of the possible complications and malignancy. Annual follow-up by a specialist until 18 years of age and then, in uncomplicated cases, annually in either primary or secondary care is suggested.

SUMMARY

Lichen sclerosus is a common chronic inflammatory dermatoses that commonly occurs in postmenopausal women, but can occur in men and prepubertal girls and boys. The disorder is usually highly responsive to ultrapotent topical steroids, but if untreated can lead to disease complications, such as scarring and loss of sexual function. In some individuals the disease can be particularly difficult to control, especially those with persistent lichenification and hyperplasia on histology. This sub-group have an increased risk of malignant transformation and need life-long follow up care. In unresponsive patients, the diagnosis of LS should always be reconsidered, with a repeat biopsy if necessary. A Cochrane systematic review will demonstrate the evidence for preexisting therapies and clearly establish areas where future clinical trials are needed.

REFERENCES

1. Hallopeau H. Lecons Clinique sur les maladies cutanees et syphilitique. L'Union Medicale 1887;43: 742–7 [in French].
2. Hallopeau H. Lichen plan sclereux. Ann Dermatol Syph 1889;10:447–9 [in French].
3. Darier J. Lichen plan sclereux. Ann Dermatol Syph 1892;3:833–7 [in French].

4. Neill SM, Tatnall FM, Cox NH. Guidelines for the management of Lichen sclerosus. Br J Dermatol 2002;147(4):640–9.
5. Clarke J, Etherington IJ, Luesley D. Response of vulvar lichen sclerosus and squamous cell hyperplasia to graduated topical steroids. J Reprod Med 1999;44:958–62.
6. Harrington CI, Dunsmore JR. An Investigation into the incidence of auto-immune disorders in patients with lichen sclerosus and atrophicus. Br J Dermatol 1981;109:661–4.
7. Meyrick Thomas RH, Ridley CM, Black MM. The association of lichen sclerosus et atrophicus and autoimmune-related disease in males. Br J Dermatol 1983;109:661–4.
8. Meyrick Thomas RH, Ridley CM, Black MM. Lichen Sclerosus et atrophicus associated with systemic lupus erythematosus. J Am Acad Dermatol 1985; 13:832–3.
9. Meyrick Thomas RH, Ridley CM, McGibbon DH, et al. Lichen Sclerosus et atrophicus and autoimmunity-a study of 350 women. Br J Dermatol 1988;118:41–6.
10. Cooper SM, Ali A, Baldo M, et al. The association of LS and erosive LP of the vulva with autoimmune disease. Arch Dermatol 2008;144:1432–5.
11. Meyrick Thomas RH, Ridley CM, McGibbon DH, et al. The development of lichen sclerosus et atrophicus in monozygotic twin girls. Br J Dermatol 1986;114:377–9.
12. Azurdia RM, Luzzi GA, Byren I, et al. Lichen sclerosus in adult men: a study of HLA associations and susceptibility to autoimmune disease. Br J Dermatol 1999;140:79–83.
13. Marren P, Yell J, Charnock FM, et al. The association between lichen sclerosus and antigens of the HLA system. Br J Dermatol 1995;132:197–203.
14. Lukowsky A, Muche JM, Sterry W, et al. Detection of expanded T cell clones in skin biopsy samples of patients with lichen sclerosus et atrophicus by T cell receptor-gamma polymerase chain reaction assays. J Invest Dermatol 2000;115:254–9.
15. Regauer S, Reich O, Beham-Schmid C. Monoclonal gamma T-cell receptor rearrangement in vulval lichen sclerosus and squamous cell carcinomas. Am J Pathol 2002;160:1035–45.
16. Regauer S. Immune dysregulation in lichen sclerosus. Eur J Cell Biol 2005;84:273–7.
17. Regauer S, Beham-Schmid C. Detailed analysis of the T-cell lymphocytic infiltrate in penile lichen sclerosus: an immunohistochemical and molecular investigation. Histopathology 2006;48:730–5.
18. Oyama N, Chan I, Neill SM, et al. Autoantibodies to extracellular matrix protein 1 in lichen sclerosus. Lancet 2003;362:118–23.
19. Howard A, Dean D, Cooper S, et al. Circulating basement membrane zone antibodies are found in lichen sclerosus of the vulva. Australas J Dermatol 2004;45(1):12–5.
20. Sander CS, Ali I, Dean D, et al. Oxidative stress implicated in the pathogenesis of lichen sclerosus. Br J Dermatol 2004;151:627–35.
21. De Vito JR, Merogi AJ, Vo T, et al. Role of Borrelia burgdorferi in the pathogenesis of morphoea/scleroderma and lichen sclerosus et atrophicus: a PCR study of thirty five cases. Br J Dermatol 2000;142:481–4.
22. Fujiwara H, Fujiwara K, Hashimoto K, et al. Detection of *Borrelia burgdorferi* DNA in (B.garinii or B afzelii) in morphoea and lichen sclerosus et atrophicus tissue of German and Japanese but not US patients. Arch Dermatol 1997;133:41–4.
23. Farrell AM, Dean D, Charnock FM, et al. Alterations in distribution of tenascin, fibronectin and fibrinogen in vulval lichen sclerosus. Dermatology 2000;201: 223–9.
24. Farrell AM, Dean D, Charnock FM, et al. Alterations in fibrillin as well as collagens I and III and elastin occur in vulval lichen sclerosus. J Eur Acad Dermatol Venereol 2001;15:212–7.
25. Ohlenbusch A, Matuschka FR, Richter D, et al. Etiology of the acrodermatitis chronica atrophicans lesion in Lyme Disease. J Infect Dis 1996;174(2):421–3.
26. Wallace HJ. Lichen Sclerosus et atrophicus. Trans St Johns Hosp Dermatol Soc 1971;57:9–30.
27. Hodgins MB, Spike RC, Mackie RM, et al. An immunohistochemical evaluation of androgen, oestrogen and progesterone receptors in the vulva and vagina. Br J Obstet Gynaecol 1998;105:216–22.
28. Clifton MM, Garner IB, Kohler S, et al. Immunohistochemical evaluation of androgen receptors in genital and extragenital lichen sclerosus: evidence for loss of androgen receptors in lesional epidermis: evidence for loss of androgen receptors in lesional epidermis. J Am Acad Dermatol 1999;41:43–6.
29. Günthert AR, Faber M, Knappe G. Early onset vulvar LS in premenopausal women and oral contraceptives. Eur J Obstet Gynecol Reprod Biol 2008;137: 56–60.
30. Powell JJ, Wojanorowska F. Lichen sclerosus. Lancet 1999;353:1777–83.
31. Lipscombe TK, Wayte J, Wojnarowska F, et al. A study of clinical and aetiological factors and possible associations of lichen sclerosus in males. Aust J Dermatol 1997;38:132–6.
32. Dalziel K. Effect of lichen sclerosus on sexual function and parturition. J Reprod Med 1995;40:351–4.
33. Marin MG, King R, Dinnerstein GI, et al. Dyspareunia and vulval disease. J Reprod Med 1998;43:952–8.
34. Powell J, Wojnarowska F. Childhood vulvar lichen sclerosus: an increasingly common problem. J Am Acad Dermatol 2001;44(5):803–6.
35. Maronn ML, Esterly NB. Constipation as a feature of anogenital lichen sclerosus in children. Pediatrics 2005;115(2):230–2.

36. Handfield Jones SE, Hinde FR, Kennedy CTC. Lichen sclerosus et atrophicus in children misdiagnosed as sexual abuse. Br Med J 1987;294:1404–5.
37. Warrington S, San Lazaro C. Lichen sclerosus and sexual abuse. Arch Dis Child 1996;75:512–6.
38. Simpkin S, Oakley A. Clinical review of 202 patients with lichen sclerosus: a possible association with psoriasis. Australas J Dermatol 2007;48:28–31.
39. Eberz B, Berghold A, Regauer S, et al. High prevalence of concomitant anogenital LS and extragenital psoriasis in adult women. Obstet Gynecol 2008;111: 1143–7.
40. Marren P, Millard PR, Wojnarowska F. Vulval Lichen Sclerosus: lack of correlation between duration of clinical symptoms and histological appearances. J Eur Acad Dermatol Venereol 1997;8:212–6.
41. Hewitt J. Histologic criteria for lichen sclerosus of the vulva. J Reprod Med 1986;31:781–7.
42. Regauer S, Liegl B, Reich O. Early vulvar lichen sclerosus: a histopathological challenge. Histopathology 2005;47:340–7.
43. Paniel B. Surgical procedures in benign vulval disease. In: Ridley CM, Neill SM, editors. The vulva. Oxford (UK): Blackwell Science; 1999. p. 288–90.
44. Derrick EK, Ridley CM, Kobza-Black A, et al. A clinical study of 23 cases of female anogenital carcinoma. Br J Dermatol 2000;143:1217–23.
45. Brisgotti M, Moreno A, Murcia, et al. Verrucous carcinoma of the vulva. A clinicopathologic and immunohistochemical study of 5 cases. Int J Gynecol Pathol 1989;8:1–7.
46. Meyrick-Thomas RH, Mc Gibbon DH, Munro DD. Basal cell carcinoma of the vulva in association with vulval lichen sclerosus et atrophicus. J R Soc Med 1985;78:16–8.
47. Friedman RJ, Kopf AW, Jones WB. Malignant melanoma in association with lichen sclerosus on the vulva of a 14 year old. Am J Dermatopathol 1984; 6:253–6.
48. Giles CG, Kneale BL. Vulvar cancer. The Cinderella of gynaecological oncology. Aust N Z J Obstet Gynaecol 1995;35:71–5.
49. Hart WR, Norris HJ, Helwig EB. Relation of lichen sclerosus et atrophicus of the vulva to development of carcinoma. Obstet Gynecol 1975;45:369–77.
50. Leibowitch M, Neill S, Pelisse M, et al. The epithelial changes associated with squamous cell carcinoma of the vulva. A review of the clinical, histologic and viral findings in 78 women. Br J Obstet Gynaecol 1990;97:1135–9.
51. Crum CP, Mc Lachlin CM, Tate JE, et al. Pathobiology of vulvar squamous neoplasia. Curr Opin Obstet Gynaecol 1997;9:63–9.
52. Carli P, Cattaneo A, De Magnis A, et al. Squamous cell carcinoma arising in lichen sclerosus: a longitudinal cohort study. Eur J Cancer Prev 1995;4: 491–5.
53. Haefner HK, Tate JE, McLachelin CM, et al. Vulvar intraepithelial neoplasia:age, morphological phenotype, papillomavirus DNA, and co-existing invasive carcinoma. Hum Pathol 1995;26:147–54.
54. Hengge W, Krause W, Hoffman H, et al. Multicentre, phase II trial on the safety and efficacy of topical Tacrolimus ointment for the treatment of lichen sclerosus. Br J Dermatol 2006;155:1021–8.
55. Helm KF, Gibson LE, Muller SA. Lichen sclerosus et atrophicus in children and young adults. Pediatr Dermatol 1991;8(2):97–101.
56. Powell J, Wojnarowska F, Winsey S, et al. Lichen sclerosus premenarche: autoimmunity and immunogenetics. Br J Dermatol 2000;142:481–4.
57. Powell J, Wojnarowska F. Childhood vulvar lichen sclerosus. The course after puberty. J Reprod Med 2002;47(9):706–9.

Treatment of Vulvovaginal Lichen Planus

Ginat W. Mirowski, DMD, MD[a,*], Allison Goddard, MD[b]

KEYWORDS

• Vulva lichen planus • Erosive disease • Scarring • Therapy

Vulvovaginal lichen planus (VVLP) is a common, complex, and frequently misdiagnosed condition characterized by pain, burning, and rawness or itching of the genitalia associated with dysuria, dyspareunia, and postcoital bleeding.[1–3] The cause of lichen planus (LP) is unknown. Evidence suggests that LP is a T cell–mediated disease, an autoimmune response to altered self-antigens.[4] On keratinzed skin, LP is characterized bya papulosquamous eruption, with pruritic, violaceous, polygonal papules and plaques associated with fine white striae. Occasionally, hypertrophic papules may be seen. When occurring on anogenital skin, scaling is rarely found because of the moist nature of the area. Thus, vulvar findings range from mild macular erythema to erythematous papules and plaques, with fine, white, lacy Wickham striae in intact epithelium, to erosions and ulcers, for which the term erosive LP is used. In VVLP, scarring occurs with both vulvar and vaginal involvement. Scarring occurs with genital, esophageal, laryngeal, and ocular involvement.[5–8] Furthermore, chronic VVLP may contribute to sexual dysfunction and psychological disability. In addition to the genitalia, other mucocutaneous sites of involvement include the buccal mucosa, tongue, gingiva, perianal area, scalp, nails, wrists, and lower legs.

DIAGNOSIS AND EVALUATION

Dermatologists diagnose skin conditions based on the morphology of the primary lesion. However, the moist environment of the genitalia and the activities of daily living (walking, wearing clothes, bathing, and engaging in sexual activity) may alter the morphology of the primary lesions on the mucosal skin (ie, lack of scales). No diagnostic laboratory studies are available because like the morphologic appearance, a biopsy is often only characteristic and not diagnostic.

Once the diagnosis is made, potential causative and exacerbating factors should be evaluated by history. A directed physical examination, medication history, and a review of systems are necessary to determine the extent of involvement. Thus, a multidisciplinary approach helps to establish the diagnosis, direct the treatment, and maximize the treatment success. Further evaluations by gynecologists, dentists, ophthalmologists, gastroenterologists, and urologists permit complete assessment of the involvement in patients with symptoms involving other organ systems. Supportive care by a psychologist, sexual therapist, and physical therapist as well as a marriage counselor is often helpful as well in some patients. Although there is no cure for LP, disease activity often can be controlled and a significant measure of pain relief achieved in nearly all patients. Ideally, patients should be able to resume the normal activities of daily living, including pleasurable sexual activity, if so desired.

CLINICAL LP

LP is a disorder that affects the skin and mucous membranes. The cause of LP is unknown. Cellular immune mechanisms seem to be primarily

[a] Department of Oral Surgery Medicine Pathology, Indiana University School of Dentistry, Indianapolis, IN, USA
[b] Division of Dermatology, Loyola University School of Medicine, 2160 South First Avenue, Maywood, IL 60526, USA
* Corresponding author. 10440 High Grove, Carmel, IN 46032.
E-mail address: gmirowsk@iupui.edu

Dermatol Clin 28 (2010) 717–725
doi:10.1016/j.det.2010.08.003
0733-8635/10/$ – see front matter

involved. Activated T cells are present in early lesions and seem to target antigenically altered basal cells. In older lesions, suppressor T cells have been shown to predominate.[4]

The onset of cutaneous lesions may occur abruptly, and pruritus is typically severe. Excoriations are rare and when present, other causes of pruritus should be sought. When occurring on extragenital skin, the primary skin lesion is a flat-topped, purple, polygonal papule with superficial, reticulated, white lines (Wickham striae). As a result, cutaneous LP is classified as a papulosquamous eruption.

Mucosal involvement may be asymptomatic, and thus patients may not seek medical treatment. However, painful erosions, erosive vaginitis, or desquamation of the gingivae are reasons for seeking care. Thus, LP with mucosal involvement (vulvar or oral) is characterized most often as an erosive rather than a papulosquamous disease.

VVLP may present in several forms, and patients may exhibit more than one form of LP concurrently or sequentially. In the largest published study on women with erosive LP (n=114), Cooper and Wojnarowska[9] reported that pain (80%), pruritus (65%), dyspareunia (61%), and irritation (48%) were the most frequent presenting symptoms. In a survey of current practices by 4 vulvar disease experts, published in 2008, on 145 patients, symptoms of soreness were reported in 72% followed by burning (66%) and pruritus (63%), and the most frequent vulvar signs were erosions (74%), red and/or purple coloration (66%), scarring (60%), and apareunia (35%).[10]

Typical papulosquamous LP of the glabrous skin is infrequently seen on the vulva (**Fig. 1**). Patients more commonly present with erythema and erosions, but peripheral reticulations may also be noted. Atrophic or erosive LP of the mucous membranes presents with erythema, tender denuded epithelium, and desquamative vulvitis or vaginitis (**Figs. 2–4**). A similar clinical presentation is noted on the gingivae (**Figs. 5** and **6**). Cooper and Wojnarowska[9] reported that most patients presented with erosions (90%) and/or white reticulations (82%). Isolated Wickham striae may be found on the labia minora and the medial aspect of the labia majora and may be asymptomatic (**Figs. 7–9**). Hypertrophic LP occurs in 20% to 25% of patients and presents with extensive, white, thickened, and hyperkeratotic plaques of the mucous membranes (**Fig. 10**).

Chronic inflammatory or erosive vulvar disease is characterized by scarring and adhesions that destroy the labia minora, the vulvar trigone, and the vaginal canal (**Figs. 11–13**). Scarring is characterized by the loss of normal architecture caused by the resorption of labia minora (agglutination) and clitoral hood, resulting in clitoral burying (68%) and narrowing of the introitus (59%). Scarring and adhesions of the vagina make sexual intercourse impossible.[1,2,9,10] A purulent discharge may be seen in 25% of patients because of the involvement of the vagina.[1,2,10]

A subset of patients with VVLP present with chronic erosive lesions of the vulva, vagina, and gingivae. This constellation of findings forms the vulvovaginal gingival or vulvovaginal penile syndromes.[11–13]

Vulvar squamous cell carcinoma is occasionally reported in women with VVLP, but the incidence of this rare condition is not known. However, one survey reports 10 of 145 patients had genital malignant neoplasm or a history of the same.[10]

In summary, the alterations or secondary changes of VVLP include atrophy, erythema, ulceration, erosion, maceration, and scarring. Thus, it is beneficial to perform a complete mucocutaneous

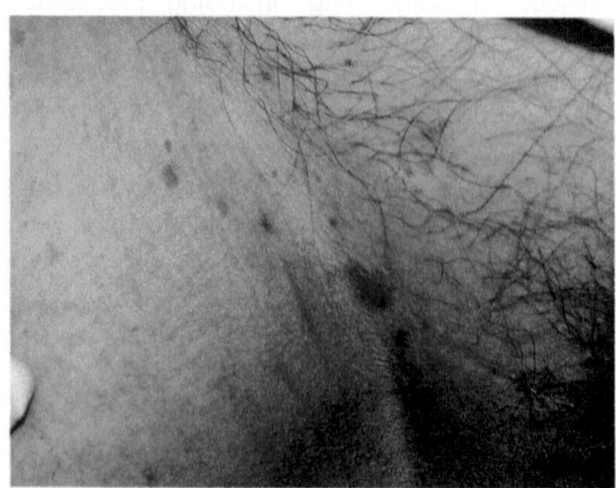

Fig. 1. LP on hair-bearing keratinized skin classically shows red or dusky, flat-topped, shiny papules.

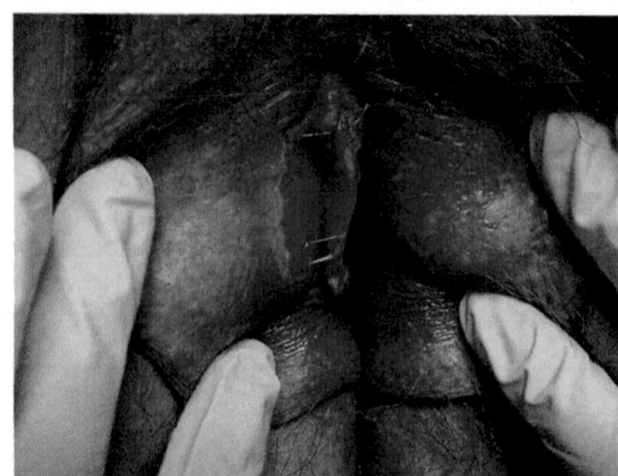

Fig. 2. Atrophic LP involving the lateral aspect of the labia minora and medial aspect of the labia majora. The rim of white epithelium is classic and useful diagnostically, when present.

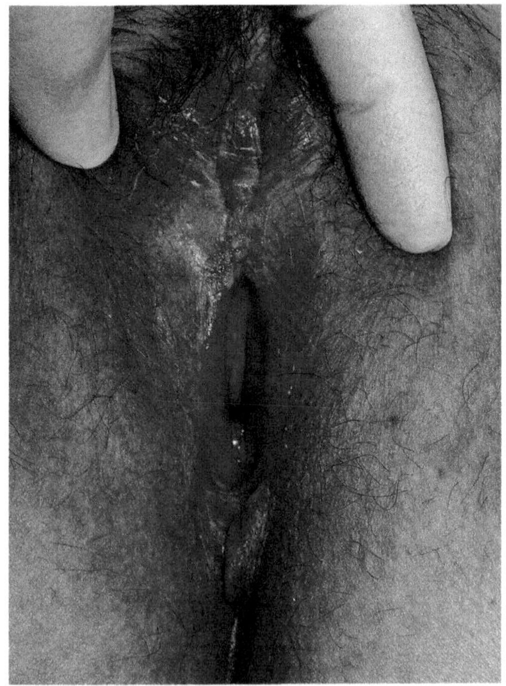

Fig. 3. Nonspecific vestibular erosions with resorption of vulvar architecture is the most common manifestation of erosive VVLP. In this patient, the white surrounding epithelium is the site most likely to yield a diagnostic biopsy.

evaluation including the scalp, glabrous and acral skin, nails, as well as the oral cavity, esophagus, larynx, and conjunctiva in order to identify other sites of involvement and potential primary lesions.

CLINICAL DIFFERENTIAL DIAGNOSIS

The differential diagnosis of anogenital LP includes papulosquamous, eczematous, atrophic, and

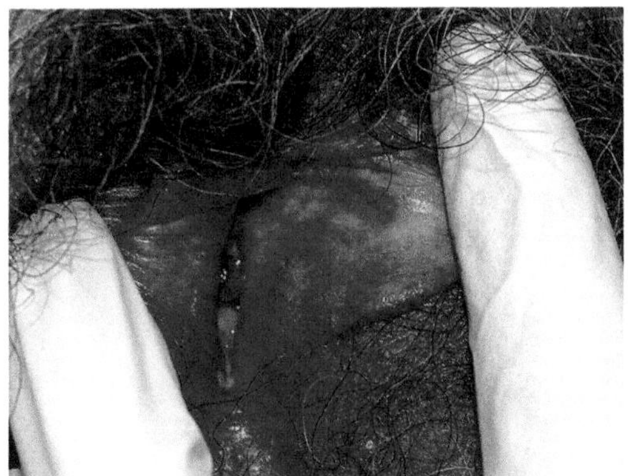

Fig. 4. Bland superficial erosions typical of erosive LP, but these erosions give no morphologic hints as to the diagnosis. Only the statistical likelihood of chronic vulvovaginal erosions representing LP suggests this diagnosis.

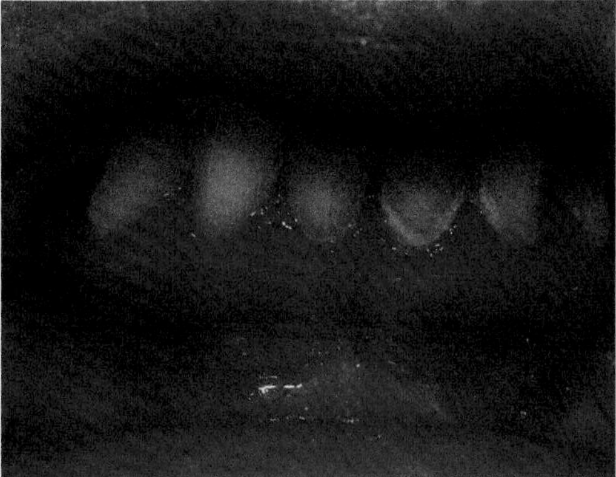

Fig. 5. Redness and bogginess of atrophic gingival LP that commonly accompanies erosive VVLP.

vesiculobullous disorders, depending on the morphologic variant of the LP present and area affected. The differential diagnosis of LP occurring on glabrous skin mimics other papulosquamous disorders, including seborrheic dermatitis, psoriasis, eczema, irritant or allergic contact, pityriasis rosea, chronic cutaneous lupus erythematosus, secondary syphilis, fungal infections and infestations, and squamous cell carcinoma. When the mucous membranes or intertriginous areas are affected, scales may be difficult or impossible to appreciate in all of these disorders.

Vesiculobullous diseases occurring on mucous membrane generally present as erosions. In addition to LP, erosive mucous membrane diseases include

- Lichen sclerosus
- Cicatricial pemphigoid
- Pemphigus vulgaris
- Lichenoid drug reaction
- Mucositis secondary to chemotherapy
- Acute graft-versus-host disease

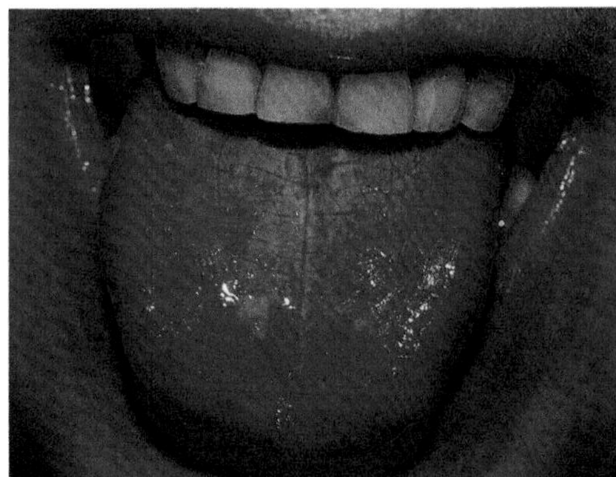

Fig. 6. VVLP is sometimes accompanied by LP of the tongue, which can be erosive or, sometimes, hypertrophic with white epithelium and loss of papillae.

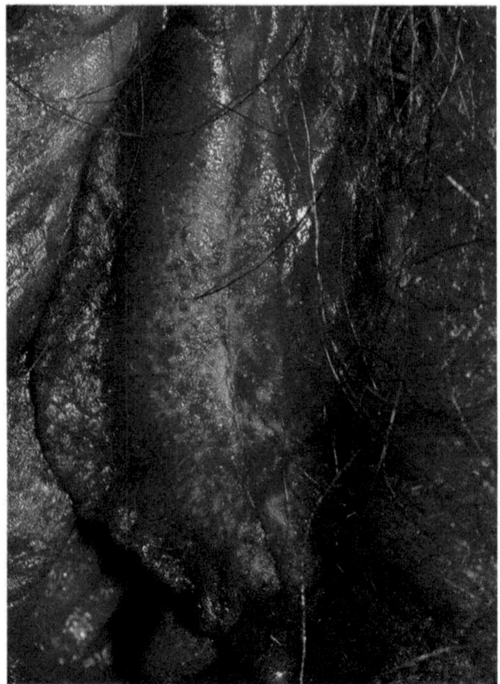

Fig. 7. The most classic and only pathognomonic findings of vulvar LP are the white, reticulate, lacy papules. Even these papules are most often accompanied by vulvar or vaginal erosions.

Infections caused by herpes or erythematous candidiasis
Acute contact dermatitis
Vulvar intraepithelial neoplasia (squamous cell carcinoma in situ)
Plasma cell mucositis (Zoon vulvitis)

The loss of normal architecture characterized by resorption of the labia minora and obliteration of the clitoris under an agglutinated clitoral hood is seen in a variety of chronic inflammatory diseases

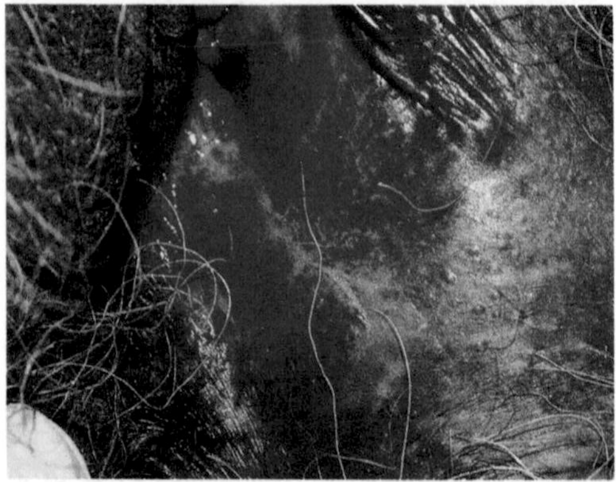

Fig. 8. Linear branching striae of LP are surrounded by bland erosions.

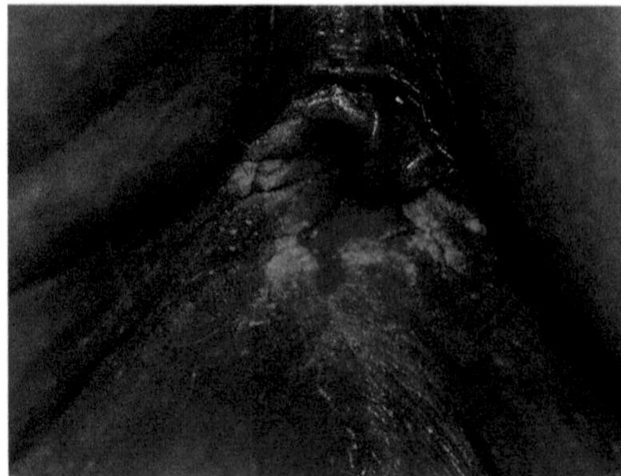

Fig. 9. Perianal and rectal LP often accompany VVLP but often are missed on examination. Nonspecific erosions and surrounding white epithelium are common in this area.

(**Fig. 14**). However, vaginal involvement is typical of LP, cicatricial pemphigoid, and pemphigus vulgaris but not of the more prevalent lichen sclerosus.

The clinical differential diagnosis of hypertrophic LP includes vulvar intraepithelial neoplasia (Bowen disease, bowenoid papulosis), squamous cell carcinoma, and condyloma acuminatum.

LABORATORY FINDINGS

The diagnosis of LP may be suspected clinically but, unless classic with white striae, should be confirmed when possible. Cytologic examination of vaginal secretions (a wet-mount examination) is characteristic but not specific (**Fig. 15**). A biopsy is sometimes diagnostic, but even when a firm diagnosis cannot be made, the histologic appearance can rule out other diseases and show characteristic findings of LP. (SEROLOGICALLY – change with page proofs) (**Table 1**).

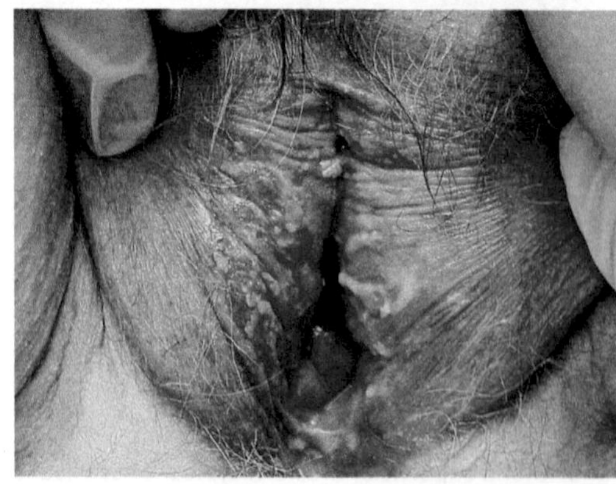

Fig. 10. Hyperkeratotic VVLP. Severe scarring that has occurred can be noted. There is complete agglutination of the labia minora and burying of the clitoris in a patient with both erosive and hypertrophic VVLP.

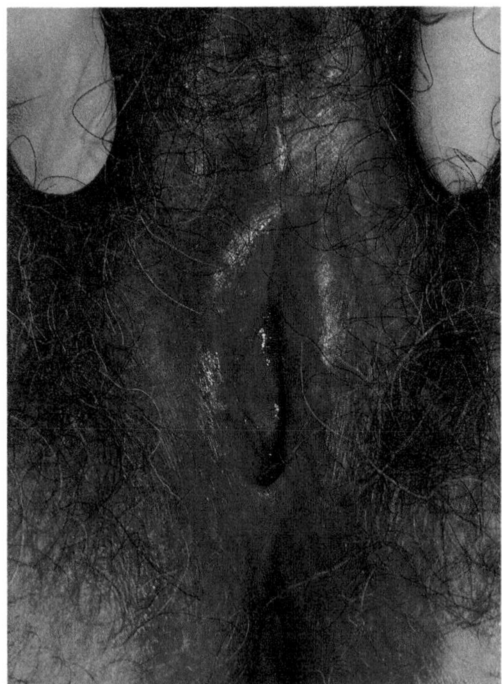

Fig. 11. Scarring with resorption of all vulvar landmarks occurs with some regularity in women with VVLP. The appearance is completely nonspecific and occurs with several inflammatory dermatoses, including lichen sclerosus, cicatricial pemphigoid, pemphigus vulgaris, and, occasionally, no underlying cause is found.

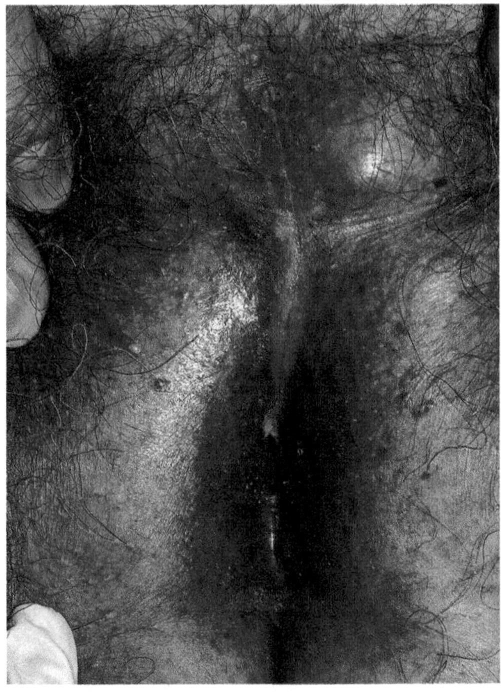

Fig. 12. Severe introital and vaginals scarring prevents sexual activity, cervical cytologic analysis, and severe stenosis can produce urinary obstruction.

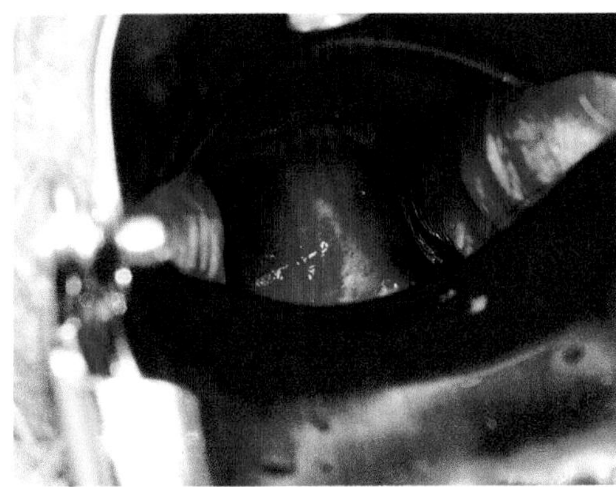

Fig. 13. Vaginal LP is generally manifested by such erosions.

In VVLP, swabs from vaginal secretions reveal sheets of lymphocytes or polymorphonuclear leukocytes, decrease in numbers of normal, large, flat, cuboidal, mature, desquamated keratinocytes, and an increase in small, round, parabasal (immature squamous) cells. These findings are shared with patients who have desquamative inflammatory vaginitis, atrophic vaginitis, and any other erosive or inflammatory vaginal disease that affects the vagina.

The biopsy, in papulosquamous LP, reveals a characteristic inflammatory reaction pattern.

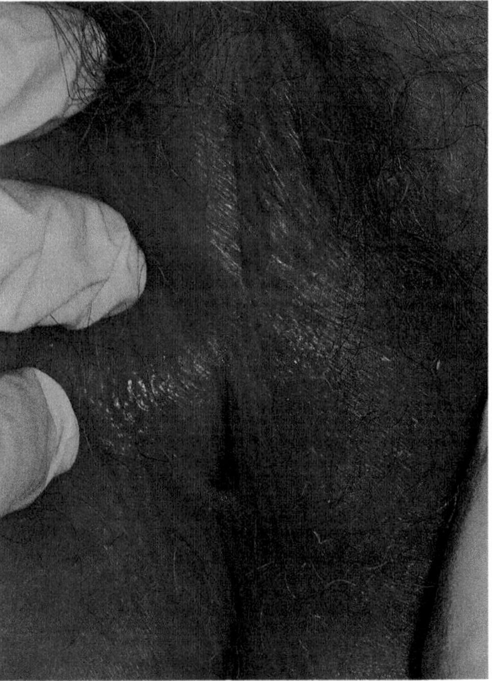

Fig. 14. Hypopigmentation and scarring of vulva is suggestive of LP; however, the lack of crinkling and typical texture change prompted a biopsy, which showed histologic findings diagnostic of LP.

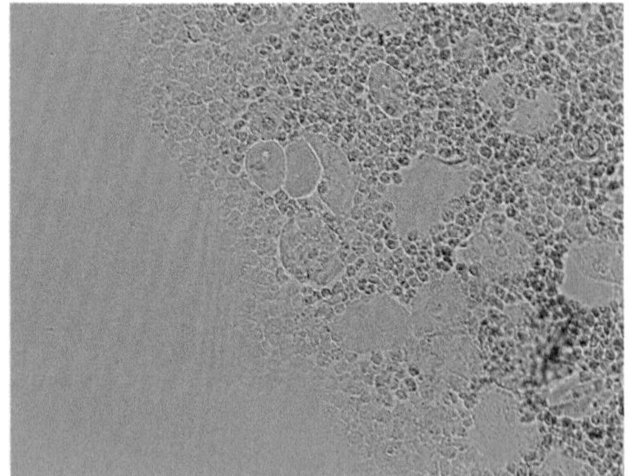

Fig. 15. A wet mount of vaginal secretions from a patient with erosive vaginal LP typically shows a marked increase in white blood cells, immature epithelial cells (parabasal cells) shed from erosions, and absent lactobacilli. These findings are also typical of atrophic vaginitis, another cause of inflammatory vaginitis seen in the postmenopausal population that is most at risk for erosive VVLP.

The epidermis is hyperkeratotic with hypergranulosis, acanthosis, sawtooth rete ridges, and dyskeratosis.[14] In both cutaneous and mucosal LP, an intense bandlike inflammatory infiltrate is seen in the dermis or submucosa. The basal cell layer shows liquefactive degeneration and loss of the basement membrane. Civatte bodies (colloid bodies, cytoid bodies, or eosinophilic hyaline spheres) are necrotic or dyskeratotic keratinocytes seen in either the lower epithelium or the submucosa. Despite these findings, the histologic findings of the more-common erosive lesions are often not specific. A mixed lymphohistiocytic infiltrate can be seen in lichen sclerosus, allergic reactions, graft-versus-host disease, cicatricial pemphigoid, or lupus erythematosus. In LP, direct immunofluorescence (IF) reveals shaggy deposition of IgG, IgM, IgA, C3, and fibrin at the basement membrane. Civatte bodies are stained in the presence of IgG, IgM, IgA, or C3. Thus, IF findings may be helpful.[14]

TREATMENT OF VVLP

In general, erosive mucosal disease is more painful and more difficult to control than extragenital cutaneous disease. Thus, therapeutic management in VVLP is challenging. Other than systemic corticosteroids, no single therapeutic regimen has been shown to be effective in all or even most patients. Review of the literature regarding the therapeutic strategy for vulvar LP is mostly limited to anecdotal observations or small series, and large randomized controlled trials do not exist. The authors discuss the various therapeutic options available and their potential side effects and pitfalls.

Once a definitive diagnosis of LP is made, the first line treatment is topical application of corticosteroids.[1,10,15,16] The addition of symptomatic relief measures can accelerate the response to treatment (see later discussion). For nonerosive disease on glabrous skin, a cream-based,

Table 1
Vulvovaginal lichen planus

Aggravating Factors	Symptomatic Treatment	Workup

Soaps, washes, and cleansers
Medications (topical)
  Antifungals, steroids, hormones
Feminine hygiene products
  Tampons/pads, vaginal douches, hygiene sprays, suppositories, lubricants
Contraception
  Condoms
  Vaginal sponge
  Spermicides
Toilet paper
Long-term moisture
  Normal vaginal secretions
  Semen
  Urinary incontinence
  Fecal incontinence
  Sweat
	Identify aggravating factors
	  History
	  Biopsy
	  Patch tests (delayed hypersensitivity reaction)
	Stop itch-scratch cycle
	  Hydroxyzine/doxepin
	Wash with water only
	Sitz baths, cool compresses, ice packs
	Pat dry (do not rub)
	Use only cotton underwear
	Avoid stockings, tight-fitting pants, and jeans
		Determine fasting blood glucose, serum iron, folate, vitamins B_6 and B_{12}, and magnesium levels, and rapid plasma reagin test
		Perform a direct cytologic examination (potassium hydroxide, cell smear)
		Obtain tissue for both histologic evaluation and immunofluorescence
		Culture for fungi such as *Candida albicans*, *C torulopsis* (*C glabrata*) and others and bacteria such as *Chlamydia* and group A streptococcus. Consider viral studies (herpes simplex virus or human papilloma virus)

mid- to low-potency, nonfluorinated corticosteroid is used. The cream vehicle minimizes maceration in the inguinal area. However, erosions or pustular disease is best treated with an ointment because the alcohol base in creams causes a burning sensation. Mucosal disease of the vulva is best treated with ointment formulations.[1,9,10] Ointments not only provide increased potency and increased absorption but also act as emollients. It is important to note that genital skin is thin and incidental occlusion increases the potency and side effect profile (atrophy and maceration) of all topical steroids. Oral disease is more responsive to gels or elixirs. As the symptoms decrease with treatment, tapering to the least-potent corticosteroid that is effective is advised. Throughout the treatment course the patient must be observed closely. Candida superinfection, dermatophyte infections, and herpes reactivation may occur secondarily to the use of steroids. An important cautionary point is that as with high-potency and even low-potency corticosteroids, atrophy, striae, and telangiectasias of noninvolved adjacent skin and mucosa can and do occur. Thus, frequent follow up of the patient is necessary.

Ultrapotent topical corticosteroids remain the mainstay first line therapy in the initial approach to the patient presenting with erosive VVLP.[1,2,10] It is common to start with twice daily application, tapering to daily or even every other day application as the symptoms improve. When prescribing topical steroids, the potency, the various vehicles available, and the affected areas to be treated are important issues to consider. Ultrahigh-potency corticosteroid ointment, such as clobetasol propionate 0.05%, can improve or resolve the symptoms of VVLP in more than 90% of patients, although scarring is irreversible.[1,2,10]

Hydrocortisone suppositories are an additional option for the treatment of vaginal LP.[17,18] A 25-mg intravaginal suppository inserted twice daily is effective but must be compounded by the pharmacy. A 25-mg rectal suppository (Anucort-HC, Anusol-HC, Cort-Dome) is available; patients must be instructed to insert this rectal suppository intravaginally. In one study, 60 women were treated with 25-mg intravaginal hydrocortisone suppositories (1/2–1) twice daily.[17] The frequency of treatment was tapered to twice weekly after several months of improvement. Overall, 81% of these women reported significant subjective improvement (burning, pruritus, dyspareunia, and vaginal discharge), and 76.8% of the women improved objectively on examination (erythema, erosion, lesions). Vaginal stenosis, however, did not significantly improve.[17]

Sometimes, particularly in localized disease, intralesional injections of triamcinolone acetonide, 3 to 10 mg/mL, can be helpful. Systemic steroids, 0.5 to 1 mg/kg, effectively and immediately treat most cases of VVLP. However, symptoms recur immediately with the cessation of this regimen. The potential side effects of the long-term use of corticosteroids necessitate the institution of alternative therapeutic agents.

Because LP is a T cell–mediated process, the use of topical calcineurin inhibitors, such as tacrolimus and pimecrolimus, has been explored with variable success in the treatment of mucosal LP.[9,10,19–22] Topical tacrolimus (compounded in a bland emollient or formulated as a 0.1% or 0.03% ointment) is applied twice daily. Symptoms typically improve in 4 weeks and continue to improve over another month. In some patients, the frequency of application can be tapered sequentially, starting with daily application, then decreasing to 3 times per week, and then tapering to weekly application of tacrolimus intravaginally and topically to the vulva. Topical tacrolimus can be associated with a burning sensation that is not tolerated by some patients. The concern with calcineurin inhibitors is increased risk of malignancy (black box warning). However, it has been found that systemic absorption is minimal. According to some investigators, the topical application of these drugs is relatively safe.[21] In a retrospective review of the medical records of 16 patients, 94% of the patients with recalcitrant symptomatic vulvar LP responded to topical treatment with tacrolimus ointment within 3 months, with partial or complete resolution of their lesions,[22] and 38% reported irritation and burning and tingling sensation, which resolved with continued use of the drug. Storing tacrolimus in the refrigerator sometimes minimizes burning sensation with application. Symptoms recurred in most patients who had responded initially, but often these symptoms were less severe. Controlled clinical trials are warranted to explore both the anecdotal success and long-term risk profile.[22–24]

When severe scarring and adhesion formation is anticipated, use of topical and systemic agents has been explored, alone or in combination with the use of a vaginal dilator. During severe flares when scarring and adhesion is a concern, intermittent intake of oral prednisone, 40 mg/d, may be prescribed. Further development of scars and adhesions can be prevented with the scheduled use of a vaginal dilator. The dilator is coated with corticosteroid or estrogen vaginal cream and used on a tapering schedule at night. Lotery and Galask[25] reported a small case series of patients (n = 3) using tacrolimus 0.1% ointment twice daily for 1 week, followed by thrice weekly. All patients reported significant improvement. Of the 3 patients, 2 used a graduated vaginal dilator coated with a vaginal estrogen cream, with increased diameter and depth of dilator insertion as well as the ability to resume sexual intercourse.[25] Another small case series from Finland reported on 5 patients with stenosing LP treated with methotrexate supplemented with ultrapotent corticosteroid cream and tacrolimus in combination with surgical dilatation. All patients reported symptomatic relief and only minimal to moderate restenosis of the vagina after 2 to 41 months.[26] Surgery is recommended only when the disease is controlled. After surgery, dilators with topical steroids and/or estrogen cream should be used to prevent new adhesions and scars from forming.

Various other systemic treatments have been tried with varied and often disappointing results. These treatments include use of griseofulvin, dapsone, minocycline combined with nicotinamide, oral retinoids, hydroxychloroquine, azathioprine, cyclophosphamide, cyclosporine, mycophenolate mofetil, methotrexate, etanercept, adalimumab, and thalidomide. Thalidomide is a systemic tumor necrosis factor inhibitor that has also been suggested for use with mixed results.[27] Systemic therapy should be considered in cases in which permanent scarring is probable or when topical therapy has failed to abort the progression of the disease. Cytotoxic and systemic immunosuppressive agents may be beneficial, but harmful side effects limit the use of these agents in cases of severe disease.

Supportive Measures

In addition to the use of topical steroids, supportive measures are an important adjunct in the armamentarium available for the care for these complex patients (see **Table 1**). Patients should be instructed to avoid using any irritating substances on the vulva (soaps, lotions, or detergents).[28] After bathing, the area should be patted dry, not rubbed. To further minimize koebnerization, irritants, potential allergens, and physical manipulation should be avoided. Burning sensation and pain may be minimized with sitz baths, ice packs, cool compresses, and application of oatmeal solutions. Systemic antihistamines help in controlling itching and rubbing. Topical emollients such as petrolatum, A and D ointment, and Aquaphor decrease friction and may be soothing to the patient.

In postmenopausal patients, hormone replacement with topical or systemic estrogen eliminates underlying atrophy caused by estrogen deficiency. Many patients report that estradiol vaginal tablets (10 or 25 μg/dose, Vagifem) are easy to use and decrease the risk of secondary irritation caused by creams. When systemic treatments are available, avoiding all topical regimens (diphenhydramine, antifungals, and estrogens) can also limit irritation or allergic reactions.

In severe or acute exacerbations, one must confirm that a secondary infection with *Candida* or herpes simplex virus is not present and that no caustic topicals were used. If an offending agent is identified, it should be treated or discontinued, or if the agent is unknown, all contacts to the area except water should be stopped. Oral prednisone, 40 mg/d, for 7 to 10 days or intramuscular administration of triamcinolone (20–40 mg) is effective in treating LP flares. Long-term suppressive therapy for candida or herpes infections, antihistamines, tricyclic antidepressants, or benzodiazepines may also be appropriate.

SUMMARY

Although a cure is not yet available for the treatment of this complex condition, many options are available. The importance of the doctor-patient relationship cannot be emphasized enough. Patients with VVLP can and do improve, and it is hoped that patients would return to normal function. More studies are necessary to further define these patients and refine the treatment options.

REFERENCES

1. Edwards L. Vulvar lichen planus. Arch Dermatol 1989;125:1677–80.
2. Torgesson RR, Edwards L. Disease and disorders of the female genitalia. Fitzpatrick's dermatology in general medicine. 7th edition. New York: McGraw Hill Medical; 2008.
3. Powell JJ, Marren P, Wojnarowska F. Erosive and vesiculobullous diseases. In: Edwards L, editor. Genital dermatology atlas. Philadelphia: Lippincott Williams & Wilkins; 2004.
4. Thornhill MH. Immune mechanisms in oral lichen planus. Acta Odontol Scand 2001;59:174–7.
5. Scully C, Eisen D, Carrozzo M. Management of oral lichen planus. Am J Clin Dermatol 2000;1:287–306.
6. Dickens DM, Heseltine D, Walton S, et al. The esophagus in LP. An endoscopic study. Br Med J 1990;300:117–32.
7. Eisen D. The clinical manifestations and treatment of oral lichen planus. Dermatol Clin 2003;21:79–89.

8. Eisen D. The evaluation of cutaneous, genital, scalp, nail, esophageal, and ocular involvement in patients with oral lichen planus. Oral Surg Oral Med Oral Pathol Oral Radiol Endod 1999;88:431–6.
9. Cooper SM, Wojnarowska F. Influence of treatment of erosive lichen planus of the vulva on its prognosis. Arch Dermatol 2006;142:289–94.
10. Cooper SM, Haefner HK, Abrahams-Gessel S, et al. Vulvovaginal lichen planus treatment: a survey of current practices. Arch Dermatol 2008;144(11):1520–1.
11. Pelisse M. The vulvo-vaginal-gingival syndrome. A new form of erosive lichen planus. Int J Dermatol 1989;28(6):381–4.
12. Eisen D. The vulvovaginal-gingival syndrome of lichen planus. Arch Dermatol 1994;130:1379–82.
13. Rogers RS, Eisen D. Erosive oral lichen planus with genital lesions: the vulvovaginal-gingival syndrome and the peno-gingival syndrome. Dermatol Clin 2003;21:91–8.
14. Fung MA, LeBoit PE. Light microscopic criteria for the diagnosis of early vulvar lichen sclerosus: a comparison with lichen planus. Am J Surg Pathol 1998;22:473–8.
15. Lewis FM. Vulval lichen planus. Br J Dermatol 1998; 138:569–75.
16. Ridley CM. Chronic erosive vulval disease. Clin Exp Dermatol 1990;15:245–52.
17. Anderson M, Kutzner S, Kaufman RH. Treatment of vulvovaginal lichen planus with vaginal hydrocortisone suppositories. Obstet Gynecol 2002;100: 359–62.
18. Mann MS, Kaufman RH. Erosive lichen planus of the vulva. Clin Obstet Gynecol 1991;34:605–14.
19. Vente C, Reich K, Rupprecht R, et al. Erosive mucosal lichen planus: response to topical treatment with tacrolimus. Br J Dermatol 1999;140: 338–42.
20. Lener EV, Brieva J, Schachter M, et al. Successful treatment of erosive lichen planus with topical tacrolimus. Arch Dermatol 2001;137:419–22.
21. Kirtschig G, Meulen AJ, Ion Lipan JW, et al. Successful treatment of erosive vulvovaginal lichen planus with topical tacrolimus. Br J Dermatol 2002; 147:604–31.
22. Byrd JA, Davis MD, Rogers RS. Recalcitrant symptomatic vulvar lichen planus: response to topical tacrolimus. Arch Dermatol 2004;140:715–20.
23. Jensen JT, Bird M, Leclair CM. Patient satisfaction after the treatment of vulvovaginal erosive lichen planus with topical clobetasol and tacrolimus: a survey study. Am J Obstet Gynecol 2004;190(6): 1759–63 [discussion: 1763–5].
24. Volz T, Caroli U, Ludtkele H, et al. Pimecrolimus cream 1% for erosive oral lichen planus- a prospective randomized double blind vehicle study. Br J Dermatol 2008;159:936–41.
25. Lotery HE, Galask RP. Erosive lichen planus of the vulva and vagina. Obstet Gynecol 2003; 101(5 Pt 2):1121–5.
26. Kortekangas-Savolainen O, Kiilholma P. Treatment of vulvovaginal erosive and stenosing lichen planus by surgical dilatation and methotrexate. Acta Obstet Gynecol Scand 2007;86:339–43.
27. Sharma NL, Sharma VC, Mahajan VK, et al. Thalidomide: experience in the therapeutic outcome and adverse reaction. J Dermatolog Treat 2007;18: 335–40.
28. Neill SM, Lewis FM. Vulvovaginal lichen planus a disease in need of a unified approach. Arch Dermatol 2008;144:1502–3.

Dermatologic Causes of Vaginitis: A Clinical Review

Libby Edwards, MD*

KEYWORDS

- Vaginitis • Vulva • Desquamative inflammatory vaginitis
- Lichen planus • Cicatricial pemphigoid
- Pemphigus vulgaris • Atrophic vaginitis

Vaginitis is a common symptom, generally characterized by introital itching or burning and vaginal discharge. Acute vaginitis most often is produced by infection, especially yeast. Candida albicans produces variable redness and, when severe, vaginal secretions containing white blood cells. Trichomonas vaginitis usually produces vaginal and cervical redness and increased white blood cells. Bacterial vaginitis is an uncommon condition with these same clinical findings. Infections are addressed elsewhere, and are not discussed in this article. However, inflammatory vaginitis is not always infectious in origin. In fact, chronic vaginitis usually is not infectious in origin, but rather produced by epithelial abnormalities.[1] Many of these are normally managed by dermatologists when occurring on other skin surfaces. Unfortunately, no specialty claims noninfectious vaginal dermatoses, and the management of most of these are not included in training programs or discussed in most venues.

ISOLATED VAGINAL DISEASE

Although rarely addressed, mucous membrane dermatoses, such as lichen planus, pemphigus vulgaris, and cicatricial pemphigoid, that affect the vagina as part of more generalized involvement are well known. Much less well understood is isolated vaginal inflammation.

Atrophic Vagina/Vaginitis

A common cause of introital burning, dryness and dyspareunia is estrogen deficiency. For years, this was an uncommon condition, because systemic estrogen replacement was supplied regularly to postmenopausal women without specific contraindications. When the results of the Women's Health Initiative were released, systemic estrogen lost favor and the use of systemic estrogen declined sharply. Clinicians often forget to address topical estrogen replacement, so that in addition to hot flashes and other menopausal symptoms, women experience thinning of the vaginal epithelium and dryness, a condition called an atrophic vagina. Occasionally, inflammation occurs when these thin, fragile vaginal walls develop erosions, producing atrophic vaginitis.

Many women with an atrophic vagina experience no symptoms of estrogen deficiency, particularly if they are not sexually active. However, the prevalence of atrophic vagina in postmenopausal women is approximately 50%, making this a very significant and common problem.[2] Patients report a sensation of uncomfortable dryness, and introital irritation occurs in some. Those who are sexually active often describe dyspareunia.

The clinical appearance of the postmenopausal vulva and vagina ranges from nearly normal to marked changes of atrophy to include diminution of the labia minora, with pallor, dryness, inelasticity, and mild narrowing of the introitus. The vagina is dry, pale, and lacking in the normal rugae, and the cervix flattens against the vaginal wall. A cotton-tipped applicator inserted to collect vaginal secretions seems completely dry in severely affected women, and a wet mount in these patients is nearly acellular. Most epithelial

Carolinas Medical Center, PO Box 32861, Charlotte, NC 29232-2861, USA
* 4335 Colwick Road, Charlotte, NC 28211.
E-mail address: LibbyEdwardsMD@gmail.com

Dermatol Clin 28 (2010) 727–735
doi:10.1016/j.det.2010.07.004
0733-8635/10/$ – see front matter

cells are parabasal cells, which are squamous epithelial cells that are immature and round, with a large nucleus compared with the cytoplasmic volume, unlike the large, flat, cuboidal, folded epithelial cells shed from a mature epithelium. Lactobacilli are absent (**Fig. 1**). Vaginal candidiasis is very uncommon in estrogen-deficient women. Less affected patients exhibit more modest findings, less dryness, and more desquamated mature squamous cells.

When the vaginal walls become irritated from the friction of sexual activity or a cystocele or rectocele protruding into the vagina, erosions sometimes develop, resulting in frank atrophic vaginitis, rather than simply an atrophic vagina. These women often experience burning and discomfort even without a trigger such as sexual activity or a gynecologic examination. Although women with an atrophic vagina report dryness rather than vaginal discharge, women with atrophic vaginitis often describe a yellow vaginal discharge. On physical examination, variable degrees of vaginal erythema and a purulent vaginal discharge are present. A wet mount shows an increase in white blood cells, so that fully developed atrophic vaginitis exhibits parabasal cells, sheets of neutrophils, no lactobacilli, and sometimes an increase in background bacteria (**Fig. 2**).

The underlying primary cause of an atrophic vagina and atrophic vaginitis is estrogen deficiency, which can occur after menopause, after delivery of a baby, with breastfeeding, and, to a variable degree, as a result of oral contraception. Obese women experience modest protection from peripheral conversion of estrogen in fat, and some clinicians believe that women who are regularly sexually active are less prone to experience an atrophic vagina.

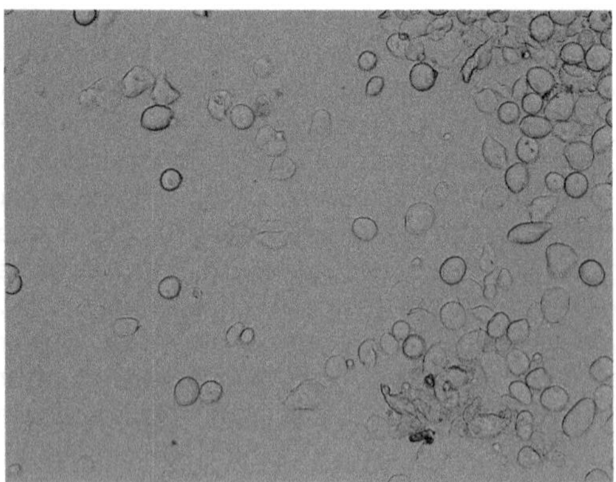

Fig. 1. The wet mount of an atrophic vagina shows rounded parabasal cells and (immature squamous epithelial cells) shed from a thin, atrophic vaginal epithelium. Results also show no lactobacilli and a correspondingly relatively high pH of greater than 5.

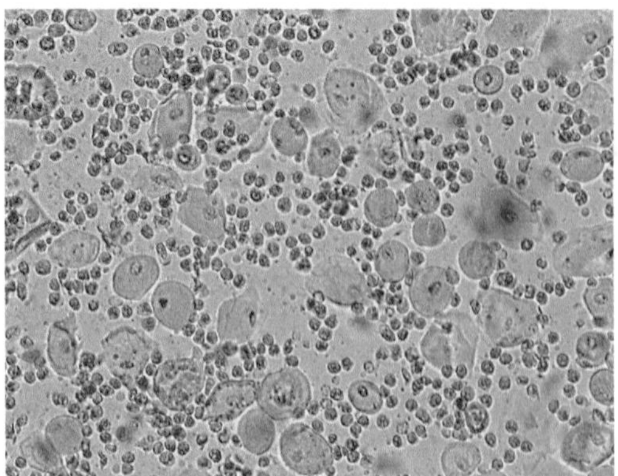

Fig. 2. This patient with atrophic vaginitis exhibits a wet mount that shows many leukocytes in addition to parabasal cells and absent lactobacilli. This wet mount is nonspecific and shared by other diseases that produce vaginal inflammation.

The treatment of an atrophic vagina and atrophic vaginitis is usually quick and rewarding. Generally, a topical estrogen effects dramatic improvement within a week. Options for estrogen replacement include estradiol cream (Estrace) or equine conjugated estrogen (Premarin) cream, 1 g inserted into the vagina 3 nights a week. Alternatively, an estradiol tablet (Vagifem), 25 or 10 mcg, is inserted into the vagina 3 nights a week. Very popular and effective is an estrogen-impregnated ring (EstRing) that is inserted into the vagina and gradually releases estradiol over 3 months. The creams are messy and, sometimes irritating, with conjugated equine estrogen sometimes more irritating than estradiol. Insertion of the rather large estrogen ring into a dry, inelastic vagina can be uncomfortable, and is more comfortable after several weeks of estrogen cream or tablets.

An estrogen-deficient vagina is somewhat protected from Candidiasis, because yeast usually only produces infection in the presence of lactobacilli. However, the addition of a topical estrogen increases the risk of yeast, particularly during the first month. Patients can be advised to call if they experience any sudden itching, or can be prescribed a 150- to 200-mg fluconazole tablet orally once a week the first month to prevent this occasional occurrence.

Occasionally patients cannot tolerate any of the topical estrogen preparations because of burning or irritation. These women can be treated initially with systemic estrogen, either in a patch or an oral formulation. Often after a few weeks, the now well-estrogenized vagina tolerates the topical preparations. In addition, estrogen can be compounded into an ointment base, which is less irritating.

Many women, because of the results of the Women's Health Initiative, are afraid of estrogen, even when prescribed topically. Other women have a personal or family history of breast cancer. Generally, these women can be reassured of the safety of topical estrogen, because the systemic absorption is low. The cream preparations have been associated with endometrial hyperplasia and breast tenderness in some patients,[3] although lower-dose preparations are less likely to produce these side effects.[4] Most oncologists permit topical estrogen in women with breast cancer. However, neutralization of the estrogen antagonists such as tamoxifen has been reported.[5]

The occasional woman with an atrophic vagina who cannot tolerate or is not permitted to use topical estrogen sometimes experiences some improvement with a vaginal moisturizer. A common choice is polycarbophil-based vaginal moisturizer Replens.[6] Although unpopular with many gynecologists, petroleum jelly is comforting to many women, and can be inserted with a finger and applied sparingly to the introitus. Women with the inflammation of atrophic vaginitis may benefit from the addition of a hydrocortisone acetate, 25 mg, rectal suppository inserted into the vagina, or a moderately potent corticosteroid ointment such as desonide ointment, 0.05%. Most recently, hyaluronic acid sodium salt, 5 mg, has been shown to be effective compared with topical estrogen.[7]

The duration of therapy is variable. Usually, postmenopausal, sexually active women benefit from ongoing estrogen replacementat at a dosing of once or twice a week. Women who are not sexually active and who experienced the sudden onset of symptoms are sometimes able to discontinue their topical estrogen replacement and remain comfortable. Patients should be advised, if their estrogen is discontinued, that recurrence of symptoms is common. Sometimes, women who are atrophic as a result of hormonal contraception, especially injectable medroxyprogesterone (DepoProvera), benefit long-term from a change of contraception.

Desquamative Inflammatory Vaginitis

First described in 1968, desquamative inflammatory vaginitis (DIV) is probably a common condition. DIV is defined by its clinical and wet mount characteristics, and is a diagnosis of exclusion.[8] Although once thought to represent lichen planus of the vagina, differences in the presentation and course of DIV indicate that it is a distinct entity.[9]

Occurring in both premenopausal and postmenopausal women, DIV typically presents with introital irritation, burning, and dyspareunia, accompanied by a clinically and microscopically purulent vaginal discharge. Women with DIV are more likely than matched controls to have had diagnoses of Candida vaginitis, bacterial vaginosis, and pelvic inflammatory disease,[10] which could be relevant or a manifestation of previous misdiagnoses by clinicians unfamiliar with this condition. Hormone replacement use is also more common in these women.[10]

An examination of the vulva shows introital redness of variable degrees; some women experience extension of erythema to the labia minora, where puffiness is often seen (**Fig. 3**). No specific vulvar lesions are present, nor is resorption of vulvar architecture seen, as occurs with lichen planus, lichen sclerosus, and the immunobullous diseases of cicatricial pemphigoid and pemphigus vulgaris. Clinicians who neglect the vaginal examination and wet mount can mistake the nonspecific vulvar findings for vestibulodynia (vulvar vestibulitis syndrome) or generalized vulvodynia, both painful syndromes sometimes associated with nonspecific erythema.

The vaginal walls are variably red. Because mucous membranes are normally somewhat red, especially in light-complexioned people, the

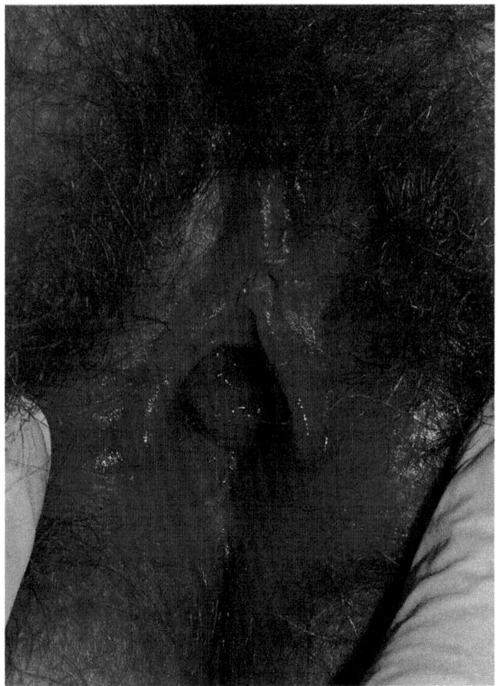

Fig. 3. The vulva of a patient with desquamative inflammatory vaginitis is characterized by redness and puffiness of the introitus and labia minora as a result of irritant contact dermatitis from irritating purulent vaginal secretions.

degree of vaginal erythema can be difficult to judge. In more marked disease, the vagina can be covered with small red macules, reminiscent of the "strawberry cervix" classic for trichomonas. Erosions and vaginal synechiae are absent. An abnormal vaginal discharge is present, usually abundant and yellowish in color, with a pH greater than 5. Green and gray discoloration of secretions also has been described.

A wet mount shows an increase in white blood cells and parabasal cells (immature squamous epithelial cells shed from a vaginal epithelium that is rapidly proliferating because of inflammation). Lactobacilli are absent, as expected with a pH greater than 5. The wet mount is identical to that for atrophic vaginitis, and basically indicates only marked inflammation of vaginal walls (see **Fig. 2**). A culture should be performed, and this will either show no pathogens, or clinical findings will persist after correction of any incidental infections. Fairly often, a culture yields group B streptococcus (*Streptococcus agalactiae*), but symptoms do not improve with appropriate antibiotic therapy. Some clinicians believe that this organism plays a role in the pathogenesis of DIV, and cite an occasional woman with this finding on culture whose vaginitis resolves with an antibiotic. Others, however, contend that an inflammatory vaginitis with *S agalactiae* on culture, and signs and symptoms that resolve while on antibiotics, should be termed *bacterial vaginitis*.[11] Most patients with inflammatory vaginitis whose culture yields group B streptococcus experience no change with antibiotic therapy, indicating the colonizing nature of this organism.

The diagnosis of DIV is made by the presence of a clinically purulent vaginal discharge; variable redness of the vaginal mucosa; a pH greater than 5; a wet mount showing an increase in leukocytes and parabasal cells and an absence of elongated rods presumed to represent lactobacilli; absence of estrogen deficiency; and cultures showing no causative organism. Exactly how many leukocytes or parabasal cells are required is not defined. Whether every one of these criteria must be present also is unknown.

The cause of DIV is unknown. Because many patients respond to topical clindamycin cream and because cultures often yield *S agalactiae* or *Escherichia coli*, some investigators have postulated infection as a factor.[12,13] However, because elimination of these organisms with alternative active antibiotics does not result in improvement in most patients, because corticosteroids also are often beneficial, and because clindamycin has nonspecific anti-inflammatory as well as antimicrobial effects, many clinicians believe that DIV is a hypersensitivity or autoimmune phenomenon. Reports of DIV occurring in women with malabsorption and vitamin D deficiency have led to a theory of vitamin D deficiency as a pathogenic factor. This author measured vitamin D levels in 20 women with DIV; although several were slightly vitamin D deficient as defined by newer guidelines, none experienced improvement in DIV with vitamin D replacement and normalization of levels (Libby Edwards, MD, unpublished data, 2008).

Biopsies have been reported only in one small series, showing either a lichenoid or a nonspecific mixed inflammatory infiltrate.[14,15] The inflammation was often mild compared that expected based on the degree of clinical redness and inflammation noted on wet mount. Direct immunofluorescence was nonspecific.

The variability of clinical findings, biopsy results, and response to therapy suggests that DIV may not be one disease, but rather may represent several, possibly related inflammatory processes. Some patients exhibit white blood cells on wet mount, but no parabasal cells, or no lactobacilli, or only a slight increase in white blood cells. Currently, no specific terminology exists to describe vaginal inflammation that does not meet all of the criteria of DIV. Vaginal inflammation in the absence of infection and specific lesions is an unexplored but common and important occurrence, and a fertile area for observational studies. In the meantime, management of all of these women is as reported for DIV.

The treatment of DIV consists of either clindamycin cream or corticosteroids.[16] Clindamycin cream, 2%, should be inserted into the vaginal nightly, presumably for its anti-inflammatory effects rather than antimicrobial actions.[13] Patients are treated for 2 to 4 weeks, and then reevaluated. Some women can discontinue their medication and remain clear for extended periods, whereas others require intermittent dosing or adjustment of dosing to the least frequent insertion that is effective.

Alternatively, topical corticosteroids can be used. Hydrocortisone acetate, 25 mg, rectal suppositories are inserted per vagina at bedtime. If this does not effect improvement, options include the compounding of 500-mg hydrocortisone suppositories, insertion of an ultrapotent topical corticosteroid such as clobetasol, or the use of combination clindamycin and a topical corticosteroid. Anecdotally, this author has found neither systemic corticosteroids nor oral antibiotics of any kind, including clindamycin, to be useful for DIV.

Many clinicians prescribe weekly fluconazole to patients receiving vaginal antibiotics or corticosteroids to prevent secondary Candidiasis. Those patients who cannot take fluconazole because of medication interactions can insert an azole suppository once or twice a week to minimize the risk of yeast.

Occasionally DIV does not respond to these therapies. These patients should be reevaluated for estrogen deficiency; cervicitis; infection to include trichomonas; any causes of erosion, including bullous or erosive mucous membrane dermatoses, complications of surgical sling placement with secondary erosion; or granulation tissue from previous surgeries. Clearly, further studies are needed to elucidate the cause and alternative therapies.

Vestibulodynia/Vulvar Vestibulitis

Vestibulodynia (previously known as vulvar vestibulitis) is a pain syndrome localized to the introitus and often mistaken for vaginitis. Currently believed to result primarily from pelvic floor dysfunction, neuropathy, and resulting anxiety and depression that worsen symptoms, vestibulodynia is not characterized by a vaginal discharge or any objective abnormalities, including inflammation, of the vagina.

THE VAGINA AS ONE SITE OF MULTIMUCOSAL EROSIVE DERMATOSES

Erosive Lichen Planus

Erosive vulvovaginal lichen planus is a common disease that usually occurs in a setting of erosions of other mucous membranes. The oral mucosa, vulva, and vagina are classically affected. Vaginal lichen planus can occur as an isolated condition, but this is extraordinarily rare. Most women with vaginal lichen planus exhibit vulvar disease and oral disease, but extragenital lichen planus of keratinizing epithelium is very uncommon in these women. Perianal and esophageal involvement are also common.

These women are usually postmenopausal, and describe pruritus, burning, soreness, and dyspareunia. The vagina exhibits patchy erosions, often within diffuse redness. Vaginal secretions are often grossly and microscopically purulent, with a wet mount showing, in addition to white blood cells, parabasal cells shed from the base of erosions and a paucity of lactobacilli. More-advanced disease is characterized by narrowing of the vagina and synechiae of the anterior and posterior walls that eventuate in complete obliteration of the vaginal space so that intercourse and the insertion of a speculum are impossible (**Fig. 4**).

The vulva typically shows vestibular erosions. Classic findings are white, fern-like striae of the modified mucous membranes, but these do not occur in most patients (**Fig. 5**). As occurs in the vagina, scarring of the vulva by lichen planus is common and can be severe.

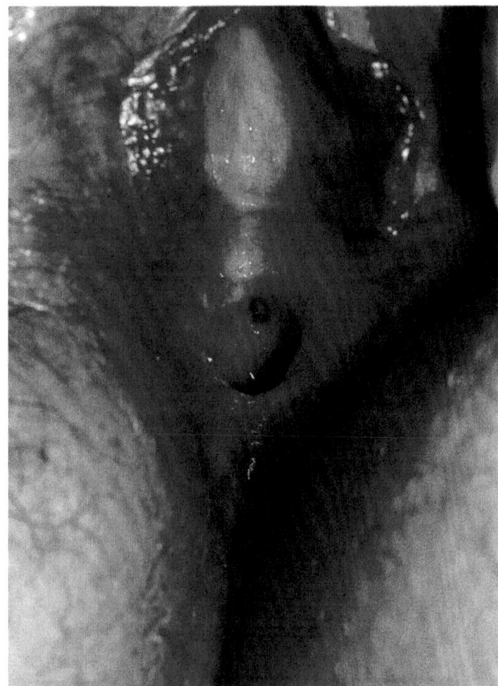

Fig. 4. Lichen planus of the vagina often produces narrowing of the introitus and synechiae. Typical redness of lichen planus can be seen on periurethral epithelium.

Oral lichen planus most often consists of erosions with surrounding white striae of the posterior buccal mucosae. However, beefy red, eroded gingivae are more common in women with erosive vulvovaginal lichen planus than in people with lichen planus of other sites.

A wet mount of vaginal secretions again shows nonspecific changes of inflammation, with parabasal cells, leukocytes, and absent lactobacilli.

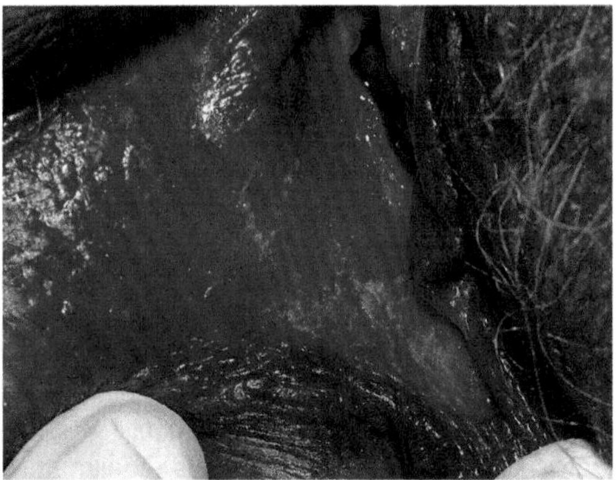

Fig. 5. Even when erosive lichen planus only affects vaginal epithelium, white striae of the vulva can indicate the diagnosis.

With lactobacilli absent, the pH is generally greater than 5 (see **Fig. 2**).

The diagnosis of lichen planus is made clinically and confirmed with biopsy, preferably with sampling taken from the white epithelium when present, or from the edge of an erosion. Often, the histology reports only lichenoid dermatitis, and therefore clinical correlation is required. The differential diagnosis of erosive vulvovaginal lichen planus includes cicatricial pemphigoid and pemphigus vulgaris. The blistering form of erythema multiforme, including Stevens-Johnson syndrome and toxic epidermal necrolysis, can appear similar but shows explosive onset and keratinized skin lesions.

The treatment of lichen planus is primarily topical corticosteroids. The vagina is a special challenge, because no formulation of corticosteroids exists for the vagina. Hydrocortisone acetate, 25 mg, rectal suppositories can be inserted at bedtime, with either 500-mg compounded hydrocortisone suppositories or clobetasol ointment substituted if the improvement is not sufficient. Calcineurin inhibitors are also used. Tacrolimus (Protopic) and pimecrolimus (Elidel) have been reported to be useful for erosive lichen planus.[17–19] This medication can be inserted into the vagina with a finger twice daily. Its use is limited by local irritation with application. In addition, these medication are labeled as possible carcinogens by the U.S. Food and Drug Administration, and chronic vulvar lichen planus is associated with an increased risk for squamous cell carcinoma.

Attention should be given to estrogen deficiency, which is common in the postmenopausal age group most prone to erosive vulvovaginal lichen planus. Estradiol cream or vaginal tablets should be provided for postmenopausal women not on systemic estrogen replacement. Patients receiving both estrogen and vaginal corticosteroids are at risk for developing a secondary yeast infection. They should either be followed carefully for this eventuality, or treated with fluconazole or an azole suppository weekly to prevent yeast. Women with active vaginal lichen planus who are not intercourse-active should be careful to insert a vaginal dilator daily to prevent closure of the vagina.

Severe disease generally is not controlled with topical agents. Systemic therapies suitable for long-term use include hydroxychloroquine, methotrexate,[20] mycophenolate mofetil,[21] tumor necrosis factor (TNF)-α antagonists (adalimumab, etanercept, and infliximab),[22] cyclosporine,[23] azathioprine,[24] cyclophosphamide,[25] and thalidomide.[26] The use of these medications for lichen planus is substantiated by case reports and small open series only. A recent report suggests benefit from an old anti-inflammatory agent, sulfasalazine.[27] None has been shown to be predictably beneficial, but each is sometimes useful in individual patients.

Vaginal lichen planus is often chronic and recalcitrant to therapy, although most women experience significant but incomplete improvement with therapy. Chronic pain, and occasionally scarring of the vagina, often prevents sexual intercourse. Squamous cell carcinoma is a known occasional sequela of oral and vulvar lichen planus, but this has not been reported for vaginal lichen planus. However, because vaginal lichen planus is regularly accompanied by vulvar and oral disease, squamous cell carcinoma remains a concern that deserves ongoing surveillance.

Cicatricial Pemphigoid

A much less common cause of inflammatory vaginitis is cicatricial pemphigoid, another multimucosal erosive disease that occurs primarily in postmenopausal women and elderly men. This immunobullous disease regularly affects the mouth and eyes, with extragenital blisters occurring in only about a third of patients. Vulvar and vaginal involvement and, as the name implies, scarring are common. Furthermore, conjunctival synechiae can result in dry, painful eyes and even blindness.

Cicatricial pemphigoid typically exhibits nonspecific erosions on mucous membranes and the modified mucous membranes of the vulva (**Fig. 6**). The blisters on thin, fragile mucous membranes generally erode as they form, and therefore the blistering nature is sometimes not appreciated except when occurring on keratinized skin (**Fig. 7**). Vaginal erosions result in inflammatory vaginitis indistinguishable from that of lichen planus and pemphigus vulgaris. Oral erosions, including erosive gingival disease, are usual.

As with wet mounts in other inflammatory vaginal conditions, parabasal cells, an increase in white blood cells, and absent lactobacilli are common (see **Fig. 2**).

The diagnosis is made through a routine biopsy of the edge of an erosion or blister, with a direct immunofluorescent biopsy of perilesional normal skin. Cicatricial pemphigoid is an autoimmune disease produced by antibodies directed against several components of the basement membrane, which causes a blister when a loss of adhesion of the epidermis to the dermis occurs.

The management of mild disease can be attempted with topical ultrapotent corticosteroids, but systemic corticosteroids are generally

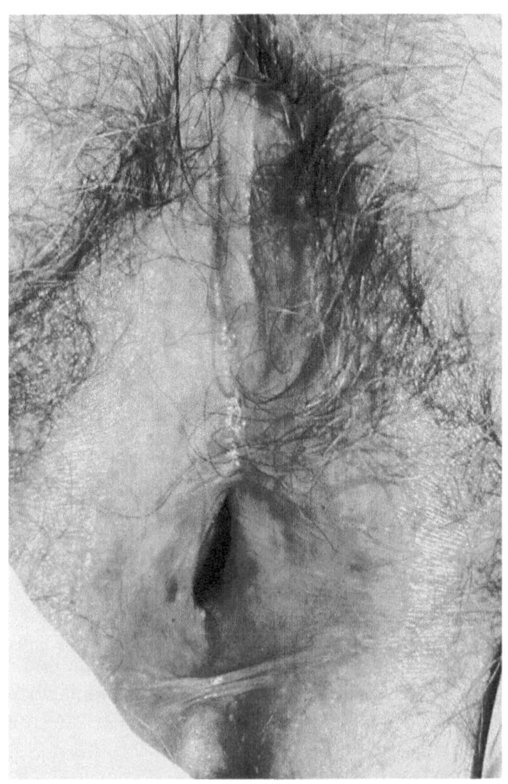

Fig. 6. The vaginal erosions and introital fragility of cicatricial pemphigoid are nonspecific. Biopsies of the edge of an erosion and a direct immunofluorescent biopsy were required to make this diagnosis.

required, often with steroid-sparing agents such as azathioprine or cyclophosphamide. Dapsone or tetracycline with niacin are sometimes beneficial, as are pulse cyclophosphamide and corticosteroids. Rituximab, an anti-CD20 antibody, is useful in some patients,[28] as are TNF-α antagonists such as etanercept.[29] Local care of the vagina should be implemented as described earlier for lichen planus, and includes estrogen replacement, use of vaginal dilators to prevent adhesions, and a high index of suspicion for secondary yeast with flares. Cicatricial pemphigoid is often very difficult to manage, and is a chronic condition that requires both ongoing medication and surveillance for scarring of the vagina, vulva, eyes, and esophagus.

Pemphigus Vulgaris

Pemphigus vulgaris is another immunobullous disease that preferentially affects mucous membranes. Pemphigus vulgaris generally occurs in younger individuals in the fourth to fifth decade. Blisters of dry, keratinized skin occur in most patients, although mucosal disease often precedes widespread disease.

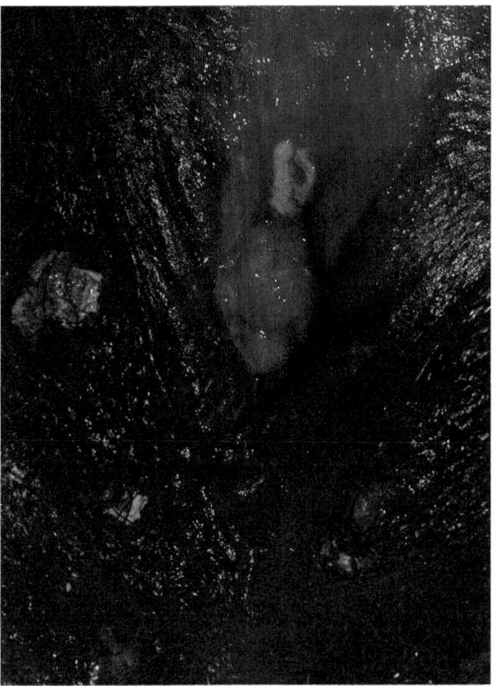

Fig. 7. These moist vulvar, fragile papules and erosions are typical of pemphigus vulgaris; the necrotic epithelium is macerated and white. Vaginal erosions consist of red erosions that are nonspecific and indistinguishable from cicatricial pemphigoid and lichen planus. Routine and direct immunofluorescent biopsies are required for diagnosis.

Patients generally complain of pain, primarily from eroded mucous membranes. Oral erosions often occur first, and patients may need to be specifically questioned about vulvovaginal symptoms, because often they do not correlate their oral and genital symptoms.

On physical examination, as with cicatricial pemphigoid and lichen planus, pemphigus vulgaris of the vagina and vulva is characterized by nonspecific red erosions of mucous membranes. Although classically considered a nonscarring condition on most epithelial surfaces, pemphigus produces vulvar and vaginal scarring, again indistinguishable from that of cicatricial pemphigoid and lichen planus. However, pemphigus vulgaris also is characterized ultimately by blisters of keratinized skin (see **Fig. 7**). These are superficial, and therefore the blisters are flaccid and erosions develop quickly.

Again, a wet mount shows increased white blood cells, parabasal cells, and absent lactobacilli (see **Fig. 2**).

The diagnosis is usually easily confirmed through a routine biopsy from the edge of an erosion or blister, with a direct immunofluorescent biopsy from adjacent normal epithelium. The cause of pemphigus vulgaris is the presence of autoantibodies directed against desmoglein 1 and 3 antigen on the surface of epithelial cells, causing them to lose adhesion. This response produces the typical histologic picture of acantholysis, in which some epithelial cells are attached only to the basement membrane and no longer to each other, and more superficial cells are single and round, producing a very superficial blister within the epidermis.

The management of pemphigus vulgaris includes local care of the vagina, involving estrogen replacement when appropriate, use of dilators to prevent synechiae, and evaluation for infections while on immunosuppressive medications. Otherwise, the management of pemphigus vulgaris of the vulvovaginal area is based on information regarding therapy of oropharyngeal disease. Systemic corticosteroids are the mainstay of therapy. Historically, steroid-sparing medications are also used, including methotrexate, azathioprine, and cyclophosphamide. Pulse cyclophosphamide and corticosteroids are also beneficial.[30] More recently, mycophenolate mofetil and rituximab have been used with success.[31,32]

Women with mild or partially controlled disease often benefit from additional local therapy in the form of topical or intralesional corticosteroids. These include hydrocortisone acetate, 25 mg, rectal suppositories inserted per vagina at bedtime. Alternatively, compounded hydrocortisone, 500 mg, suppositories can be inserted, or clobetasol ointment. Care must be taken because of systemic absorption from this mucous membrane. Intralesional triamcinolone acetate, 10 mg/mL, a very small amount injected into the base of erosions, does not produce a significant systemic effect and remains in the dermis for approximately a month.[33]

After control of the disease, medications can often be decreased to smaller doses, although the disease does not generally remit.[34]

Toxic Epidermal Necrolysis/Stevens-Johnson Syndrome

Toxic epidermal necrolysis/Stevens-Johnson syndrome is a hypersensitivity reaction to a medication or recurrent herpes simplex virus infection that consists of mucosal erosions and blisters or erosions of keratinized skin. Although the vagina is almost always affected, this is a minor aspect of a generalized blistering disease of explosive onset, so the vaginitis is not a presenting condition or diagnostic dilemma. However, care of the vagina is important during this acute disease to prevent unnecessary worse discomfort and permanent scarring. Control of secondary infection, especially candidiasis, and use of dilators to prevent vaginal closure from scarring are important.

SUMMARY

Although inflammation of the vagina is assumed to occur as a result of infection by most patients and caregivers, several noninfectious epithelial disorders affect the vagina regularly. These conditions most likely occur in a setting of chronic vaginitis. The diagnosis requires a limited history, including knowledge of estrogen administration, evaluation of a wet mount and cultures, survey of extragenital skin disease, and identification and biopsy of primary lesions.

REFERENCES

1. Nyirjesy P, Peyton C, Weitz MV, et al. Causes of chronic vaginitis: analysis of a prospective database of affected women. Obstet Gynecol 2006;108:1185–91.
2. Mac Bride MB, Rhodes DJ, Shuster LT. Vulvovaginal atrophy. Mayo Clin Proc 2010;85:87–94.
3. Suckling J, Lethaby A, Kennedy R. Local oestrogen for vaginal atrophy in postmenopausal women. Cochrane Database Syst Rev 2006;4:CD001500.
4. Bachmann G, Bouchard C, Hoppe D, et al. Efficacy and safety of low-dose regimens of conjugated estrogens cream administered vaginally. Menopause 2009;16:719–27.
5. Kendall A, Dowsett M, Folkerd E, et al. Caution: vaginal estradiol appears to be contraindicated in postmenopausal women on adjuvant aromatase inhibitors. Ann Oncol 2006;17:584–7.
6. Biglia N, Peano E, Sgandurra P, et al. Low-dose vaginal estrogens or vaginal moisturizer in breast cancer survivors with urogenital atrophy: a preliminary study. Gynecol Endocrinol 2010;26(6):404–12.
7. Ekin M, Yaşar L, Savan K, et al. The comparison of hyaluronic acid vaginal tablets with estradiol vaginal tablets in the treatment of atrophic vaginitis: a randomized controlled trial. Arch Gynecol Obstet 2010. [Epub ahead of print].
8. Gardner HL. Desquamative inflammatory vaginitis: a newly defined entity. Am J Obstet Gynecol 1968;102:1102–5.
9. Edwards L, Friedrich EG Jr. Desquamative vaginitis: lichen planus in disguise. Obstet Gynecol 1988;71:832–6.
10. Newbern EC, Foxman B, Leaman D, et al. Desquamative inflammatory vaginitis: an exploratory case-control study. Ann Epidemiol 2002;12(5):346–52.

11. Clark LR, Atendido M. Group B streptococcal vaginitis in postpubertal adolescent girls. J Adolesc Health 2005;36:437–40.
12. Donders GG, Vereecken A, Bosmans E, et al. Definition of a type of abnormal vaginal flora that is distinct from bacterial vaginosis: aerobic vaginitis. BJOG 2002;109(1):34–43.
13. Sobel JD. Desquamative inflammatory vaginitis: a new subgroup of purulent vaginitis responsive to topical 2% clindamycin therapy. Am J Obstet Gynecol 1994;171:1215–20.
14. Peacocke M, Djurkinak E, Thys-Jacobs S. Treatment of desquamative inflammatory vaginitis with vitamin D: a case report. Cutis 2008;81:75–8.
15. Murphy R, Edwards L. Desquamative inflammatory vaginitis: what is it? J Reprod Med 2008;53: 124–8.
16. Murphy R. Desquamative inflammatory vaginitis. Dermatol Ther 2004;17(1):47–9.
17. Byrd JA, Davis MD, Rogers RS 3rd. Recalcitrant symptomatic vulvar lichen planus: response to topical tacrolimus. Arch Dermatol 2004;140: 715–20.
18. Voltz T, Caroli U, Ludtkele H, et al. Pimecrolimus cream 1% in erosive oral lichen planus—a prospective randomized double-blind vehicle study. Br J Dermatol 2008;159:936–41.
19. Al Johani KA, Hegarty AM, Porter SR, et al. Calcineurin inhibitors in oral medicine. J Am Acad Dermatol 2009;61:829–40.
20. Jang N, Fischer G. Treatment of erosive vulvovaginal lichen planus with methotrexate. Australas J Dermatol 2008;49:216–9.
21. Frieling U, Bonsmann G, Schwarz T, et al. Treatment of severe lichen planus with mycophenolate mofetil. J Am Acad Dermatol 2003;49:1063–6.
22. O'Neill ID. Off-label use of biologicals in the management of inflammatory oral mucosal disease. J Oral Pathol Med 2008;37:575–81.
23. Madan V, Griffiths CE. Systemic ciclosporin and tacrolimus in dermatology. Dermatol Ther 2007;20: 239–50.
24. Verma KK, Mittal R, Manchanda Y. Azathioprine for the treatment of severe erosive oral and generalized lichen planus. Acta Derm Venereol 2001;81:378–9.
25. Paslin DA. Sustained remission of generalized lichen planus induced by cyclophosphamide. Arch Dermatol 1985;121:236–9.
26. Sharma NL, Sharma VC, Mahajan VK, et al. Thalidomide: an experience in therapeutic outcome and adverse reactions. J Dermatolog Treat 2007;18: 335–40.
27. Omidian M, Ayoobi A, Mapar M, et al. Efficacy of sulfasalazine in the treatment of generalized lichen planus: randomized double-blinded clinical trial on 52 patients. J Eur Acad Dermatol Venereol 2010;24: 1051–4.
28. Taverna JA, Lerner A, Bhawan J, et al. Successful adjuvant treatment of recalcitrant mucous membrane pemphigoid with anti-CD20 antibody rituximab. J Drugs Dermatol 2007;6:731–2.
29. Kennedy JS, Devillez RL, Henning JS. Recalcitrant cicatricial pemphigoid treated with the anti-TNF-alpha agent etanercept. J Drugs Dermatol 2010;9: 68–70.
30. Zivanovic D, Medenica L, Tanasilovic S, et al. Dexamethasone-cyclophosphamide pulse therapy in pemphigus: a review of 72 cases. Am J Clin Dermatol 2010;11:123–9.
31. Beissert S, Mimouni D, Kanwar AJ, et al. Treating pemphigus vulgaris with prednisone and mycophenolate mofetil: a multicenter, randomized, placebo-controlled trial. J Invest Dermatol 2010;130(8):2041–8.
32. Schmidt E, Goebeler M, Zillikens D. Rituximab in severe pemphigus. Ann N Y Acad Sci 2009;1173: 683–91.
33. Mignogna MD, Fortuna G, Leuci S, et al. Adjuvant triamcinolone acetonide injections in oropharyngeal pemphigus vulgaris. J Eur Acad Dermatol Venereol 2010. [Epub ahead of print].
34. Mignogna MD, Fortuna G, Leuci S, et al. Oropharyngeal pemphigus vulgaris and clinical remission: a long-term, longitudinal study. Am J Clin Dermatol 2010;11:137–45.

Erosive Diseases of the Vulva

Clare Pipkin, MD

KEYWORDS

• Vulvar • Dermatosis • Genital • Erosive • Lichen planus
• Vulvitis

Erosive diseases in the vulvovaginal area are often chronic, painful, progressive, and debilitating conditions that frequently result in considerable patient anxiety and frustration. These conditions, which represent a mixture of inflammatory, infectious, and neoplastic processes, are often difficult to diagnose and treat. The morphology of erosive disease is often nonspecific and therefore a thorough knowledge of the differential diagnosis is important (**Box 1**). This article provides an overview of the clinical features, causes/associations, histology, and treatment of some of the more commonly encountered conditions causing erosive vulvar disorders. Particular emphasis is given to lichen planus (LP), which is the most common cause of erosive vulvitis.

GENERAL APPROACH TO THE EVALUATION OF EROSIVE VULVAR DISEASE

In approaching the patient with erosive vulvar disease, a spectrum of disease processes must be considered. Consequently, the clinician must be attuned to a range of details both in history and physical examination to arrive at the correct diagnosis (**Box 2**). Occam's razor often does not apply to genital skin; multiple problems may coexist. For example, a patient with lichen sclerosus (LS) may also have an irritant dermatitis from urinary incontinence as well as fissures from a yeast infection. In addition, when the patient continues to complain of pain despite a normal examination, the diagnosis of vulvodynia should be entertained.

The first step in the evaluation of these disorders is a detailed history focusing not only on clinical symptoms but also on precipitating factors and relevant comorbidities. Symptom history should be sufficiently detailed. For example, symptoms of itching versus burning may be helpful in distinguishing a contact dermatitis versus an irritant dermatitis.

Many exposures may precipitate erosive disease in the vulvovaginal skin. The presence of incontinence should be ascertained, because this may cause an irritant dermatitis. A detailed history of all hygiene practices is necessary, because many agents can produce an irritant contact dermatitis. Patients should be directly questioned about all topicals they apply to the area, particularly those containing benzocaine, because of the high frequency of allergic contact dermatitis. Sexual practices should be reviewed (including the use of condoms, spermicides, or lubricants). Estrogen status should be ascertained because an estrogen deficiency can predispose to atrophy in the vulvovaginal area, which may compromise the barrier function of the skin. The use of topical immunosuppressives may increase the risk of infections, such as candidiasis or herpes. Oral medication exposures, both prescription and over-the-counter, may also be relevant because some erosive conditions can be induced by medications.

Past medical history and review of symptoms should concentrate on identifying conditions that may predispose to or are associated with specific vulvovaginal disorders. For example, a history of an abnormal Pap smear may raise suspicion for vulvar intraepithelial neoplasia (VIN). A review of systems (ROS), including oral, ocular, aural, genitourinary, and gastrointestinal systems, may

Department of Dermatology, Duke University, DUMC 3643, Durham, NC 27710, USA
E-mail address: clare.pipkin@duke.edu

Dermatol Clin 28 (2010) 737–751
doi:10.1016/j.det.2010.08.005
0733-8635/10/$ – see front matter

Box 1
Differential diagnosis of erosive vulvar diseases

Inflammatory dermatoses with possible erosion

- Lichen planus
- Lichen sclerosus
- Fixed drug eruption
- Stevens-Johnson syndrome/toxic epidermal necrolysis
- Irritant/allergic contact dermatitis
- Plasma cell (Zoon) vulvitis
- Lichen simplex chronicus

Inflammatory vesiculobullous diseases

- Subepidermal blistering diseases
  - Bullous pemphigoid
  - Cicatricial pemphigoid
  - Linear IgA disease
  - Bullous systemic lupus erythematosus
  - Epidermolysis bullosa acquisita
- Intraepidermal blistering diseases
  - Pemphigus vulgaris
  - Benign familial pemphigus (Hailey-Hailey disease)

Nutritional

- Vitamin B_2 deficiency
- Acrodermatitis enteropathica

Infections

- Candidiasis
- Impetigo
- Herpes simplex
- Herpes zoster

Malignancies

- Vulvar intraepithelial neoplasia
- Squamous cell carcinoma
- Basal cell carcinoma
- Extramammary Paget disease
- Langerhans cell histiocytosis

Paraneoplastic diseases

- Necrolytic migratory erythema
- Paraneoplastic pemphigus

Box 2
Specific elements of history and physical examination to assist in making a diagnosis

History

- Itching versus burning
- Hygiene practices
- Use of sanitary pads
- Estrogen status (eg, posttotal hysterectomy, postmenopausal, postpartum)
- Incontinence problems
- Underlying immunosuppressive disease
- Related symptoms: abnormal vaginal discharge, vaginal bleeding, dyspareunia/apareunia, dysuria, oral symptoms, ocular symptoms, dysphagia, hearing difficulties
- History of abnormal Pap smear
- Previous abdominal surgery

Medications

- Review of all topical agents (especially benzocaine-containing products) that come into contact with genital skin
- Review all prescription and over-the-counter oral medications

Review of systems

- Screen for symptoms associated with autoimmune disorders such as hypothyroidism, diabetes, connective tissue disease
- Screen for depression and anxiety

Physical examination

- Full cutaneous examination with attention to oral, ocular, and perianal skin
- Vulvar examination: make a checklist for presence or absence of all normal structures, examine for evidence of scarring
- Vaginal examination with wet mount of secretions

suggest a systemic diagnosis such as LP. In performing the ROS, it should also be kept in mind that both LP and LS have been associated with a greater frequency of autoimmune diseases.[1]

Attention to psychological status is particularly important when evaluating patients with vulvovaginal disease. There may be fear about the cause of the disease. Many patients suffer with dyspareunia or apareunia and this may adversely affect the relationship with their significant other. For some patients, it may take years to arrive at a diagnosis and they may have a great deal of frustration. As a result, the psychosocial effect of these disorders is considerable and appropriate screening for depression and anxiety should be performed.[2]

A full skin examination including all mucous membrane surfaces may be helpful in making a diagnosis. Many inflammatory conditions have a predilection for mucosal surfaces and special emphasis should be given to the oral cavity, conjunctiva, and anus, as well as vagina. A speculum examination to directly visualize the vagina should be attempted; however, in patients with erosive vaginal disease with or without scarring, this examination may not be possible because of discomfort. A wet mount of vaginal secretions to assess for changes suggestive of inflammation can be of great value.

In assessing the vulva, a checklist for normal structures, including the labia minora and clitoris, should be performed.[3] Some conditions may lead to resorption of the labia minora and/or scarring or adhesions, which can result in a burrowed clitoris or narrowed introitus. The location of the erosive changes should be documented.

Morphology in the vulva can be nonspecific and a skin biopsy is often necessary to make a diagnosis. If an erosion is present, it is best to take a biopsy sample from intact skin at the edge of the erosion. Biopsy for direct immunofluorescence (DIF) should also be performed in the same area. Possible pitfalls in diagnosis include biopsy into an eroded area that lacks the epidermis necessary to make the correct diagnosis. Similarly, biopsy into any advanced scarring process may lead to a nonspecific result if the active inflammation has subsided. Multiple biopsies from different regions may be necessary to show diagnostic findings. Because of the complexity of histopathologic interpretation in the skin, biopsy specimens should be sent to a dermatopathologist for evaluation. For any fissures or pustules, fungal or bacterial culture should be considered. Polymerase chain reaction (PCR) for herpes simplex virus (HSV) or varicella zoster virus may be appropriate in certain cases.

Disease-specific treatments are discussed later; however, a few general treatment recommendations can be made. For immediate care of eroded skin, soaking in plain water or Sitz bath followed by application of plain petrolatum may be helpful. Topical anesthetics, such as lidocaine 2% jelly may also provide immediate, if short-lasting, relief of symptoms. As a general rule when selecting topical treatment of erosive disease, ointments are preferred to creams because they are less irritating. Cleansing practices should be minimal, often with water sufficing. Estrogen deficiency should be addressed if present. Dilator use should be considered for erosive vaginal disease. If pruritus is a significant feature, oral medications such as hydroxyzine, doxepin, or a low-dose tricyclic antidepressant may be appropriate.

When patients are undergoing treatment of their erosive disease, patient education and close follow-up are necessary. This strategy includes monitoring for atrophy if patients are treated with superpotent topical steroids. Proper patient education on how and where to apply topical steroids should be provided, preferably with a written diagram. The vulvar trigone is relatively resistant to steroid atrophy, whereas application in other areas in the groin may lead to striae formation. When patients flare or seemingly do not respond as expected, follow-up evaluation to assess for possible infection or contact dermatitis is needed. The development of malignancy remains a concern in certain conditions such as LP and LS, and thus long-term follow-up to monitor for this complication is also essential.

LP

In diagnosing the patient with erosive disease, a familiarity with erosive LP is critical because it is one of the most common erosive conditions encountered in vulvar specialty clinics.[4,5]

Clinical Features

LP is the most common chronic erosive vulvar dermatosis. LP is generally a disease of postmenopausal women, and, although this occasionally occurs before menopause, erosive vulvar LP does not occur in children.

Usually unassociated with extragenital LP, there are 3 primary vulvar morphologies: bland, nonspecific erosions; white, interlacing striae; and white plaques/patches of epithelium that mimic LS (**Fig. 1**). All 3 forms sometimes occur together. With more advanced disease, scarring to include loss of labia minora, narrowing of the introitus, and scarring of the clitoral hood to the clitoris occur in some.

The most frequent complaints of vulvar LP are genital soreness, burning, pruritus, and dyspareunia. Vulvar LP most often is associated with oral and vaginal LP, so that reports of abnormal vaginal discharge or bleeding, and oral pain are common. The vagina can scar closed, and gingival disease progresses in some to loss of teeth.

Causes/associations

LP is believed to be a T-cell–mediated autoimmune response to an unknown antigen.[6] Patients with LP have an increased incidence of autoimmune disorders. Many different medications have been implicated in the development of lichenoid drug eruptions. Medications that are commonly implicated in cutaneous LP include angiotensin-converting enzyme inhibitors, nonsteroidal antiinflammatory drugs (NSAIDs), hydrochlorothiazide, β-blockers, antimalarials, allopurinol, and many

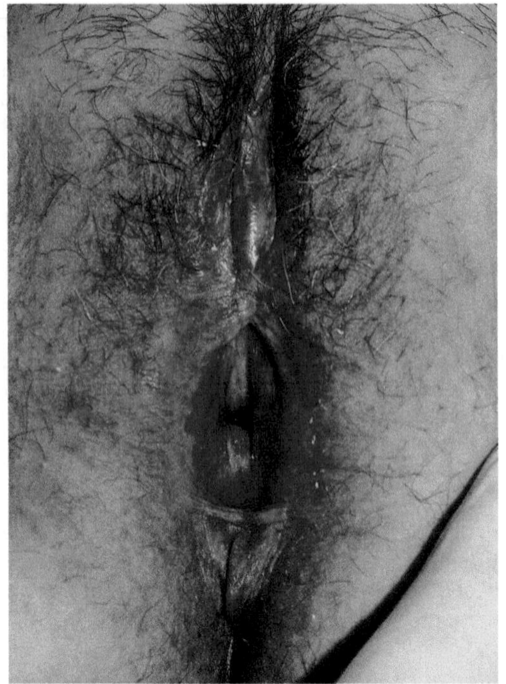

Fig. 1. Erosive vulvar LP most often presents with nonspecific erosions, particularly in the vestibule, sometimes with surrounding white epithelium or pathognomonic white, interlacing, lacy papules.

others, including tumor necrosis factor α (TNF-α) antagonists.[7,8]

Making the Diagnosis

If the lacy white surface changes known as Wickham striae are present, it may be simple to make the diagnosis by clinical examination and a skin biopsy to confirm the diagnosis. In selecting the best area to biopsy, an area of Wickham striae or white epithelium surrounding an erosion is best. However, many patients do not show white lesions. If only erosive disease is present, a biopsy from intact skin at the edge of an erosion is recommended.[9] It may be necessary to perform several biopsies in different areas if the morphology is not classic. If the biopsy is nonspecific, a biopsy for DIF should be performed as described earlier.

Histology

Routine histology shows an interface dermatitis, which is typically a lymphocytic predominant infiltrate that occurs at the dermoepidermal junction. The basal cell damage that occurs takes the form of Civatte bodies (apoptotic keratinocytes). Colloid bodies are eosinophilic structures found in the papillary dermis. In mucosal biopsies, plasma cells may also be prominent. Wedge-shaped areas of hypergranulosis, variable acanthosis, and a saw-tooth appearance of the lower epidermis may be present. DIF of involved skin shows colloid bodies in the papillary dermis with nonspecific staining for complement (C3) and immunoglobulins (Ig). An irregular band of fibrin is present along the basal layer in most patients and may extend into the papillary dermis.[10]

Disease Course

Erosive mucosal LP typically runs a chronic course with a waxing and waning pattern. Progression to scarring, particularly in patients with vulvovaginal-gingival syndrome, is common. The development of squamous cell carcinoma (SCC) is a recognized but rare phenomenon in patients with LP. The incidence of SCC with vulvar LP is uncertain but may be estimated to be between 1% and 2%.[11] Based on this malignant potential, all patients should have long-term follow-up, and any new and/or nonresponsive lesions should be biopsied.

Treatment

Treatment is crucial for these patients not only to relieve the symptoms associated with the disease but also to prevent disease progression and long-term complications such as scarring. There is a paucity of data regarding optimal management in genital LP, and most studies are limited by nonrandomized study designs and small sample size. Because LP of the genital region is not generally curable, the goals of treatment are induction and maintenance of remission. LP can often be treated with topical agents, whereas oral agents are reserved for more severe cases. Oral and topical agents are often used in tandem.

Topical steroids are considered the first-line treatment of LP. A superpotent steroid such as clobetasol propionate 0.05% ointment can be used once or twice a day as an initial treatment. For vaginal involvement, hydrocortisone 25-mg suppositories may be inserted into the vagina every other day for the first month and tapered down as able.[9] During intensive topical steroid treatment, monthly evaluation is recommended. Some experts suggest prophylaxis for candidiasis with a weekly oral dose of fluconazole 150 mg when intravaginal steroids are used.[9] For more resistant areas, intralesional triamcinolone, using a concentration between 3.3 and 10 mg/mL, may be injected locally. Pretreatment with a topical anesthetic is suggested. When the disease is under control, topical steroids are commonly used for long-term maintenance. The optimal strength of steroid and frequency of application remains to be determined. Topical calcineurin inhibitors, including tacrolimus 0.1% ointment and pimecrolimus 1% cream, are considered second-line agents when topical steroids fail.[12]

Patients with severe erosive LP often achieve insufficient benefit from topical medications. These women require systemic treatment in addition to topical corticosteroids. Other than systemic corticosteroids, there are no systemic medications that produce predictable improvement, but many have show occasional benefit. These medications include azathioprine, methotrexate, TNF-α antagonists, cyclophosphamide, cyclosporine, retinoids, hydroxychloroquine, and mycofenolate mofetil (MMF). Treatment with low-molecular-weight heparin, oral metronidazole, alefacept, and thalidomide has also been reported.[13–16] Although used in the past, griseofulvin and dapsone are considered not generally helpful.[17,18]

Surgery

Surgical intervention for scarring should be considered only when active disease is under control. Attempts at adhesiolysis should be performed only by a surgeon with expertise in caring for these patients.

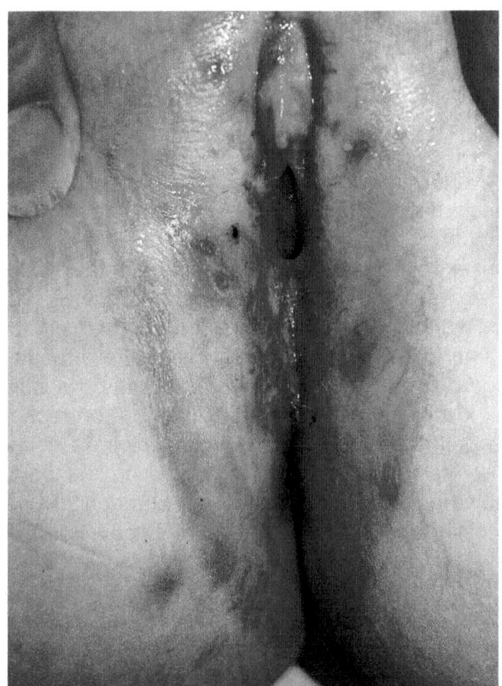

Fig. 2. LS is not primarily an erosive disease, but it is characterized by fragility and itching, so that secondary erosions and maceration are common.

LS

Clinical Features

LS is a chronic disorder that primarily affects the vulva of postmenopausal women, but occasionally occurs in premenopausal women and prepubertal girls. Patients typically complain of itching, and the fragility of LS allows purpura and tearing with scratching, with resulting pain and dyspareunia. Dysuria and pain with defecation often occur as well, particularly in pediatric patients. The classic appearance is that of white to ivory papules coalescing into plaques with a crinkled or waxy texture. LS occurs primarily on periclitoral skin and the perineal body initially but also affects the labia minora, medial labia majora, and perianal skin. Extragenital cutaneous involvement occurs occasionally, but almost never affects the mouth or vagina. Long-standing LS can lead to either resorption or fusion of the labia minora, obliteration of the clitoris, and narrowing of the introitus. Erosions occur, but are primarily from mild trauma of scratching or sexual activity, so these are most often angular or irregular, and they are migratory rather than stable and nonhealing, as occurs with LP and immunobullous disease (**Fig. 2**).

Causes/associations

LS seems to be a disease produced by multiple factors, with autoimmunity being the major cause.

Histology

Routine histology of early lesions shows an interface dermatitis with vacuolar change of the basal layer of the epidermis and may mimic LP. In addition, broad zones of subepidermal edema with homogenization of the collagen are seen. With time, the upper dermis becomes more sclerotic and the epidermis develops atrophy. Hyperkeratosis may also be seen.[10] Features favoring a diagnosis of LS rather than LP include basilar epidermotropism, basement membrane thickening, epidermal atrophy, loss of papillary dermal elastic fibers, paucity of cytoid bodies, and lack of wedge-shaped hypergranulosis.[10]

Treatment

Successful treatment of LS is typically achieved with a superpotent topical steroid, such as clobetasol proprinate 0.05% used twice a day initially and then tapered as control of symptoms is achieved. When skin normalizes, either the frequency or potency of the corticosteroid can be decreased, but discontinuation is regularly associated with recurrence. Topical tacrolimus and pimecrolimus may be used as a second-line treatment. SCC is a recognized development in about 3% of patients. The risk is greater in areas with thick, white irregular plaques, erosions, or ulcers. Patients require lifelong follow-up.

FIXED DRUG ERUPTION

Clinical Features

Several variants of fixed drug eruption (FDE) have been described, including classic and nonpigmenting.[19] FDE is characterized by the sudden onset of one or more oval, edematous, dusky red plaques on the skin or mucous membranes. The hallmark is the reappearance of the lesions in the same location with rechallenge of the offending agent. It may take about 2 weeks after the initial exposure to develop the reaction, but on rechallenge the lesions usually develop within 24 hours. The lesions may occur anywhere on the body; however, lips, face, hands, feet, and genitalia are most common. Some patients may develop vesicles or bullae that rupture, causing erosions. Patients may complain of burning or itching. Classic FDE heals with postinflammatory hyperpigmentation; nonpigmenting FDE lacks this feature. Although data are limited, vulvar FDE may more commonly present as a nonpigmenting FDE.[20] Patients with vulvar nonpigmenting FDE typically present with a symmetric vulvitis with erosive changes, with inflammation extending into the inguinal creases.[20]

Causes/associations

This dermatosis is the direct result of medication ingestion. Some of the more common causative agents include trimethoprim-sulfamethoxazole, NSAIDs, barbiturates, tetracyclines, metronidazole, griseofulvin, and carbamazepine.[21] In a case series focused specifically on vulvar FDE, ibuprofen, cyclooxygenase-2 inhibitors, 3-hydroxy-3-methylglutaryl-coenzyme reductase inhibitors, and pseudoephedrine, among others, were found to be causative.[20] There has also been a case report of fluconazole causing a vulvar FDE.[22]

Histology

Routine histology of classic FDE shows a lichenoid reaction pattern with prominent vacuolar change and Civatte body formation. In patients with nonpigmenting FDE, these findings are absent.[19,20] Nonpigmenting FDE findings may be nonspecific and include epidermal spongiosis and/or a mild perivascular and interstitial mixed inflammatory infiltrate in the dermis.[20]

Treatment

Discontinuation of the offending agent and future avoidance is the recommended treatment. Lesions typically resolve within a few weeks of medication discontinuation. Topical steroids may be used for symptomatic treatment.

STEVENS-JOHNSON SYNDROME/TOXIC EPIDERMAL NECROLYSIS

Clinical Features

The presentation of either Stevens-Johnson syndrome (SJS) or toxic epidermal necrolysis (TEN) is typically dramatic. Controversy regarding classification of these 2 syndromes remains ongoing but many believe they represent a spectrum of disease. Initial symptoms of both TEN and SJS can be fever, stinging in the eyes, and pain with swallowing.[23] These symptoms are followed by an abrupt onset of symmetric red macules, which progress to central blister formation and extensive areas of epidermal necrosis. The skin may be tender. The oral mucosa is always involved. For the diagnosis of SJS, patients must have 2 or more mucosal surfaces involved and most have some degree of skin involvement. Purulent conjunctivitis with photophobia may be present. Genital involvement with erosions of vulva or vagina may be observed (**Fig. 3**).[23] In classifying the disease, the percentage of cutaneous epidermal detachment has been used: less than 10% is consistent with SJS, 10% to 30% is considered SJS/TEN overlap, and greater than 30% is consistent with TEN. To assess degree of epidermal necrosis in early cases, tangential pressure on erythematous areas may be applied to see if epidermal detachment occurs (giving a so-called positive Nikolsky sign). In addition, generalized lymphadenopathy, enlarged liver and spleen, pneumonia, and hepatitis may be present. Electrolyte imbalances and dehydration may develop. Patients with significant skin necrosis are at risk of sepsis.

Causes/associations

Medications are commonly implicated in TEN and less so in SJS. Medications that are associated include sulfonamides, NSAIDs, and anticonvulsants.

Histology

Routine histology shows an interface reaction pattern with prominent epithelial cell necrosis. In TEN, typically there are sheets of necrosis. In SJS, the necrosis is more focal.

Treatment

Treatment remains controversial for these disorders. Supportive care is the mainstay of treatment. Patients with significant skin necrosis benefit from

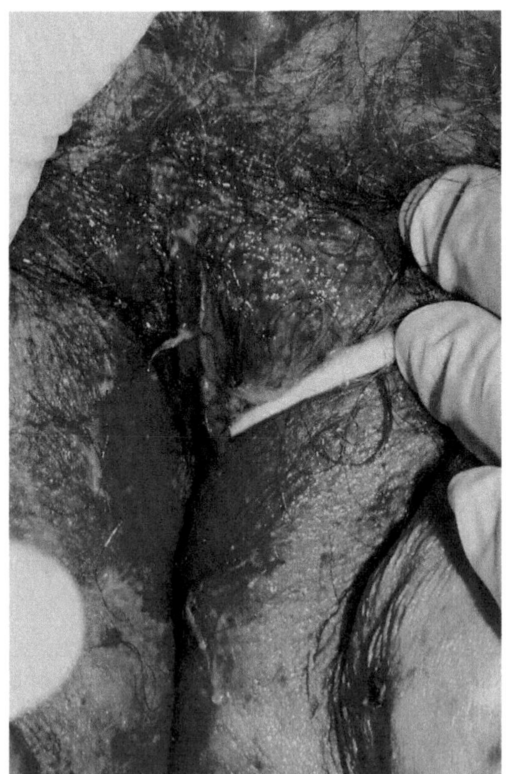

Fig. 3. This patient with TEN had bullae of keratinized skin, oral and conjunctival erosions, and sloughing of the modified mucous membranes of the vulva.

care in an intense care unit, one preferably with expertise in burns. Depending on area/organs involved, specialist care should be sought for specific recommendations. Adequate hydration, repletion of electrolytes, and nutritional support are mandatory. Simple wound care of eroded areas may include petrolatum-impregnated gauze. Any identified offending medication should be discontinued. Systemic treatment with steroids is sometimes used in SJS but remains highly controversial in TEN. Intravenous immunoglobulin used in high doses also remains controversial in the treatment of TEN.

IRRITANT AND ALLERGIC CONTACT DERMATITIS

Vulvar tissue is particularly vulnerable to irritation and sensitization. The skin of the labia shows increased hydration, occlusion, and frictional properties, which may increase susceptibility to irritants and contact sensitizers. Furthermore, the nonkeratinized vulvar vestibule is likely to be more permeable than keratinized regions.[24] Patients with an impaired barrier function, occurring in the setting of estrogen deficiency or any other underlying skin condition, are at increased risk for these complications.

Clinical Features

Typically both irritant and allergic contact dermatitis produce erythema and edema. However, severe reactions in both cases may cause erosion, or erosions may occur secondarily from scratching. Irritant contact dermatitis typically presents with stinging or burning rather than itching. Allergic contact dermatitis is a delayed immune response that typically occurs several days after allergen presentation. Itching is a typical complaint. Localized erythema with associated vesicles, bullae, and sometimes weeping is typical in the acute phase (**Fig. 4**). With repeated rubbing, the skin may become lichenified.

Causes/associations

With regards to irritant dermatitis, hygiene practices are often to blame, and the patient should be directly questioned on all cleansing routines. In addition, incontinence, sweat, douches, and topical medications, such as 5-fluorouracil, can all cause irritation. For allergic contact dermatitis, commonly reported allergens include benzocaine, diphenhydramine, neomycin, preservatives (such as benzalkonium chloride, quaternium-15, formaldehyde, and parabens), fragrances, lanolin, tea tree oil, latex, spermicides, and chlorhexidine among others.[3,24,25] Vagisil (Combe Inc, White Plains, NY), an over-the-counter topical agent marketed for vaginal itching (which contains benzocaine and resorcinol), has been shown in one series to be the most common relevant agent in causing contact dermatitis.[25] Although topical steroid allergy is a recognized phenomenon, only low reaction rates from topical steroids have

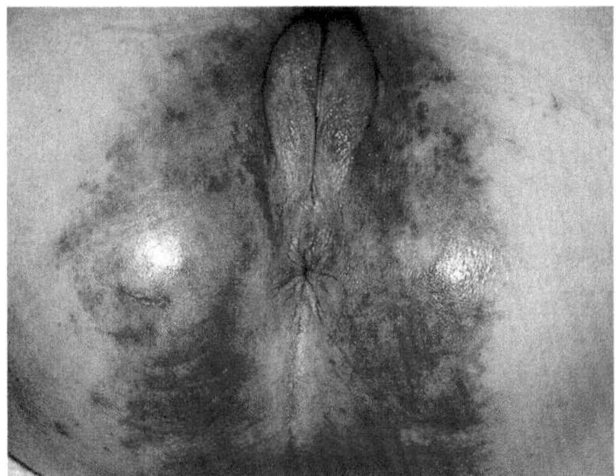

Fig. 4. This young woman with intellectual disability has an erosive irritant contact dermatitis from constant contact with urine, with superimposed linear excoriations from scratching.

been found in patch-test studies focusing on vulvar dermatoses.[26]

Histology

Biopsy is not typically indicated in these patients.

Treatment

Treatment is aimed at identifying and discontinuing the irritant or allergen. To control inflammation, a medium- to high-potency topical steroid can be used in most cases or an oral steroid in severe cases. Any factors contributing to abnormalities in barrier function such as low estrogen or underlying dermatosis must be addressed.

BULLOUS PEMPHIGOID

Clinical Features

Bullous pemphigoid (BP) is the most common autoimmune bullous disease. It is characterized by tense bullae that develop on normal and erythematous skin. Eczematous or urticarial lesions may precede the development of bullous lesions. Pruritus can be intense, and peripheral eosinophilia may be present. The mean age of onset is 65 years.[27] Lesions are typically nonscarring. Involvement of the vulva seems to be more common in children, either as a localized variant or in association with generalized BP, than in adults, based on the few case series that have been reported.[28,29]

Causes/associations

Medications that have been associated include furosemide, ibuprofen, captopril, penicillamine, and other antibiotics.[27]

Histology

Routine histology shows a subepidermal blister with variable dermal inflammatory infiltrate that usually includes eosinophils. DIF of perilesional skin shows deposition of IgG and/or C3 along the epidermal basement membrane zone. For all immunobullous diseases, DIF of biopsied skin processed using the salt-split technique and/or obtaining patient serum for indirect immunofluorescence studies may be useful when the diagnosis is in doubt. In BP, target antigens include BPAG2 (180 kDa) and BPAG1 (230 kDa).

Treatment

Treatment includes topical steroids, oral steroids, minocycline with niacinamide, dapsone, as well as azathioprine and cyclophosphamide.

CICATRICIAL PEMPHIGOID

Clinical Features

Cicatricial pemphoid (CP), also called mucous membrane pemphigoid, is a rare condition characterized by primarily mucosal vesicles, erosions, and scar formation at various sites. The typical age of presentation is 60 to 80 years. However, childhood disease is well documented.[30,31] The most commonly involved sites are oral and ocular. Genital involvement is estimated to be between 17% and 54%.[28,32] Genital lesions typically present as erosions, rather than intact vesicles, because of friction (**Fig. 5**). Cutaneous lesions may be present in about 25% of patients.[32] The cutaneous lesions often present as flaccid bullae and erosions on an erythematous base but can also resemble lesions of BP, with tense vesicles and bullae.[33] Scarring alopecia may be also present. Patients generally complain of pain and/or pruritus in the affected areas.

Causes/associations

HLA DQB1*301 allele has been shown to be increased in both oral and ocular CP.[33]

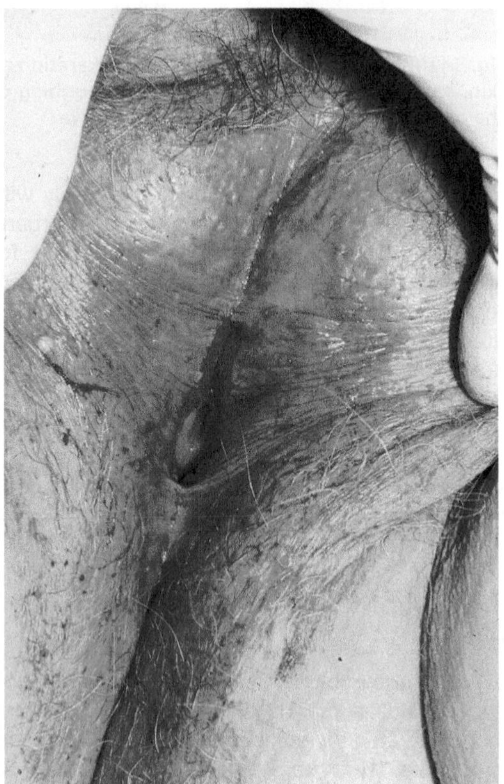

Fig. 5. Cicatricial pemphigioid produces nonspecific erosions and remarkable scarring of vulvar architecture, hence the name of cicatricial, which means scarring. This clinical picture is indistinguishable from erosive, scarring LP.

Histology

Routine histology of an intact lesion shows a subepidermal blister and a diffuse perivascular mixed inflammatory infiltrate. DIF biopsy of perilesional skin in most cases shows a linear continuous band at the basement membrane zone, comprised of IgG, C3, and to a lesser degree IgA and IgM.[33] The DIF findings are not specific and may be seen with BP, pemphigoid gestationis, epidermolysis bullosa acquisita (EBA), and bullous systemic lupus erythematosus.[33] The major antigens that are targeted are BPAG 2, β_4-integrin, and laminin-5 and 6, although others have also been described.[33]

Treatment

Successful treatment of CP presents a significant challenge. The choice of treatment is typically based on the severity, the site involved, and the rapidity of progression.[34] A classification system to stratify high- and low-risk groups has been developed. Low-risk groups include those with lesions in the oral mucosa or cutaneous surface. High-risk groups include those with disease occurring in ocular, genital, nasopharyngeal, esophageal, and laryngeal mucosa.[34] Low-risk patients may be treated with a combination of topical steroids, topical tacrolimus, or tetracycline hydrochloride (1–2 g/d) and niacinamide (2–2.5 mg/d). A consensus group[34] has recommended for rapidly progressive, high-risk patients, oral prednisone (1–1.5 mg/kg/d) plus cyclophosphamide (1–2 mg/kd/d) as an initial treatment. Alternatively, azathioprine (1–2 mg/kg/d) may be substituted. However, as the clinical efficacy of azathioprine may take several months, cyclophosphamide is preferred for acute management. Cyclophosphamide may be given as intravenous pulse therapy or continuous oral therapy.[35] Dapsone (50–200 mg/d) may be considered as an alternative and should be given for at least 3 months to determine efficacy. MMF has been anecdotally reported as helpful as well, often at a dose of 2 g/d.[35] Cyclosporine and methotrexate have been believed to be not effective.[35] Intravenous immunoglobulin has shown preliminary promise as well for treatment-resistant ocular disease.[33]

Patients with antibodies to laminin-5, termed antiepiligrin CP, have been shown to have a higher incidence of both solid cancers as well as a possible association with B-cell lymphoma and cutaneous T-cell lymphoma.[36–38] An age-appropriate cancer screening is indicated in this particular subgroup.

LINEAR IGA DISEASE

Clinical Features

Linear IgA disease (LAD) is an autoimmune vesicobullous dermatosis. This disease occurs either in children older than 5 years (previously called chronic bullous disease of childhood) or in adults older than 60 years.[38] The lesions are typically tense vesicles and bullae in clusters. In children, involvement of the genitalia is common.[38] The lesions often consist of an urticarial plaque surrounded by vesicles at the periphery, giving an appearance that has been likened to a string of pearls.[27] Oral involvement is common but ocular involvement is rare.[33]

Causes/associations

Medications that have been implicated in this disorder include lithium, vancomycin, and diclofenac.[27]

Histology

Routine histology is nonspecific and shows a subepidermal blister with a mixed inflammatory infiltrate. Papillary microabscesses are seen in about half of patients. On DIF of perilesional skin, a linear band of IgA can be seen along the epidermal basement membrane zone.[33] Other immunoreactants, such as C3 and IgG, have been reported. Target antigens include a 97-kd antigen that is identical to a portion of BPAG2 and collagen VII.[33]

Treatment

The most common treatments are dapsone or sulfapyridine. When alternative treatment is needed, systemic steroids, tetracycline with niacinamide, and intravenous immunoglobulin can be considered.[27]

BULLOUS SYSTEMIC LUPUS ERYTHEMATOSUS

Clinical Features

Bullous systemic lupus erythematosus is an uncommon variant of lupus that is most commonly described in young African American women with systemic lupus erythematosus.[33] Patients present with a nonscarring, diffuse vesiculobullous eruption on normal or inflamed skin. Erythematous plaques with annular configuration, urticarial papules, and targetoid lesions have been described.[39] A second phenotype, which is similar to classic EBA, has also been described.[39] Lesions generally occur in areas of sun exposure; however, oral and pharyngeal as well as vulvar involvement have been reported.[40] Lesions of chronic, cutaneous lupus (discoid lupus) may occur in genital skin.[41,42] However, these lesions are less likely to cause erosive changes.

Histology

Routine histology of a vesicle shows a subepidermal blister with mixed inflammatory cell infiltrate that is typically neutrophil predominant.[43] The histology of primary lupus lesions, such as epidermal atrophy, basal cell keratinocyte vacuolization, basement membrane thickening, is absent.[43] DIF of perilesional skin shows a broad, linear, or mixed linear and granular pattern at the epidermal basement membrane zone, comprised of IgG and C3. IgA and IgM may also be present.[33] The target antigen is typically type VII collagen.

Treatment

A dramatic therapeutic response to dapsone is typically seen within the first 2 to 4 days of initiation of therapy.[39]

EBA

Clinical Features

There are 2 recognized forms of EBA. The classic form is characterized by skin fragility, vesicles, and erosions that localize to mechanically stressed surfaces that tend to heal with scarring and milia formation.[44] Inflammatory variants mimicking CP, BP, and LAD disease have been described[44] and in some patients features of both forms may occur. EBA has been described in both adults and children but most cases begin in the fourth to fifth decade.[43] Mucous membrane involvement has been reported in 50% of patients.[45]

Causes/associations

Several systemic diseases have been anecdotally reported in association with EBA, including collagen vascular diseases, inflammatory bowel disease, and autoimmune disorders.

Histology

Routine histology of an intact lesion shows a subepidermal blister with or without dermal inflammation. DIF of perilesional skin shows linear IgG and/or C3 deposits along the epidermal basement membrane zone. Type VII collagen is the target antigen.

Treatment

Treatment can be challenging and often provides only temporary relief. Initial treatment may consist of high-dose systemic steroids plus other antiinflammatory or immunosuppressive agents, which may include dapsone, colchicine, methotrexate, azathioprine, cyclophosphamide, or cyclosporine. Intravenous immunoglobulin has shown some promise,[27] and rituximab has been reported helpful in case reports.[46]

PEMPHIGUS VULGARIS

Clinical Features

Pemphigus vulgaris (PV) is an autoimmune blistering disorder of the skin and mucous membranes that presents with flaccid bullae or erosions that heal without scarring (**Fig. 6**). The Nikolsky sign is often positive.[27] Age of onset is usually between 50 and 60 years. The oral mucosa is almost always affected. Lesions may also occur in the pharynx, larynx, esophagus, conjunctiva, and anal mucosa. Involvement of the female genital tract is present in about half of the patients.[47] A study of 77 women with genital PV showed that almost all patients had lesions occurring in labia minora, 36% had vaginal involvement, and 15% had cervical involvement.[47] Pap smears obtained from patients with cervical PV may show acantholytic suprabasal cells showing dyskeratotic changes indistinguishable from cervical intraepithelial neoplasia.[6] It is recommended that a conventional Pap smear be performed to follow up any abnormality found on the newer and more

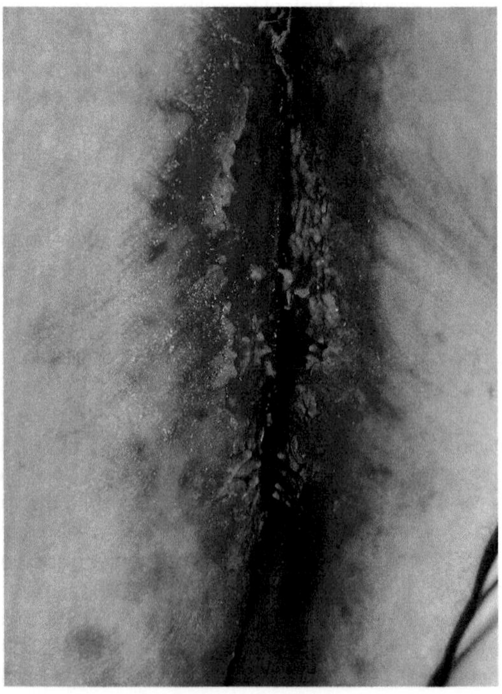

Fig. 6. PV produces flaccid bullae that quickly erode, as has occurred in the gluteal cleft of this woman, producing maceration and recurrent infection.

commonly performed liquid-based Pap smears.[47] True malignant change also remains a concern. There are reports of microinvasive SCC of the cervix in association with cervical PV.[48]

Causes/associations

Drug-induced pemphigus may occur and has been associated with penicillamine, captopril, penicillin, ceftazidime, rifampin, β-blockers, progesterone, heroin, and pyrazole compounds.[27]

Histology

Routine histology of a lesion shows suprabasal acantholysis of keratinocytes. However, the basal cells remain attached to the basement membrane, which can give the appearance of a tombstone row. DIF of perilesional skin shows IgG bound to the keratinocyte cell surface. The presence of autoantibodies varies on the areas involved. Mucosal involvement is associated with antibodies to desmoglein 3 when cutaneous involvement is associated with antibodies to desmoglein 1.

Treatment

For limited disease, topical steroids may be used. For more widespread disease, systemic treatment with high-dose steroids alongside dapsone, azathioprine, cyclophosphamide, methotrexate, and MMF should be considered. Intravenous immunoglobulin and rituximab have been used in refractory cases.[27,46]

PARANEOPLASTIC PEMPHIGUS

Clinical Signs and Symptoms

Paraneoplastic pemphigus (PNP) is an autoimmune syndrome that occurs in patients with an underlying neoplasm, usually lymphoreticular in origin. PNP is characterized by severe oral and ocular erosions. Genital involvement is a common feature.[49] The cutaneous lesions may be polymorphic and may present as target lesions suggestive of erythema multiforme, vesicobullous lesions suggestive of BP, or LP-like violaceous papules.

Causes/association

PNP is associated with underlying neoplasms. Lymphoma, chronic lymphoid leukemia, Castleman tumor, and thymoma have all been associated.[50]

Histology

Routine histology may show a variety of features that may include an interface dermatitis, keratinocyte necrosis, or intraepidermal acantholysis. On DIF, deposition of IgG and C3 on the keratinocyte cell surface is always seen and a granular/linear deposition of C3 along the basement membrane zone can sometimes be seen. In contrast to other forms of pemphigus, indirect immunofluoresence study using rat bladder as a substrate is typically positive. Target antigens include desmoplakin I and II, BPAG1, envoplakin, periplakin, plectin, desmoglein 1 and 3, and an uncharacterized 170-kd protein.[33]

Treatment

Treatment includes oral steroids as well as adjuvant immunosuppressive/immunomodulatory agents (cyclophosphamide, dapsone, plasmapheresis, and rituximab). Treating the underlying neoplasm should also be attempted. The prognosis is generally poor when associated with malignancy.

INFECTIONS

Candidiasis

Candidal infections are usually caused by the yeast *Candida albicans*. Local factors such as incontinence, sweat, and heat provide a favorable environment. Diabetes, administration of oral antibiotics, and immunosuppression (including topical steroids, which may be used to treat many of the conditions described earlier) can all be risk factors. Typically, red plaques within skin folds are seen (**Fig. 7**). Satellite pustules may be present. When

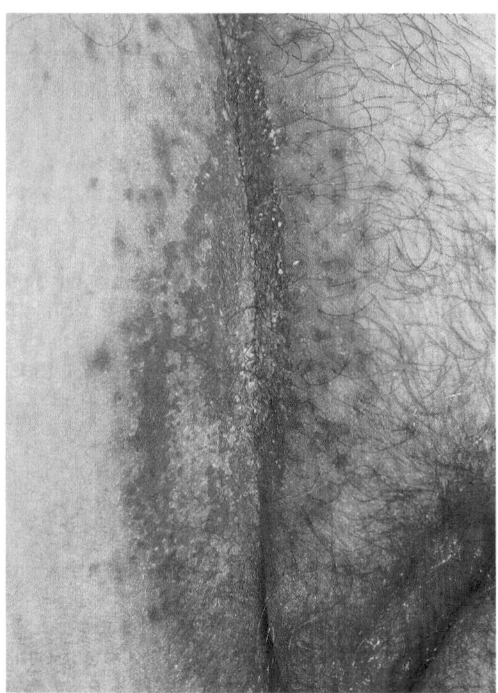

Fig. 7. Severe candidiasis presents as eroded plaques with satellite papules and pustules.

superficial pustules coalesce and rupture, an erosion may be seen. Fissures may also be present. One series found approximately 25% of patients had fissures present.[51] Vulvovaginal candidal infections are typically found in estrogenized tissue and are thus uncommon in prepubertal girls.[52] A skin scraping shows hyphae, pseudohyphae, and budding yeast. Depending on affected areas, a topical antifungal such as nystatin or an azole may be used. For eroded areas, nystatin may be preferable because this is the only available antifungal that comes as an ointment. Oral treatment with fluconazole is an alternative.

Herpetic Infections

Herpetic infections are characterized by grouped vesicles that may rupture, causing erosion. There may be a prodrome of local burning or itching. Genital herpes infections (which may be caused by HSV type 2 and less commonly type 1) are common, and most clinicians are familiar with their presentation. Rarely, morphologically atypical forms may be seen such as a single ulcer, single erosion, or fissure.[53] The possibility of herpes zoster, caused by the varicella zoster virus, should also be kept in mind. Diagnosis is most rapidly made with PCR performed on a swab taken from the base of a ruptured vesicle. Treatment of HSV includes patient education, early treatment of lesions with oral antivirals such as acyclovir, and suppressive treatment when appropriate. Treatment of herpes zoster includes oral antiviral if treatment can be initiated within 72 hours of development of lesions, with the hope that postherpetic neuralgia may be prevented.

Impetigo

Impetigo is a superficial bacterial infection that may be caused by *Staphylococcus aureus* or *Streptococcus pyogenes*. It may present with honey-colored crusted areas or it may be bullous. The bullous lesions are fragile and often a collarette of scale may be the only finding seen. Diagnosis may be confirmed by skin swab culture. Treatment is either with mupirocin 2% ointment or oral antibiotic, such as cephalexin.

MALIGNANCY

In the setting of malignancy, the skin may become more friable, leading to erosive or ulcerative changes. SCC accounts for most genital cancers and is often associated with a chronic inflammatory disorder such as LP or LS. The lesion may appear as a firm red or skin-colored papule or plaque that may erode or ulcerate. VIN may present in a variety of forms. It may appear similar to viral warts or it may be a pigmented or erythematous eroded plaque (**Fig. 8**). Basal cell carcinoma rarely occurs in genital skin. It typically presents as pearly translucent papule with telangiectasias. A rolled border may be present. Extramammary Paget disease is an uncommon neoplasm that develops in areas of high density of apocrine glands. It presents as a slow-growing red plaque, which may erode. Pruritus is a prominent feature.

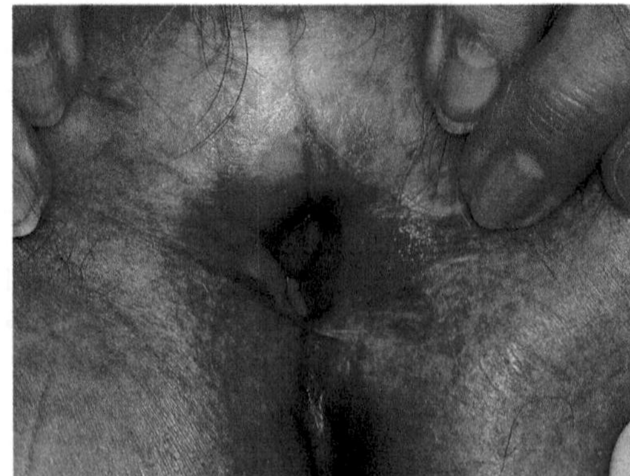

Fig. 8. VIN often presents with deep red, glistening plaques that appear eroded, as has occurred in this patient with underlying LS.

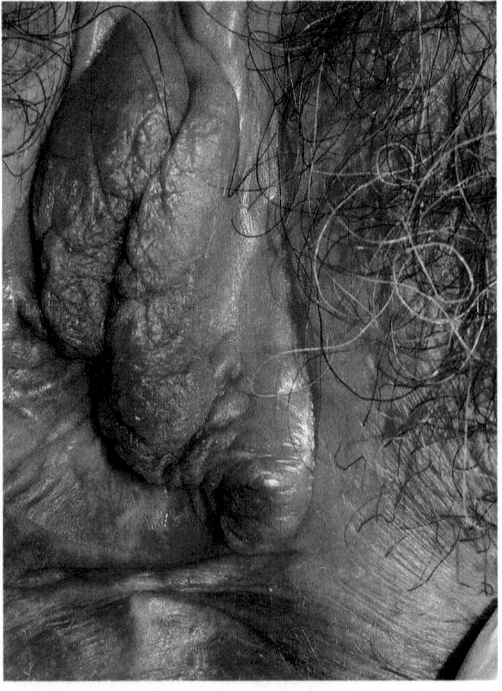

Fig. 9. Fine, linear fissures in skin folds occur with any inflammatory process; *Candida* is the most common cause.

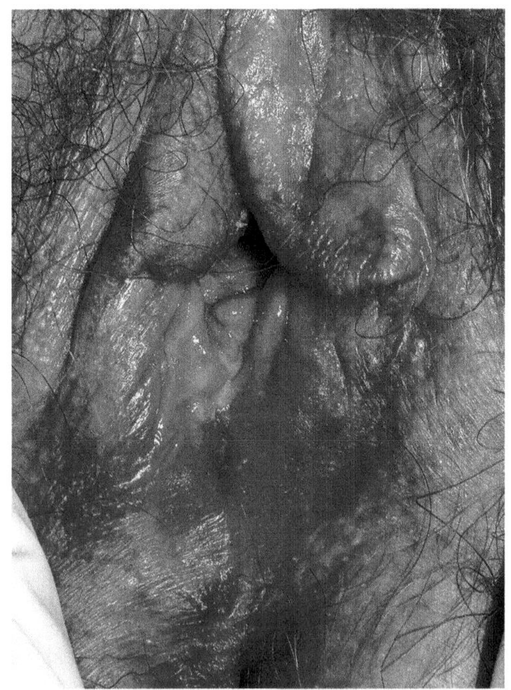

Fig. 10. Recurrent posterior fourchette fissuring with sexual intercourse is a common, painful condition of unknown cause; this generally requires surgery in the form of a perineoplasty, because simple excision with suture closure worsens the splitting.

In some patients, an underlying adenocarcinoma is found. Surgical excision is the mainstay for all invasive malignancies. Imiquimod has shown promise for usual VIN.[54] Langerhans cell histiocytosis is a rare disorder that typically presents in children younger than 2 years. Erythematous papules, pustules, and vesicles occur in the scalp, flexural areas, and perineum.

FISSURES

Fissures are fine linear erosions, which can be painful. These fissures can occur in the setting of infection, lichen simplex chronicus, inadequate estrogen, or trauma (**Fig. 9**).[55] Candidiasis is the most common infection, and typical associated erythema and pustules may or may not be present. Infection with *Streptococcus pyogenes* as well as less commonly *Staphylococcus aureus* or *Streptococcus agalactiae* may be causative.[45] In the setting of lichen simplex chronicus (which may be secondary to any number of causes), the skin is hyperkeratotic and in moist areas appears white. Fissuring may develop within these areas. Posterior fourchette fissuring may occur in the setting of sexual intercourse (**Fig. 10**). Increasing lubrication during sexual activity, topical estrogen cream when appropriate, or surgical treatment are options in this setting.

SUMMARY

This article provides an overview of the most common conditions that present with erosive disease in the vulva. Diagnostic evaluation includes a detailed history and complete physical examination. These conditions sometimes have a nonspecific appearance and skin biopsy is often required. More than one problem can occur in the vulva, with infection, contact dermatitis, and estrogen deficiency complicating treatment. Patients with erosive disease require close follow-up to monitor for side effects of treatment, disease progression, and malignancy.

REFERENCES

1. Cooper SM, Ali I, Baldo M, et al. The association of lichen sclerosus and erosive lichen planus of the vulva with autoimmune disease: a case-control study. Arch Dermatol 2008;144:1432.
2. Lundqvist EN, Wahlin YB, Bergdahl M, et al. Psychological health in patients with genital and oral erosive lichen planus. J Eur Acad Dermatol Venereol 2006; 20:661.
3. Margesson LJ. Vulvar disease pearls. Dermatol Clin 2006;24:145.
4. Hansen A, Carr K, Jensen JT. Characteristics and initial diagnoses in women presenting to a referral center for vulvovaginal disorders in 1996–2000. J Reprod Med 2002;47:854.
5. Micheletti L, Preti M, Bogliatto F, et al. Vulval lichen planus in the practice of a vulval clinic. Br J Dermatol 2000;143:1349.
6. Batta K, Munday PE, Tatnall FM. Pemphigus vulgaris localized to the vagina presenting as chronic vaginal discharge. Br J Dermatol 1999;140:945.
7. Asarch A, Gottlieb AB, Lee J, et al. Lichen planus-like eruptions: an emerging side effect of tumor necrosis factor-alpha antagonists. J Am Acad Dermatol 2009;61:104.
8. Boyd AS, Neldner KH. Lichen planus. J Am Acad Dermatol 1991;25:593.
9. Buell C, Koo J. Long-term safety of mycophenolate mofetil and cyclosporine: a review. J Drugs Dermatol 2008;7:741.
10. Weedon D, Strutton G. Skin pathology. New York. 2nd edition. London: Churchill Livingstone; 2002.
11. Kirtschig G, Wakelin SH, Wojnarowska F. Mucosal vulval lichen planus: outcome, clinical and laboratory features. J Eur Acad Dermatol Venereol 2005; 19:301.

12. Goldstein AT, Thaci D, Luger T. Topical calcineurin inhibitors for the treatment of vulvar dermatoses. Eur J Obstet Gynecol Reprod Biol 2009;146:22.
13. Buyuk AY, Kavala M. Oral metronidazole treatment of lichen planus. J Am Acad Dermatol 2000;43:260.
14. Camisa C, Allen CM. Treatment of oral erosive lichen planus with systemic isotretinoin. Oral Surg Oral Med Oral Pathol 1986;62:393.
15. Fivenson DP, Mathes B. Treatment of generalized lichen planus with alefacept. Arch Dermatol 2006;142:151.
16. Pacheco H, Kerdel F. Successful treatment of lichen planus with low-molecular-weight heparin: a case series of seven patients. J Dermatolog Treat 2001;12:123.
17. Rogers RS 3rd, Eisen D. Erosive oral lichen planus with genital lesions: the vulvovaginal-gingival syndrome and the peno-gingival syndrome. Dermatol Clin 2003;21:91.
18. Smith YR, Haefner HK. Vulvar lichen sclerosus: pathophysiology and treatment. Am J Clin Dermatol 2004;5:105.
19. Shelley WB, Shelley ED. Nonpigmenting fixed drug eruption as a distinctive reaction pattern: examples caused by sensitivity to pseudoephedrine hydrochloride and tetrahydrozoline. J Am Acad Dermatol 1987;17:403.
20. Fischer G. Vulvar fixed drug eruption. A report of 13 cases. J Reprod Med 2007;52:81.
21. Sehgal VN, Srivastava G. Fixed drug eruption (FDE): changing scenario of incriminating drugs. Int J Dermatol 2006;45:897.
22. Wain EM, Neill S. Fixed drug eruption of the vulva secondary to fluconazole. Clin Exp Dermatol 2008;33:784.
23. Bolognia J, Jorizzo JL, Rapini RP. Dermatology. New York. London: Mosby; 2003.
24. Farage MA. Vulvar susceptibility to contact irritants and allergens: a review. Arch Gynecol Obstet 2005;272:167.
25. Haverhoek E, Reid C, Gordon L, et al. Prospective study of patch testing in patients with vulval pruritus. Australas J Dermatol 2008;49:80.
26. Marren P, Wojnarowska F, Powell S. Allergic contact dermatitis and vulvar dermatoses. Br J Dermatol 1992;126:52.
27. Yeh SW, Ahmed B, Sami N, et al. Blistering disorders: diagnosis and treatment. Dermatol Ther 2003;16:214.
28. Marren P, Wojnarowska F, Venning V, et al. Vulvar involvement in autoimmune bullous diseases. J Reprod Med 1993;38:101.
29. Urano S. Localized bullous pemphigoid of the vulva. J Dermatol 1996;23:580.
30. Farrell AM, Kirtschig G, Dalziel KL, et al. Childhood vulval pemphigoid: a clinical and immunopathological study of five patients. Br J Dermatol 1999;140:308.
31. Hoque SR, Patel M, Farrell AM. Childhood cicatricial pemphigoid confined to the vulva. Clin Exp Dermatol 2006;31:63.
32. Ahmed AR, Hombal SM. Cicatricial pemphigoid. Int J Dermatol 1986;25:90.
33. Fleming TE, Korman NJ. Cicatricial pemphigoid. J Am Acad Dermatol 2000;43:571.
34. Chan LS, Ahmed AR, Anhalt GJ, et al. The first international consensus on mucous membrane pemphigoid: definition, diagnostic criteria, pathogenic factors, medical treatment, and prognostic indicators. Arch Dermatol 2002;138:370.
35. Sacher C, Hunzelmann N. Cicatricial pemphigoid (mucous membrane pemphigoid): current and emerging therapeutic approaches. Am J Clin Dermatol 2005;6:93.
36. Gibson GE, Daoud MS, Pittelkow MR. Anti-epiligrin (laminin 5) cicatricial pemphigoid and lung carcinoma: coincidence or association? Br J Dermatol 1997;137:780.
37. Sadler E, Lazarova Z, Sarasombath P, et al. A widening perspective regarding the relationship between anti-epiligrin cicatricial pemphigoid and cancer. J Dermatol Sci 2007;47:1.
38. Patricio P, Ferreira C, Gomes MM, et al. Autoimmune bullous dermatoses: a review. Ann N Y Acad Sci 2009;1173:203.
39. Vassileva S. Bullous systemic lupus erythematosus. Clin Dermatol 2004;22:129.
40. Kettler AH, Bean SF, Duffy JO, et al. Systemic lupus erythematosus presenting as a bullous eruption in a child. Arch Dermatol 1988;124:1083.
41. Burge SM, Frith PA, Juniper RP, et al. Mucosal involvement in systemic and chronic cutaneous lupus erythematosus. Br J Dermatol 1989;121:727.
42. Jolly M, Patel P. Looking beyond the ordinary: genital lupus. Arthritis Rheum 2006;55:821.
43. Gammon WR, Briggaman RA. Epidermolysis bullosa acquisita and bullous systemic lupus erythematosus. Diseases of autoimmunity to type VII collagen. Dermatol Clin 1993;11:535.
44. Schmidt E, Hopfner B, Chen M, et al. Childhood epidermolysis bullosa acquisita: a novel variant with reactivity to all three structural domains of type VII collagen. Br J Dermatol 2002;147:592.
45. Edwards L. Genital dermatology atlas. Philadelphia: Lippincott Williams & Wilkins; 2004.
46. Schmidt E, Hunzelmann N, Zillikens D, et al. Rituximab in refractory autoimmune bullous diseases. Clin Exp Dermatol 2006;31:503.
47. Akhyani M, Chams-Davatchi C, Naraghi Z, et al. Cervicovaginal involvement in pemphigus vulgaris: a clinical study of 77 cases. Br J Dermatol 2008;158:478.
48. Dvoretsky PM, Bonfiglio TA, Patten SF Jr, et al. Pemphigus vulgaris and microinvasive squamous-cell carcinoma of the uterine cervix. Acta Cytol 1985;29:403.

49. Tilakaratne W, Dissanayake M. Paraneoplastic pemphigus: a case report and review of literature. Oral Dis 2005;11:326.
50. Joly P, Richard C, Gilbert D, et al. Sensitivity and specificity of clinical, histologic, and immunologic features in the diagnosis of paraneoplastic pemphigus. J Am Acad Dermatol 2000;43:619.
51. Eckert LO, Hawes SE, Stevens CE, et al. Vulvovaginal candidiasis: clinical manifestations, risk factors, management algorithm. Obstet Gynecol 1998;92:757.
52. Fischer G, Rogers M. Vulvar disease in children: a clinical audit of 130 cases. Pediatr Dermatol 2000;17:1.
53. Lautenschlager S, Eichmann A. The heterogeneous clinical spectrum of genital herpes. Dermatology 2001;202:211.
54. van Seters M, van Beurden M, ten Kate FJ, et al. Treatment of vulvar intraepithelial neoplasia with topical imiquimod. N Engl J Med 2008;358:1465.
55. Lynch PJ, Edwards L. Genital dermatology. New York: Churchill Livingstone; 1994.

Diagnosis and Management of Vulvar Ulcers

Grace D. Bandow, MD[a,b]

KEYWORDS

- Genital ulceration • Aphthae • Vulva • Ulcers
- Behçet's disease • Crohn's disease

ULCERS VERSUS EROSIONS

Ulcers should be differentiated from erosions both clinically and histologically. This is accomplished on the basis of depth. An erosion is a defect in the epidermis only, resulting in a red, smooth, moist, superficial, atrophic plaque. Ulcers are deeper, extending into the underlying dermis, and appear necrotic at the base with either yellow, fibrinous material or an eschar adherent to it. Large, deep, or long-standing ulcers heal with scarring, while erosions and superficial ulcers typically heal without scarring. Erosive diseases of the vulva are reviewed elsewhere.

TYPES OF ULCERS

Causes of vulvar ulcers are diverse and can be divided into infectious and noninfectious categories. Infectious causes include primary syphilis, lymphogranuloma venereum (LGV), chancroid, granuloma inguinale (GI), and herpes simplex virus (HSV). In the United States, HSV is the most common of these. Noninfectious ulcers include those caused by drug reactions or adverse effects, autoimmune or inflammatory disease, trauma, and aphthous ulcers.

Aphthous Ulcers

Oral aphthae (aphthosis, aphthous stomatitis, recurrent aphthous ulcers) have similar characteristics to vulvar aphthae. Commonly known as cancer sores, they are painful, recurring lesions of the oral mucous membranes. This is the most common lesion affecting oral mucosa, occurring in up to 20% of the general population and 60% of select groups.[1–3] They are typically very tender and can become painful enough to interfere with speech, mastication, or swallowing.[4]

Both oral and vulvar aphthae have been classified into three groups: minor, major, and herpetiform.[5] Minor aphthae are smaller than 1 cm and heal within 7 to 10 days without scarring. Major aphthae are greater than 1 cm, deep, extremely painful, and heal with scarring in 10 to 30 days. Herpetiform aphthae are multiple, grouped, small ulcers that heal without scarring, and despite the name, are not associated with HSV.

Aphthae are classified further based on clinical course, as either simple or complex. Most patients have simple aphthosis, or several episodes per year of either minor, major, or herpetiform aphthae separated by disease-free periods. Complex aphthosis is defined as either almost constant presence of three or more ulcers, or recurrent oral and genital aphthae and exclusion of Behçet's disease (BD).[6]

Vulvar aphthae are thought to be relatively rare, and they are reported infrequently. Clinicians who specialize in caring for women and girls with vulvar disease, however, believe that vulvar aphthae are, in fact, not rare. Although studies looking at incidence and characteristics of vulvar aphthae are few, authors agree that most cases meet criteria for major aphthae (>1 cm). Some patients can further be classified as having complex aphthosis, because they have recurrent vulvar ulcers and concurrent oral ulcers in the absence of other features of BD.

This work was not supported by a grant or other funding source.
[a] Dermpath Diagnostics, 100 Midland Avenue, Port Chester, NY 10573, USA
[b] Department of Dermatology, Columbia University, 161 Fort Washington Avenue, 12th Floor, New York City, NY 10032, USA
E-mail address: gracebandow@gmail.com

Dermatol Clin 28 (2010) 753–763
doi:10.1016/j.det.2010.08.008
0733-8635/10/$ – see front matter

In the case of vulvar aphthae, keratinized, hair-bearing, as well as mucosal skin can be involved. Reported sites include the vagina, introitus, forchette, labia minora, labia majora, and perineal body. The most common location is the medial aspect of the labia minora, often presenting bilaterally on opposing labial surfaces as "kissing aphthae" (**Figs. 1** and **2**).[7,8] Ulcers are typically 1 to 2 mm deep with well-demarcated, ragged borders. Borders can become overhanging and heaped up, sometimes simulating an ulcerated malignant tumor. The base of the ulcer ranges from black, necrotic tissue, to gray or yellow adherent exudates. The surrounding skin is usually erythematous, edematous, warm, and tender. Associated regional lymphadenopathy and cellulitis can occur.

As with the oral variant, the cause of vulvar aphthae is not known and even less well studied. They can occur in adult women, but are more common in adolescent or premenarchal girls who are neither sexually active/abused, nor immunocompromised. Their discovery can be alarming and often precipitates an anxiety-provoking, costly, and unsuccessful search for sexual abuse or sexually transmitted infections. Patients and even many clinicians do not recognize noninfectious causes of vulvar ulcers; education about this entity is essential.

Lipschutz first reported vulvar aphthae in 1913 in adolescent girls in whom no specific cause was identified.[9] Many authors have questioned the association with a viral infection, based on frequently associated antecedent fever, myalgias, and malaise. Epstein-Barr virus (EBV) has been most commonly implicated. Halvorsen and colleagues identified and reviewed 26 individual case reports of EBV-associated aphthae, a diagnosis which was supported by initial and convalescent antibody titers and Monospot testing.[10] Few reports describe isolation of EBV directly from the base of the ulcer either by culture or by polymerase chain reaction (PCR).[8,10,11]

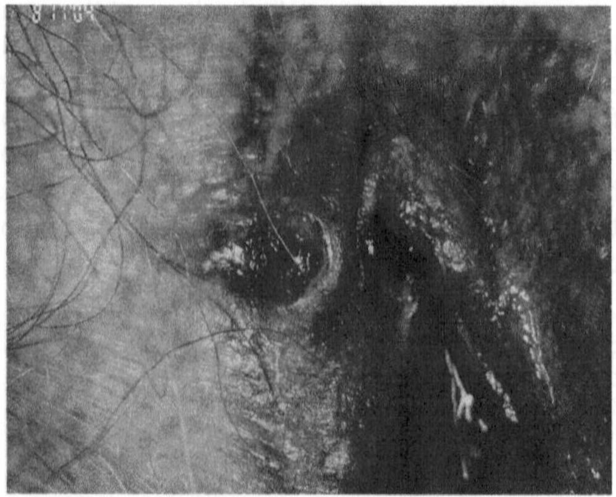

Fig. 1. Vulvar aphthous ulcer in a teenage girl.

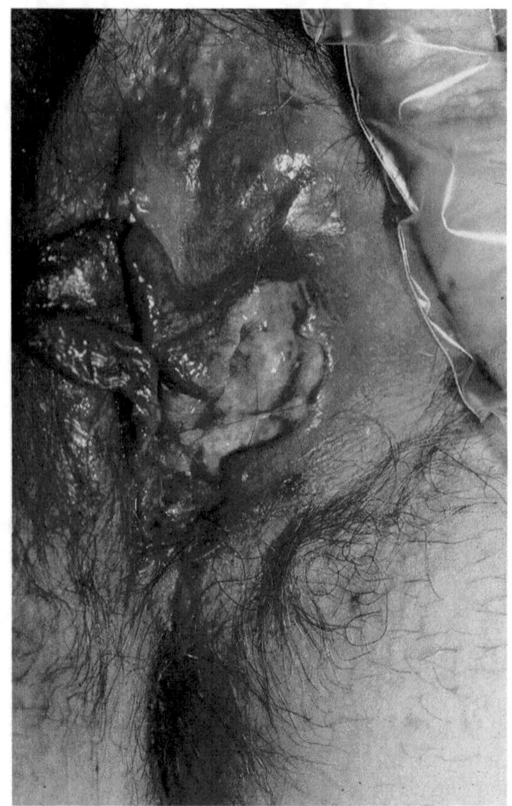

Fig. 2. Vulvar aphthous ulcer in a woman.

Various theories have been postulated to explain the development of vulvar ulcers associated with EBV. EBV is a ubiquitous virus, and both the oropharynx and genital tract have been shown to harbor EBV even in the absence of symptoms.[12] Therefore, direct transmission from sexual partners, either by genital–genital or orogenital contact, has been suggested as the cause.[13] Many of the reported cases, however, occurred in patients before the onset of any kind of sexual activity. Of 26 reported cases, only 6 reported prior sexual activity.[10] It has been postulated, based on these cases, that either autoinoculation or hematogenous spread from the patient's own oropharyngeal infection is the source for these vulvar lesions.[8,14,15]

Efforts to prove an association with specific viruses or other infections in larger cohorts have failed to confirm this theory. In a retrospective review of nine patients with nonsexually transmitted vulvar ulcers, eight of whom were premenarchal, none had evidence for EBV infection.[16] In a larger review 2 years later, Huppert and colleagues[7] studied 20 patients with vulvar aphthae, 5 of whom were premenarchal. Although 7 out of 20 patients appeared ill on initial examination, and 19 out of 20 had systemic complaints compatible with a viral illness (the most common being fever, malaise, and headache); only 2 had acute EBV and 2 had possible (equivocal) cytomegalovirus (CMV) infections. A thorough search for bacterial and fungal infections was negative in all study participants.

Other viruses have been implicated in vulvar aphthae. One author reported the case of a 13-year-old girl with influenza A and concomitant major vulvar aphthae. However, the patient had a recurrence of the lesions 2 months after the initial infection without a systemic viral illness.[17] There is one report of a large ulcer of the labium minus associated with typhoid fever (*Salmonella paratyphi*) in a 25-year-old woman with a recent travel history.[18] Most likely, many different viral infections, either respiratory or gastrointestinal, can precipitate vulvar aphthae, making a specific search extremely difficult.

Noninfectious causes have also been sought to explain vulvar aphthae in young girls. Friction and occlusion from tight-fitting clothing has been proposed as a physical cause in this group. Cebesoy and colleagues[19] noted that 10 out of 10 premenarchal girls between the ages of 9 and 13 with vulvar aphthae associated with no known cause or underlying systemic illness reported frequently wearing tight-fitting pants or polyester underwear. Seven out of 10 had kissing ulcers, and authors proposed that chronic irritation was possibly playing a role.

Evaluation of Vulvar Aphthae

The most important aspect of the evaluation of a patient with vulvar aphthae is a complete history and physical examination, with particular attention to signs or symptoms of an underlying associated systemic condition: BD human immunodeficiency virus (HIV), malabsorption, ulcerative colitis, Crohn's disease (CD), celiac disease, cyclic neutropenia, periodic fever syndromes, and leukemia. Regardless of the debate over a true association with a recent viral infection, signs and symptoms such as fever, malaise, myalgias, upper respiratory disease, and gastrointestinal symptoms should be elicited. Questions pertaining to triggering factors or exposures such as trauma, abuse, and sexually transmitted infections should be posed carefully. Excluding BD becomes important in patients who have recurrent oral and vulvar ulcers, and may not be possible on the first episode. This is discussed in greater detail. Obtaining a detailed history may not reveal an underlying etiology, and this should not discourage the patient or physician. Patients and parents should be reassured that vulvar aphthae are similar to oral aphthae in that a cause is often not identified.

An extensive laboratory work-up is often undertaken, creating great anxiety on the part of the patient and parents, and generating enormous, unnecessary medical expense. These searches are usually futile and should be tailored to the history and examination. Excluding HSV with viral culture or PCR is prudent. In sexually active or high-risk patients, screening for syphilis and HIV is appropriate. LGV, GI and chancroid are rare in the United States and should only be pursued in cases with a high index of suspicion. Based on current literature, search for EBV and CMV is not recommended. Routine bacterial and fungal cultures reveal skin flora or nonpathogenic bacteria and do not add benefit.

Obtaining a biopsy may be difficult, particularly in a young patient. Results are typically nonspecific: chronic active inflammation and necrosis without vasculitis.[15,20] If a biopsy is performed, care should be taken to obtain a full-thickness punch or incisional specimen that includes skin from the periphery of the ulcer, rather than from the center of the lesion. In a high-risk patient in whom infection is suspected, biopsy with special staining for organisms can be a helpful way to make the diagnosis.

Chronic or recurrent vulvar aphthae in the absence of HIV, cyclic neutropenia, inflammatory bowel disease, or BD (primary complex aphthosis) is rare. Therefore, search for an underlying cause (secondary complex aphthosis) should be thorough. Continuous management to assess for the evolution for BD is essential, since patients may initially present with vulvar aphthae, and later meet criteria for BD. Similar to the evaluation for primary, isolated episode of vulvar aphthae, history and physical examination are the most important components of a work-up for chronic or recurrent aphthae.

Laboratory evaluation of chronic vulvar aphthae should include HSV PCR or culture and HIV testing. Neutropenia and hematologic deficiencies should be ruled out with a complete blood count with differential, serum iron, folate, zinc, and vitamin B12.[1] Consider searching for celiac with antibody testing and HLA-B27 for BD.[21,22]

Treatment of Vulvar Aphthae

Many treatments for oral aphthae have not been rigorously studied and for vulvar aphthae have not been studied at all. Therefore, treatment of vulvar aphthae is based on that of oral aphthae, case reports, and mostly anecdotal experience. National registries and randomized trials are needed to assess the benefit of various treatment modalities.

The main components of treatment are supportive care, including adequate pain management, and the reduction of ulcer duration. Treatment of recurrent or chronic ulcers is directed at resolution and prevention.

Supportive care begins with patient and parent reassurance that aphthae are not infectious, communicable, or sexually transmitted. Making the comparison with more commonly known "canker sores" can be helpful. Rest and proper fluid and nutrition are recommended, especially in the setting of systemic symptoms. Twice daily sitz baths in plain, warm water are the best method for gentle cleansing. Cleansing with a hand-held shower head is a good alternative. Soaps and other topical over-the-counter agents are not tolerated and should be discouraged because of their irritant or allergic potential.

Pain can be severe and must be addressed adequately. Barrier agents are helpful in managing painful ulcers. Orabase (carmellose sodium) is a denture adhesive paste that provides a barrier. It can be used either alone or compounded with a topical corticosteroid.

Developed in the 1980s, sucralfate is a basic aluminum salt of sucrose octasulfate, which binds preferentially to proteins on ulcerated tissue and promotes healing by multiple different mechanisms. It has antibacterial properties,[23,24] stimulates fibroblast and keratinocyte proliferation,[25] and promotes angiogenesis.[26] Sucralfate has been extensively studied for use in disease of the gastrointestinal tract, mostly peptic ulcer disease. Given its success in this area, clinicians have adopted it for treating a myriad of other erosive and ulcerative conditions including burns,[27] chronic venous ulcers,[28] and severe adult erosive diaper dermatitis.[29] There is one published report of its successful use in three patients with vaginal ulcerations caused by pessary use, laser ablation, and an ulcer of unknown etiology.[30] These patients were treated with sucralfate 10% suspension douches twice daily and experienced complete resolution of long-standing ulcers that had been refractory to previous treatments. Similar to Orabase, sucralfate also can be compounded with a topical steroid.

Polyvinylpyrrolidone–sodium hyaluronate gel (Gelclair) is a viscous oral gel with two barrier-forming ingredients that adhere to mucosal surface. It is a class 1 medical device approved in 2001. Since that time, multiple studies have shown its efficacy in relieving pain secondary to oral mucositis from chemotherapy.[31] One open trial of 30 patients, including 4 with severe diffuse aphthae of unknown cause and 10 with severe acquired immunodeficiency syndrome (AIDS)-associated oral lesions noted significant reduction in pain scores at 5 to 7 hours and at 1 week after use.[32] This is a novel and interesting agent that could also be evaluated for pain control in vulvar ulcers.

Topical anesthesia is the second important component of pain management, and can be delivered in a number of formulations. Various compounded topical "caine" anesthetics are effective. Lidocaine can be dispensed to the patient for use at home up to four times daily in various preparations and vehicles: 2% gel, spray, or viscous solution; 4% cream; or 5% ointment. Gel or ointment is preferred. Huppert describes success with benzocaine 20% oral gel.[7]

External dysuria can be severe. Voiding under water in a bathtub and use of topical anesthetics and barrier agents before micturition are helpful solutions.

Pain can be managed with nonsteroidal anti-inflammatory drugs or oral narcotic agents. Some patients, particularly young girls, may require short hospitalization for effective pain management, placement of a Foley catheter, rest, and wound care. Patients who appear to have secondary cellulitis of surrounding tissue warrant antibiotics.

While the immunopathogenesis of aphthae is poorly understood, medical treatment is directed at diminishing inflammation. Of the topical agents available, a potent inhibitor of inflammatory mediators, amlexanox 5% oral paste (Aphthasol), is the most extensively studied. For oral aphthae, it is superior to both placebo paste and to no treatment at all for reduction of pain, ulcer size, and ulcer duration.[33] Additional benefit can be obtained by starting the paste at the onset of prodromal symptoms rather than waiting for active ulceration.[34] Using this method, Murray and colleagues found that only 35% of patients who treated mucosa with prodromal symptoms went on to develop an ulcer, and healing time was 4.1 days faster in those who did develop an ulcer. Efficacy of amlexanox paste is equal to clobetasol ointment for the treatment of oral aphthae.[35] Amlexanox is another agent that should be evaluated for use in vulvar aphthae.

The mainstay of topical therapy for vulvar aphthae is corticosteroids. Double-blind, placebo-controlled trials showed that topical corticosteroids significantly reduce oral ulcer duration and pain when compared with placebo.[36,37] Class 1 topical steroids should be used in their ointment form to reduce exposure to irritant or allergic components of creams, gels, or foams. Physicians should not hesitate to use ultrapotent steroids on the vulva in this circumstance, presuming the patient or parent understands appropriate focal application. Although lacking supportive data both for oral and vulvar aphthae, intralesional and oral steroids also may have benefit, and studies are needed to assess their use over current topical agents.

Tetracycline antibiotics have been used in various formulations for treating oral aphthae.[38,39] In trials, the mouthwashes are dosed four times daily for 1 to 2 minutes. They significantly reduce pain and duration of recurrent ulcers compared with placebo. Formulas for compounding mouthwashes have been described.[40] Use of topical antibiotics for vulvar ulcers has not been studied; however, many case reports describe using oral antibiotics for presumed infection during management of acute vulvar aphthae. The failure of antiseptic mouthwashes[41,42] to improve pain or ulcer duration for oral aphthae suggests that the antimicrobial effect is not as important as perhaps the anti-inflammatory effect of these antibiotics. Trials exploring the use of either oral or topically applied antibiotics for vulvar ulcers are warranted.

Treatment of Chronic/Recurrent Aphthae

Chronic vulvar aphthae unassociated with an underlying illness (primary complex aphthosis) is rare, and studies to support therapeutic decisions do not exist. Physicians who manage these patients must extrapolate from experience in the treatment of chronic oral aphthae. Because the mechanism of ulcer formation is likely similar in these two anatomic sites and can occur simultaneously in the same patient, the data on treatment of chronic oral aphthae are reviewed here.

The approach to managing complex aphthosis is different from managing a solitary episode or simple aphthae. Complex aphthosis, by definition, is chronic and recurrent, thus requiring systemic agents to heal long-standing lesions, reduce recurrences, and induce remission. The main systemic agents used include thalidomide, dapsone, colchicine, pentoxifylline, and tumor necrosis factor (TNF) inhibitors. Treatment choice is based on patient profile, medical history, and previous treatment trials. As with any chronic dermatologic condition requiring ongoing systemic therapy, rotating agents to reduce adverse effects is helpful.

Comparisons of systemic therapeutic modalities for chronic aphthae are rare. Letsinger and colleagues published one of the first reports of a large series of this kind. This paper reviewed treatment of 42 patients with primary complex oral aphthosis. The authors proposed a therapeutic strategy starting with colchicine 0.6 mg two to three times daily as tolerated, progressing to dapsone dosed from 25 to 100 mg daily, and then to a combination of these two agents at full tolerated doses. The authors found that the two drugs combined were much more effective than either one alone, and nearly as effective as thalidomide, the final step in their suggested therapeutic ladder. Fifty-seven percent and 59% of patients achieved at least 50% improvement in these last two treatment groups, respectively.

Since the publication of this study, a second review of systemic treatments for 21 patients with severe recurrent oral aphthae has been published.[20] Patients initially were treated with prednisone for 2 weeks starting at 0.5 mg/kg/d, which was reduced to half that dose for a second week. Simultaneously, one of four systemic agents was started and maintained for 6 months: thalidomide, dapsone, colchicine, or pentoxifylline. The authors found that thalidomide was the most efficient and best-tolerated drug, with seven out of eight (87.5%) patients experiencing complete remission. Eight of nine patients treated with dapsone (89%) and eight of nine patients treated with colchicine (89%) experienced excellent-to-moderate improvement in their disease. Three out of five (60%) patients treated with Pentoxifylline had excellent-to-moderate improvement. Dapsone was best for inducing remission, with three patients remaining ulcer free for up to 9 months after discontinuation of the drug. Otherwise, most patients relapsed within weeks to several months of cessation of therapy.

Introduced in the 1950s as a sedative, thalidomide was subsequently banned worldwide in 1962 after the discovery of its devastating teratogenic effects. Thalidomide saw a renewed acceptance for its use in erythema nodosum leprosum (ENL) and was approved and classified as an orphan drug for this indication by the US Food and Drug Administration in 1998.[43] ENL remains the only approved indication for this drug; however, it has re-emerged as an alternative off-label therapy for many other dermatologic conditions.[44] Careful monitoring using the System for Thalidomide Education and Prescribing Safety (STEPS) program is mandatory to ensure appropriate use and prevent pregnancy. The mechanism of action of thalidomide is multifactorial and poorly understood, but in the case of aphthae, is probably mediated in part by its anti-TNF effect.[45,46]

Its effectiveness in complex aphthosis initially was shown in three open-label trials using thalidomide doses ranging from 100–400 mg/d. Most patients had significant improvement or complete resolution of lesions and pain within several weeks of starting therapy.[47–49] Larger randomized trials definitively established the efficacy of this drug. On 100 mg/d, 48% and 44% of patients experienced complete remission compared with only 9% and 8% of patients receiving placebo.[50,51] These studies reported relapse times of 20 to 30 days after stopping therapy.

Successful use of TNF inhibitors in BD has led to their off-label use in complex aphthosis. Scheinberg reported success using etanercept for two patients with chronic recurrent aphthous stomatitis, one meeting criteria for BD.[52] Both patients discontinued thalidomide, despite its effectiveness, because of adverse effects, and were subsequently treated with etanercept. Complete remission occured in both patients within 3 and 5 weeks of therapy. Recurrence was noted after discontinuation within 5 and 7 weeks. Each patient quickly responded after a second reintroduction of etanercept. Robinson and colleagues subsequently reported success using etanercept for another case of severe, recalcitrant oral aphthae.[53] Treatment with adalimumab led to complete resolution of a 7-year history of recalcitrant, severe major aphthae in an 18-year-old.[54] Such encouraging reports are increasing in number, and larger trials using these agents are desperately needed for this disabling condition.

Behçet's Disease

BD is a multisystem disease of unknown etiology, with the highest prevalence in the Mediterranean, particularly Turkey, with a rate of 1 case per 250 people in the population over 12 years old.[55] A pathognomonic test for BD does not exist; therefore the diagnosis is made based on the satisfaction of established criteria. International study group criteria for BD were established in 1990.[56] By this consensus, patients must have recurrent oral aphthae at least three times in 1 year, plus two of the following:

- Recurrent genital aphthae
- Uveitis or retinal vasculitis
- Erythema nodosum-like lesions or papulopustular skin lesions
- Positive pathergy test.

Ulcers involving oral and genital skin and mucosa are a hallmark of the disease. Second to oral ulcers, genital ulcers are the next most common feature of BD, occurring in 57% to 93% of patients.[57] Recognizing these lesions is essential, because they may precede other features of the disease. Overlooking this association may result in delay in diagnosis and an increase in mortality.[58] Aphthae associated with BD typically occur more frequently and more often in crops compared with recurrent aphthous stomatitis (RAS).[59] Genital ulcers of BD typically start as a tender nodule, become deep and painful, and eventually heal with scarring. Searching for scars on genital skin, even in the absence of active, clinical disease, is an important part of the examination.[58] Ulcers typically are found on the labia majora, but can occur anywhere on the vulva, perineum, or perianal skin. They can also occur intravaginally, potentially leading to fistula formation with the urethra or bladder.[58] Exceptionally deep external genital ulcers can lead to labial destruction.[58]

Treatment of aphthae of BD is based on experience in treating RAS and has been reviewed in detail elsewhere.[59] In the opinion of Alpsoy, who has written extensively about this disease, colchicine alone or plus benzathine penicillin is a good starting point for women with genital ulcers. Thalidomide and dapsone are second choices with immunosuppressive agents (cyclosporine, azathioprine, and TNF inhibitors) to follow for unresponsive patients. Topical barriers, antibiotics, anesthetics, and corticosteroids can be used as described for treating primary aphthosis.

TNF-alpha, derived from gamma–delta Th-1 lymphocytes, is postulated to play a role in the pathogenesis of BD. Accordingly, off-label use of TNF inhibitors is increasingly being used for BD.[60,61] Although primarily used for ophthalmic, gastrointestinal, and other more severe systemic manifestations, there are multiple reports of successful use of TNF inhibitors, particularly infliximab, for treating severe oral and genital aphthae of BD.[62–66] Complete remission is observed with maintenance therapy. A representative case is illustrated by Robertson and colleagues, who successfully used infliximab to treat severe orogenital aphthae associated with BD. The patient was a 65-year-old woman who had failed treatment with dapsone, thalidomide, azathioprine, cyclosporine, and colchicine. There was marked improvement after the first infusion with infliximab (scheduled at 0, 2, and 6 weeks at 5 mg/kg). By the third infusion, she was completely clear of ulcerations for the first time in 10 years.[64]

Likewise, etanercept has shown to be useful for treating aphthae of BD. Two female patients enjoyed complete remission of oral and vulvar ulcers when etanercept, 25 mg twice weekly, was added to their regimens of methotrexate in one case and methotrexate and prednisolone in the second.[67,68] Other data indicate that etanercept may be best reserved for clearing oral aphthae rather than genital aphthae. A recent randomized controlled trial comparing 25 mg twice weekly etanercept with placebo for mucocutaneous BD in 40 men showed that the drug had little effect on genital ulcers, while oral ulcers began clearing within 1 week of treatment.[69]

Infliximab was effective in a case resistant to etanercept.[70] This is most likely due to the effect of infliximab on both soluble and membrane-bound TNF, and therefore, more powerful TNF blockade. With this in mind, a reasonable approach is to treat patients with etanercept as a first-line agent, due to its excellent safety profile, and move to infliximab if response is suboptimal.

HIV-Associated Aphthous Ulcers

Most studies examining HIV-associated ulcers are conducted in Africa and involve the risk of transmission and coinfection with herpes simplex, syphilis, or chancroid. The literature investigating vulvar aphthae associated with HIV is scant, consisting primarily of case reports. HIV-associated aphthae are similar to ulcers that affect the oral mucosa, esophagus, and rectum in these patients, and pathogenesis may be the same.

They are typically large, painful, and recurrent (**Fig. 3**). Patients are generally severely immunocompromised with a low CD4 count and AIDS-defining infections.[71] Thirty-seven percent have coexistent oral ulcers.[71] HIV-associated aphthae can persist for weeks or months, becoming necrotic and causing disabling pain. Local destruction by nonhealing ulcers can be severe, with formation of a recto-vaginal fistula reported in one woman and a labial–vaginal fistula extending to the ischiorectal fossa in another.[72,73] Five fistulas resulting from HIV-associated aphthae were reported in a national survey involving 29 severely immunocompromised women: four recto-vaginal fistulas requiring diverting colostomies and one vaginal–perineal fistula.[71]

The pathogenesis of HIV-associated aphthae remains unknown. Immunosuppression, altered host response, and direct infection by HIV are proposed etiologies. In support of these theories is the fact that the CD4 count is typically low, and some women respond to antiretroviral therapy.[71,74] In one retrospective review of 307 HIV-positive women, 14% were found to have vulvar ulcers, 60% of which were classified as aphthae of unknown etiology. By definition, neither malignant nor ulcer-causing infections was identified on work-up of these patients.[73]

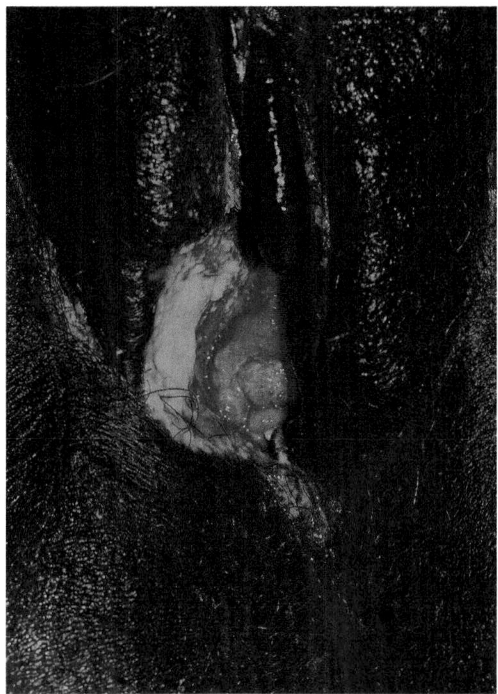

Fig. 3. Large, destructive genital ulcer associated with HIV.

Although biopsies are usually nondiagnostic, obtaining one as part of the evaluation is nevertheless recommended in patients with HIV-associated aphthae both to rule out malignancy and as a method of searching for potentially treatable infectious causes such as CMV, HSV, and mycobacterial infections. All women presenting with HIV-associated ulcers should additionally be screened for HSV and syphilis. Screening for chancroid, LGV, and GI in select patients with high-risk behavior or from endemic regions is also prudent.

Early identification and treatment of HIV-associated vulvar aphthae are essential given the potentially crippling sequelae. Variably favorable response typically is seen with either topical, intralesional, or oral corticosteroids.[71] High-dose corticosteroids are reported to promote healing of individual patients,[72] although the ideal dosing regimen has not been studied. Antiviral therapy with acyclovir is not beneficial.[71] Given the successful use of thalidomide for the treatment of complex aphthosis and aphthae of BD, this drug has been used to treat HIV-associated ulcers. The largest trial is a randomized controlled trial of 57 HIV-positive patients with oral aphthae. The treatment group received 200 mg/d. After 4 weeks of treatment, 55% of these patients had complete healing of ulcers compared with only 7% of the placebo group.[75]

Crohn's Disease

CD is an inflammatory bowel disease characterized by noncaseating granulomatous lesions, occurring in a skip pattern at any location along the gastrointestinal tract from the mouth to the anus. Mucocutaneous manifestations occur in up to 44% of patients,[76] but they do not necessarily mirror intestinal involvement.[77] Skin manifestations can be categorized as either histologically specific or nonspecific (reactive). Histologically specific lesions have noncaseating granulomas similar to those seen in the intestinal lesions. Nonspecific or reactive skin manifestations include entities such as pyoderma gangrenosum, erythema nodosum, and oral aphthae.[76]

Of those who present with cutaneous CD, 70% present with genital involvement.[78] Therefore, CD initially may present to the dermatologist in the form of vulvar ulcerations, and recognition of these findings should prompt an investigation for the disease.

Vulvar CD presents most commonly with erythema and unilateral or bilateral labial swelling. Chronic edema leads to firm coalescing papules and fibrotic nodules, which could be confused with lymphatic obstruction.[5] Ulcers associated with CD are classically long "knife cut" lesions in the genitocrural folds or interlabial creases. This presentation is almost pathognomonic for CD (**Fig. 4**). Other genital findings are skin tags, abscesses, draining fistulas, and eventually scarring.[78] Perianal fistulae form by direct extension of rectal CD, and can extend to the vagina or vulva.

Histologic findings of noncaseating granulomas help establish the diagnosis. The differential diagnosis of granulomatous vulvar lesions includes conditions such as sarcoidosis, foreign body implantation, hidradenitis supperativa (HS), mycobacterial or deep fungal infections, and sexually transmitted infections such as granuloma inguinale. The ulcerations and occasionally the presence of vasculitis histologically can help differentiate CD from sarcoidosis. Polarizing microscopy should be performed in search of foreign body material. Tuberculin skin test, chest radiograph, tissue culture, PCR, and special stains can help identify mycobacterial and deep fungal infections. Classic HS usually can be distinguished based on clinical appearance alone; however, differentiation from CD can be difficult. Clinical features of abscesses, fistulae, webbed scars, and comedomes involving skin along the milk line in a recurrent nature are typical of HS. The presence or history of other follicular occlusive entities adds support to the diagnosis: severe cystic acne, pilonidal cyst, and dissecting cellulitis of the scalp.

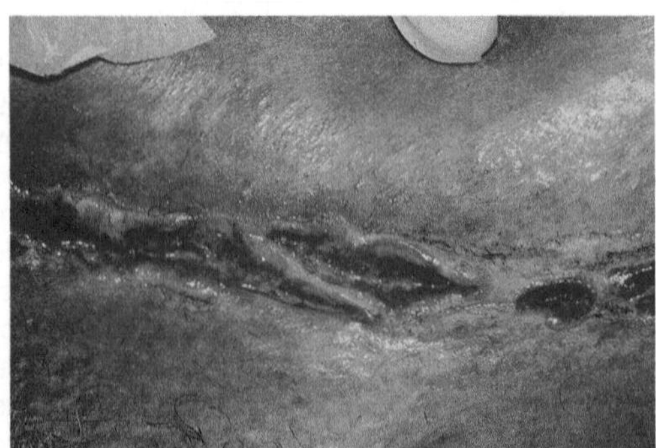

Fig. 4. "Knife-cut" ulceration associated with Crohn's disease.

Treatment of CD requires systemic administration of various antibiotics, immunosuppressive agents, and anti-inflammatory agents such as metronidazole, corticosteroids, azathioprine, sulfasalazine, or 6-mercaptopurine. Cutaneous CD is rare, and treatment trials have not been performed. A small series showed that infliximab is very effective in healing pyoderma gangrenosum and aphthous stomatitis associated with CD.[79] Infliximab and adalimumab have both been used successfully to treat individual cases of cutaneous CD.[80–82] Cyclosporine and mycophenolate mofetil have been reported to be successful in individual cases of cutaneous CD.[83,84] Other cutaneous directed therapy includes intralesional corticosteroids, incision and drainage for abscesses, and surgical repair for fistulae.[5]

REFERENCES

1. Jurge S, Kuffer R, Scully C, et al. Mucosal disease series. Number VI. Recurrent aphthous stomatitis. Oral Dis 2006;12(1):1–21.
2. Rogers RS. Recurrent aphthous stomatitis in the diagnosis of Behcet's disease. Yonsei Med J 1997; 38(6):370–9.
3. Ship JA. Recurrent aphthous stomatitis. An update. Oral Surg Oral Med Oral Pathol Oral Radiol Endod 1996;81(2):141–7.
4. Disorders of the mucous memebranes. In: James WD, Berger TG, Elston EM, editors. Andrews' diseases of the skin, clinical dermatology. 10th edition. Philadelphia: WB Sanders; 2006. p. 810–2.
5. Lynch P. Vulvar ulcers. In: Black M, editor. Obstetric and gynecologic dermatology. 3rd edition. China: Elsevier; 2008. p. 241–56.
6. Ghate JV, Jorizzo JL. Behcet's disease and complex aphthosis. J Am Acad Dermatol 1999;40(1):1–18.

7. Huppert JS, Gerber MA, Deitch HR, et al. Vulvar ulcers in young females: a manifestation of aphthosis. J Pediatr Adolesc Gynecol 2006;19(3):195–204.
8. Taylor S, Drake SM, Dedicoat M, et al. Genital ulcers associated with acute Epstein-Barr virus infection. Sex Transm Infect 1998;74(4):296–7.
9. Lipschutz B. Uber eine eigenartige Geschwursform des weiblichen Genitales (ulcus vulvae actum). Arch Dermatol Syph (Berlin) 1913;114:363 [in German].
10. Halvorsen JA, Brevig T, Aas T, et al. Genital ulcers as initial manifestation of Epstein-Barr virus infection: two new cases and review of the literature. Acta Derm Venereol 2006;86(5):439–42.
11. Portnoy J, Ahronheim GA, Ghibu F, et al. Recovery of Epstein-Barr virus from genital ulcers. N Engl J Med 1984;311(15):966–8.
12. Naher H, Gissmann L, Freese UK, et al. Subclinical Epstein-Barr virus infection of both the male and female genital tract: indication for sexual transmission. J Invest Dermtol 1992;98(5):791–3.
13. Brown ZA, Stenchever MA. Genital ulceration and infectious mononucleosis: a report of a case. Am J Obstet Gynecol 1977;127(6):673–4.
14. Sisson BA, Glick L. Genital ulceration as a presenting manifestation of infectious mononucleosis. J Pediatr Adolesc Gynecol 1998;11(4):185–7.
15. Hudson LB, Perlman SE. Necrotizing genial ulcerations in a premenarcheal female with mononucleosis. Obstet Gynecol 1998;92:642–4.
16. Deitch HR, Huppert J, Adams Hillard PJ. Unusual vulvar ulcerations in young adolescent females. J Pediatr Adolesc Gynecol 2004;17(1):13–6.
17. Wetter DA, Bruce AJ, Maclaughlin KL, et al. Ulcus vulvae acutum in a 13-year-old girl after influenza A infection. Skinmed 2008;7(2):95–8.
18. Pelletier F, Aubin F, Puzenat E, et al. Lipschutz genial ulceration: a rare manifestation of paratyphoid fever. Eur J Dermatol 2003;13(3):297–8.
19. Cebesoy FB, Balat O, Inaloz S. Premenarchal vulvar ulceration: is chronic irritation a causative factor? Pediatr Dermatol 2009;26(5):514–8.
20. Mimura MAM, Hirota SK, Sugaya NN, et al. Systemic treatment in severe cases of recurrent aphthous stomatitis: an open trial. Clinics (Sao Paulo) 2009;64(3):193–8.
21. Pastore L, Carroccia A, Compilato D, et al. Oral manifestations of celiac disease. J Clin Gastroenterol 2008;42(3):224–32.
22. Letsinger JA, McCarty MA, Jorizzo JL. Complex aphthosis: a large case series with evaluation algorithm and therapeutic ladder from topical to thalidomide. J Am Acad Dermatol 2005;52:500–8.
23. Bergmans D, Bonten M, Gaillard C, et al. In vitro antibacterial activity of sucralfate. Eur J Clin Microbiol Infect Dis 1994;13(7):615–20.
24. Tryba M, Mantey-Stiers F. Antibacterial activity of sucralfate in human gastric juice. Am J Med 1987;83(3B):125–7.
25. Burch RM, McMillan BA. Sucralfate induces proliferation of dermal fibroblasts and keratinocytes in culture and granulation tissue formation in full-thickness skin wounds. Agents Actions 1991;34:229–31.
26. Folkman J, Szabo S, Shing Y. Sucralfate affinity for fibroblast growth factor. J Cell Biol 1990;111:223a.
27. Banati A, Cowdhury SR, Mazumder S. Topical use of sucralfate cream in second and third-degree burns. Burn 2001;27(5):465–9.
28. Tumino G, Masuelli L, Bei R, et al. Topical treatment of chronic venous ulcers with sucralfate: a placebo controlled randomized study. Int J Mol Med 2008;22(1):17–23.
29. Markham T, Kennedy F, Collins P. Topical sucralfate for erosive irritant diaper dermatitis. Arch Dermatol 2000;136(10):1199–200.
30. Lentz SS, Barrett RJ, Homesley HD. Topical sucralfate in the treatment of vaginal ulceration. Obstet Gynecol 1993;81(5):869–71.
31. Buchsel PC, Murphy PJM. Polyvinylpyrrolidone–sodium hyaluronate gel (Gelclair): a bioadherent oral gel for the treatment of oral mucositis and other painful oral lesions. Expert Opin Drug Metab Toxicol 2008;4(11):1449–54.
32. Innocenti M, Moscatelli G, Lopez S. Efficacy of Gelclair in reducing pain in palliative care patients with oral lesions: preliminary findings from an open pilot study. J Pain Symptom Manage 2002;24(5):456–7.
33. Khandwala A, Van Inwegen RG, Alfano MC, et al. 5% Amlexanox oral paste, a new treatment for recurrent minor aphthous ulcers. I. Clinical demonstration of acceleration of healing and resolution of pain. Oral Surg Oral Med Oral Pathol Oral Radiol Endod 1997;83(2):222–30.
34. Murray B, McGuinness N, Biagioni P. A comparative study of the efficacy of Aphtheal in the management of recurrent minor aphthous ulceration. J Oral Pathol Med 2005;34(7):413–9.
35. Rodriguez M, Rubio JA, Sanchez R. Effectiveness of two oral pastes for the treatment of recurrent aphthous stomatitis. Oral Dis 2007;13(5):490–4.
36. Merchant HW, Gangarosa LP, Glassman AB, et al. Betamethasone-17-benzoate in the treatment of recurrent aphthous ulcers. Oral Surg 1978;45(6):870–5.
37. Thompson AC, Nolan A, Lamey J. Minor aphthous oral ulceration: a double-blind cross-over study of beclomethasone dipropionate aerosol spray. Scott Med J 1989;34(5):531–2.
38. Guggenheimer J, Brightman VJ, Ship II. Effect of chlortetracycline mouth rinses on the healing of recurrent aphthous ulcers: a double-blind controlled trial. J Oral Ther Pharmacol 1968;4(5):406–8.

39. Graykowski EA, Kingman A. Double-blind trial of tetracycline in recurrent aphthous ulceration. J Oral Pathol 1978;7(6):376–82.
40. Altenburg A, Zouboulis CC. Current concepts in the treatment of recurrent aphthous stomatitis. Skin Therapy Lett 2008;13(7):1–4.
41. Meiller TF, Kutcher MJ, Overholser CD, et al. Effect of an antimicrobial mouth rinse on recurrent aphthous ulcerations. Oral Surg Oral Med Oral Pathol 1991;72(4):425–9.
42. Hunter L, Addy M. Chlorhexidine gluconate mouthwash in the management of minor aphthous ulceration. A double-blind, placebo-controlled cross-over trial. Br Dent J 1987;162(3):106–10.
43. Radomsky CL, Levine N. Thalidomide. Dermatol Clin 2001;19(1):87–103.
44. Wu JJ, Huang DB, Pang KR, et al. Thalidomide: dermatological indications, mechanisms of action, and side-effects. Br J Dermatol 2005;153(2):254–73.
45. Sampaio EP, Sarno EN, Galilly R, et al. Thalidomide selectively inhibits tumor necrosis factor alpha production by stimulated human monocytes. J Exp Med 1991;173(3):699–703.
46. Moreira AL, Sampaio EP, Zmuidzimas A, et al. Thalidomide exerts its inhibitory action on tumor necrosis factor alpha by enhancing mRNA degradation. J Exp Med 1993;177(6):1675–80.
47. Torras H, Lecha M, Mascaro JM. Thalidomide treatment of recurrent necrotic giant mucocutaneous aphthae and aphthosis. Arch Dermatol 1982;118(11):875.
48. Jenkins JS, Powell RJ, Allen BR, et al. Thalidomide in severe orogenital ulceration. Lancet 1984;22(2): 1424–6.
49. Grinspan D. Significant response of oral aphthosis to thalidomide treatment. J Am Acad Dermatol 1985;12(1):85–90.
50. Ranselaar CG, Boone RM, Kluin-Nelemans HC. Thalidomide in the treatment of neuro-Behcet's syndrome. Br J Dermatol 1986;115(3):367–70.
51. Revuz J, Guillaume JC, Janier M, et al. Crossover study of thalidomide vs placebo in severe recurrent aphthous stomatitis. Arch Dermatol 1990;126(7):923–7.
52. Scheinberg MA. Treatment of recurrent oral aphthous ulcers with etanercept. Clin Exp Rheumatol 2002;20(5):733–4.
53. Robinson ND, Guitart J. Recalcitrant, recurrent aphthous stomatitis treated with etanercept. Arch Dermatol 2003;139(10):1259–62.
54. Vujevich J, Zirwas M. Treatment of severe, recalcitrant, major aphthous stomatitis with adalimumab. Cutis 2005;76(2):129–32.
55. Azizlerli G, Kose AA, Sarica R, et al. Prevalence of Behcet's disease in Istanbul, Turkey. Int J Dermatol 2003;42(10):803–6.
56. Criteria for diagnosis of Behcet's disease. International study group for Behcet's disease. Lancet 1990;335(8697):1078–80.
57. Zouboulis CC. Epidemiology of adamantiades—Behçet's disease. Ann Med Interne (Paris) 1999;150(6):488–98.
58. Alpsoy E, Zouboulis CC, Ehrlich GE. Mucocutaneous lesions of Behçet's disease. Yonsei Med J 2007;48(4):573–85.
59. Alpsoy E, Akman A. Behçet's disease: an algorithmic approach to its treatment. Arch Dermatol Res. 2009;301(10):693–702.
60. Graves JE, Nunley K, Heffernan MP. Off-label uses of biologics in dermatology: rituximab, omalizumab, infliximab, etanercept, adalimumab, efalizumab, and alefacept (part 2 of 2). J Am Acad Dermatol 2007;56(1):e55–79.
61. O'Neill ID. Off-label use of biologicals in the management of inflammatory oral mucosal disease. J Oral Pathol Med 2008;37(10):575–81.
62. Goossens PH, Verburg RJ, Breedveld FC. Remission of Behçet's syndrome with tumour necrosis factor alpha blocking therapy. Ann Rheum Dis 2001;60(6):637.
63. Almoznino G, Ben-Chetrit E. Infliximab for the treatment of resistant oral ulcers in Behçet's disease: a case report and review of the literature. Clin Exp Rheumatol 2007;25:S99–102.
64. Robertson LP, Hickling P. Treatment of recalcitrant, orogenital ulceration of Behcet's syndrome with infliximab. Rheumatology (Oxford) 2001;40(4):473–4.
65. Haugeberg G, Velken M, Johnsen V. Successful treatment of genital ulcers with infliximab in Behcet's disease. Ann Rheum Dis 2004;63(6):744–5.
66. Connolly M, Armstrong JS, Buckley DA. Infliximab treatment for severe orogenital ulceration in Behçet's disease. Br J Dermatol 2005;153(5):1073–5.
67. Curigliano V, Giovinale M, Fonnesu C, et al. Efficacy of etanercept in the treatment of a patient with Behçet's disease. Clin Rheumatol 2008;27(7):933–6.
68. Atzeni F, Sarzi-Puttini P, Capsoni F, et al. Successful treatment of resistant Behçet's disease with etanercept. Clin Exp Rheumatol 2005;23(5):729.
69. Melikoglu M, Fresko I, Mat C, et al. Short-term trial of etanercept in Behçet's disease: a double-blind, placebo-controlled study. J Rheumatol 2005;32(1):98–105.
70. Estrach C, Mpofu S, Moots RJ. Behçet's syndrome: response to infliximab after failure of etanercept. Rheumatology 2002;41(10):1213–4.
71. Anderson J, Clark RA, Watts DH, et al. Idiopathic genital ulcers in women infected with human immunodeficiency virus. J Acquir Immune Defic Syndr Hum Retrovirol 1996;13(4):343–7.
72. Schuman P, Christensen C, Sobel JD. Aphthous vaginal ulceration in two women with acquired immunodeficiency syndrome. Am J Obstet Gynecol 1996;174(5):1660–3.
73. LaGuardia KD, White MH, Saigo PE, et al. Genital ulcer disease in women infected with human immunodeficiency virus. Am J Obstet Gynecol 1995;172:553–62.

74. Covino JM, McCormack WM. Vulvar ulcer of unknown etiology in a human immunodeficiency virus-infected woman: response to treatment with zidovudine. Am J Obstet Gynecol 1990;163:116–8.
75. Jacobson JM, Greenspan JS, Spritzler J, et al. Thalidomide for the treatment of oral aphthous ulcers in patients with human immunodeficiency virus infection. N Engl J Med 1997;336:1487–93.
76. Lester LU, Rapini RP. Dermatologic manifestations of colonic disorders. Curr Opin Gastroenterol 2008; 25(1):66–73.
77. Chalvardijan A, Nethercott JR. Cutaneous granulomatous vasculitis associated with Crohn's disease. Cutis 1982;30(5):645–55.
78. Ploysangam T, Heubi JE, Eisen D. Cutaneous Crohn's disease in children. J Am Acad Dermatol 1997;36:697–704.
79. Kaufman I, Caspi D, Yeshurun D, et al. The effect of infliximab on extraintestinal manifestations of Crohn's disease. Rheumatol Int 2005;25(6):406–10.
80. Van Dullemen H, De Jong E, Slors F, et al. Treatment of therapy-resistant perineal metastatic Crohn's disease after proctectomy using antitumor necrosis factor chimeric monoclonal antibody, cA2: report of two cases. Dis Colon Rectum 1998;41(1):98–102.
81. Petrolati A, Altavilla N, Cipolla R, et al. Cutaneous metastatic Crohn's disease responsive to infliximab. Am J Gastroenterol 2009;104(4):1058.
82. Miller FA, Jones CR, Clarke LE, et al. Successful use of adalimumab in treating cutaneous metastatic Crohn's disease: report of a case. Inflamm Bowel Dis 2009;15(11):1611–2.
83. Carranza DC, Young L. Successful treatment of metastatic Crohn's disease with cyclosporine. J Drugs Dermatol 2008;7(8):789–91.
84. Nousari HC, Sragovich A, Kimyai-Asadi A, et al. Mycophenolate mofetil in autoimmune and inflammatory skin disorders. J Am Acad Dermatol 1999; 40:265–8.

Vulvar Edema

Yaa Amankwah, MB, ChB[a,*], Hope Haefner, MD[b]

KEYWORDS

- Vulvar edema • Vulvar swelling • Crohn disease
- Hidradenitis suppurativa

Vulvar edema is associated with a variety of medical conditions. There are also several other vulvar conditions that closely mimic edema making it difficult at times to clearly differentiate these conditions from edema. Vulvar edema can be a diagnostic dilemma and a treatment challenge for health care providers as well a significant frustration for affected individuals.

PATHOPHYSIOLOGY

Edema is defined as abnormal and excessive accumulation of fluid within the skin. The amount of interstitial fluid is a result of the balance of fluid hemostasis. Increased secretion or impaired removal of fluid results in edema. Edema is facilitated by any of the following factors: increased intravascular hydrostastic pressure, reduced plasma oncotic pressure, increased blood vessel wall permeability, obstructed lymphatic clearance of fluids, and, finally, changes in the water retention properties of tissue. Body areas with distensible and loose skin, including the genitalia, are common sites for edema formation. Depending on the underlying cause of edema, the resultant fluid accumulation is either of plasma or lymphatic origin and at times both. Fluid of plasma origin often results in pitting edema (soft on palpation producing an indentation of the skin) whereas fluid of lymphatic origin is nonpitting (firm to palpation and nonindenting). Edema can develop acutely on exposure to allergens, including topical medications, infections, and toxins, and in certain medical conditions, such as lupus, leukemia, and lymphoma. The resulting edema in these situations is termed, *angioedema*. This is a result of increased vascular permeability in response to mediators of inflammation. Angioedema, a rare condition, may be hereditary (C1 esterase inhibitor deficiency). Generally, when acute angioedema occurs, onset of symptoms is often within minutes to hours and effects may last up to several days. Edema may be generalized or occasionally restricted to specific body sites, such as the vulva.

Any inflammatory or obstructive process can produce edema. At times, remarkable vulvar edema can occur without obvious inflammatory disease or trauma (**Box 1**).

INFLAMMATORY CONDITIONS

Contact Dermatitis

Contact dermatitis of the vulva is inflammation occurring as a result of contact of the skin with

Box 1
Diseases that can be subtle but produce isolated vulvar edema

- Contact dermatitis
- Crohn disease
- Hidradenitis suppurativa
- Primary herpes simplex virus (HSV) infection
- Recurrent vulvovaginal candidiasis (RVVC)
- Pelvic obstruction due to tumor, radiation, or surgery
- Edema associated with pregnancy/prolonged delivery
- Subcutanous tumors that mimic edema (lipomas, cysts, and so forth)

[a] Department of Obstetrics, Gynecology and Newborn Care, The Ottawa Hospital, University of Ottawa, 1965 Riverside Drive, 7th Floor, Box 503, Ottawa, Ontario K1H7W9, Canada
[b] Department of Obstetrics and Gynecology, The University of Michigan Hospitals, 1500 East Medical Center Drive, L 4000 Women's Hospital, Ann Arbor, MI 48109, USA
* Corresponding author.
E-mail address: yamankwah@ottawahospital.on.ca

Dermatol Clin 28 (2010) 765–777
doi:10.1016/j.det.2010.08.001
0733-8635/10/$ – see front matter

a variety of substances and can manifest as either an acute dermatitis or a chronic dermatitis after prolonged exposure (**Fig. 1**).[1] The presentation of contact dermatitis is variable and this impairs diagnosis. Often the cause is multifactorial. There are two types of contact dermatitis, irritant and allergic contact dermatitis. Strong or caustic irritants cause an immediate irritant contact dermatitis that corresponds to the area of contact, as in the use of trichloroacetic acid for anogenital warts or an azole cream used in already inflamed vulvovaginal candidiasis (VVC). This is characterized by immediate pain on contact and well-circumscribed skin changes, which make diagnosis easy. More common is a delayed, chronic irritant contact dermatitis due to prolonged or frequent exposure to milder irritants. Common contact irritants include overwashing, laundry detergent, fabric softener, dyes in clothing,[2] soaps, body washes, hygiene sprays, bubble bath, bath oils, tampons, panty liners, menstrual and incontinence pads, urine, sweat, semen, feces, douches, spermicides (nonoxynol-9 and benzalkonium chloride), and condoms.[3] The clinical presentation consists of irritation and burning in a setting of poorly demarcated erythema, and more severe disease manifests edema, and, sometimes, superficial erosions, within glazed erythema.

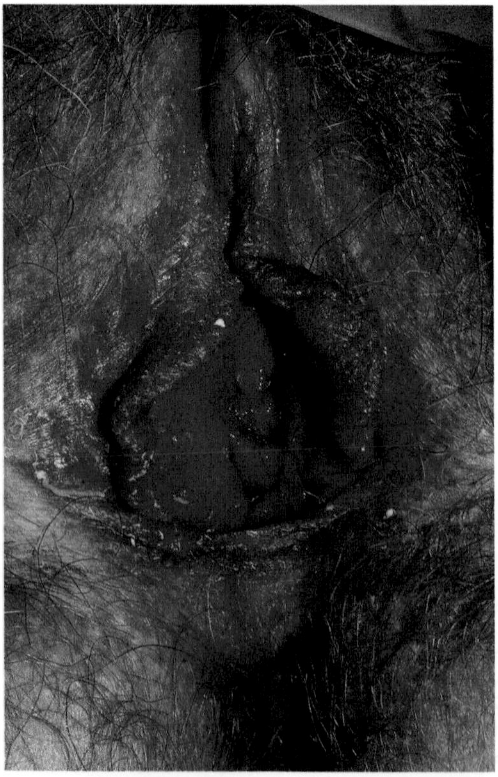

Fig. 1. Contact dermatitis showing well-demarcated erythematous patches involving the vestibule, labia minora, and interlabial sulci.

Allergic contact dermatitis is usually a type IV delayed hypersensitivity reaction and only occurs in those patients previously sensitized to the antigen. Vulvar allergens include anesthetics (benzocaine and diphenhydramine), antibiotics (neomycin sulfate and sulfa), antimycotics (clotrimazole), nonsteroidal anti-inflammatory drugs (bufexamac), antivirals (acyclovir), corticosteroids, chlorhexidine, fragrances, preservatives (parabens and propylene glycol), and lanolin.[1] It may be difficult to differentiate chronic irritant contact dermatitis from allergic contact dermatitis; however, allergic contact dermatitis is extremely pruritic, and skin changes follow exposure by 1 to 2 days. The appearance of affected skin ranges from normal to erythema, vesicles, and, in severe cases, edema. Treatment of contact vulvitis includes eliminating the offending agent and symptomatic relief with cool gel packs applied to the vulvar skin for comfort. Nighttime scratching should be prevented with sedation, because there are no medications with inherently anti-itch properties. Elimination of the itch-scratch cycle is essential, and sedation with medications, such as amitriptyline (25 to 50 mg at bedtime) or hydroxyzine (10 to 50 mg) usually is helpful. Corticosteroids ointment of high to mid potency are used in a taper to reverse inflammation and subsequently the vulvar edema. At times, oral steroid tapers are required; prednisone (40 mg for small adults to 60 mg for large adults) each morning for 7 to 10 days can be discontinued without a taper other than transition to a topical corticosteroid. Allergic contact dermatitis requires up to a month of corticosteroid therapy, and irritant contact requires less.

Crohn Disease

Crohn disease, a chronic relapsing and remitting inflammatory bowel condition, can affect the entire length of the gastrointestinal tract from the oral cavity to the anus. Extraintestinal disease with or without continuity to the intestine sometimes occurs. Fifteen percent of patients have disease involving the mucocutaneous tissues.[4] Extraintestinal Crohn disease, also called metastatic Crohn disease, may present with gynecologic manifestations, which often are not recognized and are difficult to treat. In 85% of cases, the diagnosis of gastrointestinal Crohn disease precedes vulvar involvement. Vulvar lesions occur in approximately 2% of women with Crohn disease.[5] More common is perianal disease, with fistulae, tags, and edema. Fairly often, the only manifestation of vulvar Crohn disease is asymmetric labial edema, without other skin signs that suggest this diagnosis. More severe disease is characterized by labial edema with linear knife-like ulcerations, abscesses, or fissures located in the interlabial sulcus, perineum, or crural folds (**Fig. 2**). Rectovaginal, anocutaneous, and recto-Bartholin fistulae can occur. Development of enterovaginal fistulas leads to vaginal scarring. Vulvar fistulae and abscess formation may precede active intestinal disease by years, making diagnosis of anorectal Crohn difficult.[6–8] At times, repeat gastrointestinal screening for Crohn disease may be required for diagnosis. The diagnosis also is suggested by the presence of noncaseating granulomas on skin biopsy, but granulomatous inflammation is characteristic of hidradenitis suppurativa (HS) as well, another cause of anogential edema (discussed later).

The first-line treatment of vulvar Crohn disease can vary from the usual gastrointestinal treatment regimen. Generally, for initial treatment, oral metronidazole is used. Ciprofloxacin, both for its antimicrobial and its nonspecific anti-inflammatory properties, may also be used. Metronidazole and ciprofloxacin may be combined if needed for better response. For resistant disease or for the treatment of open, draining fistulas, infliximab (Remicade), etanercept (Enbrel), or adalimumab (Humira) may be used. These are anti–tumor necrosis factor (TNF) substances. TNF is a protein produced by the immune system that may cause the inflammation associated with Crohn disease. Corticosteroids and the 5-aminosalicylic acid drugs are generally effective only for bowel disease rather than for perineal disease; however, an occasional patient with vulvar Crohn disease has responded well to corticosteroids. Immunosuppressants, such as 6-mercaptopurine and azathioprine, have also been used at times.

Hidradenitis Suppurativa (Inverse Acne)

HS is a chronic, noninfectious, follicular occlusive condition resulting in painful nodules and abscesses in characteristic locations of the axillae and groin (**Fig. 3**). After occlusion of hair follicles with desquamated keratin debris, the distending follicle enlarges with accumulating trapped keratin,

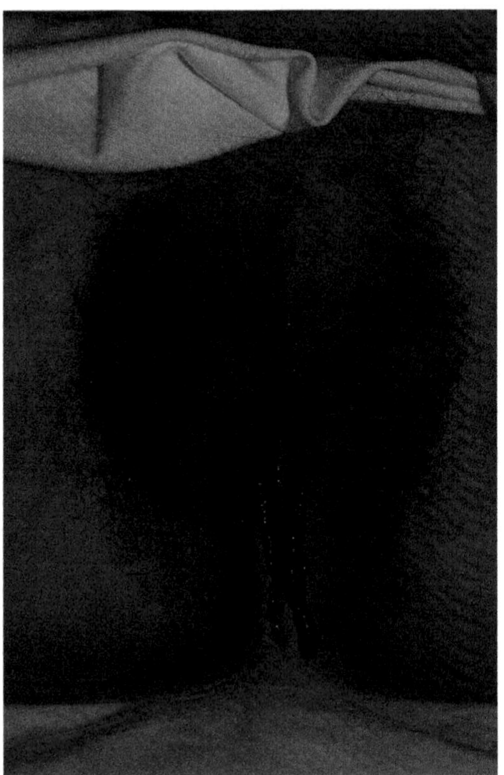

Fig. 2. Crohn disease of the vulvar: edema on the right labium majus, more prominent than on the left side and likely overlying a developing abscess.

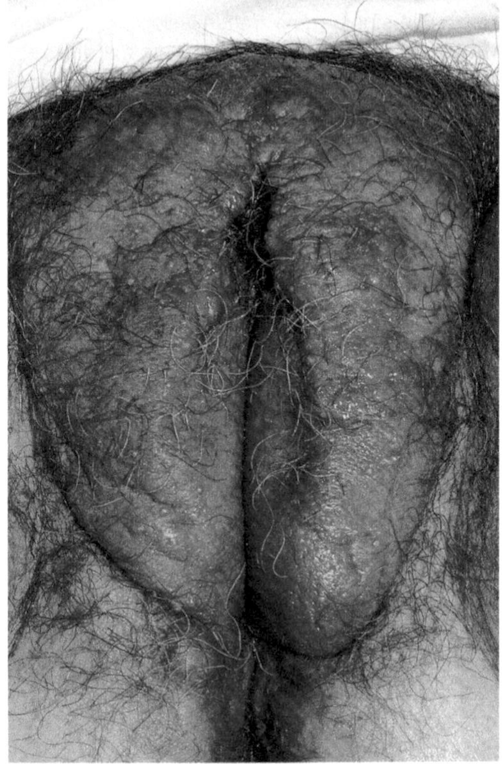

Fig. 3. Hidradenitis suppurativa: multiple vulvar abscesses with edema of the mons pubis and labia majora.

until there is rupture of the distended follicle, with a resulting foreign body reaction to the keratin producing folliculitis. This results in noninfectious abscess formation. The abscesses drain, forming chronic sinus tracts and hypertrophic scarring with decreased mobility, lymphedema, and deformity. HS occurs on a spectrum of severity, from an occasional dermal nodule to severe, foul-smelling, draining skin with deformity, pain, and dysfunction. Even extremely mild disease is sometimes manifested by edema that is far out of proportion to subtle scarring noted on examination. Affected body areas include one or more of the apocrine gland-containing areas; the axillae, groin, and inframammary, periareola, perianal, and perineal regions. Aprocrine glands are not found on the inner aspects of the labia minora and vestibule. The presence of abscess formation in these areas should raise suspicion of other conditions, such as anorectal Crohn disease.

The prevalence of HS is described as from 1% to 4% of the population. It often begins after menarche and improves after menopause with peak incidence at ages 20 to 30 years. Women are more commonly affected than men, with female/male ratios ranging from 2:1 to 5:1. Predisposing factors include smoking, diabetes mellitus, and obesity. There are several reports of familial involvement with a possible single gene transmission.[9] Chronic HS with draining sinuses and abscesses is difficult to differentiate from Crohn disease, lymphogranuloma venereum (LGV), pyoderma gangrenosum, and squamous cell carcinoma. Biopsy specimens looking for follicular hyperkeratosis, active folliculitis, sinus tracts, apocrine, and eccrine stasis may help clarify the diagnosis. Biopsies generally are not required for the diagnoses of hidradenitis suppurativa, however. There have been reports of squamous cell carcinoma in up to 3.2% of patients with perineal hidradenitis suppurativa.[10] HS is staged by Hurley's criteria (I–III) based on the severity of tissue involvement with abscesses and scarring. Generally, 75% remain in stage I, 24% progress to stage II, and 1% progress to stage III.

The goal of treatment is to prevent the progression of the disease and decrease existing disease to the mildest form. General treatment measures include education, support, reduction of friction heat and sweating in the area, and the use of antiseptic washes and cleansers. Weight loss and smoking cessation should be advised. Medical treatment uses antiandrogens, such as spirinolactone- or aldactone-containing oral contraceptive pills, in an extended cycle regimen to decrease end organ sensitivity. Chronic administration of antibiotics with anti-inflammatory effects minimizes the activity of this disease; these include doxycycline (100 mg twice daily), clindamycin (150 mg twice daily), and trimethoprim-sulfamethoxyzole (double strength twice daily). Measures to reduce the duration of flares and secondary infection include clindamycin 1% lotion twice daily and a 7- to 10-day course of tetracycline (250–500 mg orally 4 times daily), doxycycline (100 mg orally twice daily), amoxicillin/clavulinic acid (875/125 mg twice daily), or clindamycin (300 mg orally twice daily).[11] Zinc gluconate tablets (50 mg orally twice daily) have anti-inflammatory and wound-healing purposes and are used as an adjunct to treatment.[12] Intralesional triamcinolone acetonide (0.5 to 1 mL of a 10 mg/mL concentration) injected into the center of painful early papules and nodules is also helpful in suppressing inflammation. Dapsone (50–100 mg orally once a day chronically) can also be used. Monitoring parameters for dapsone include a weekly complete blood cell count ×4, then monthly ×6, then every 6 months. Liver function tests should be obtained as a baseline, then periodically. Long-term suppression of lesions is maintained with tetracyclines, clindamycin, or trimethoprim-sulfamethoxyzole, dapsone, and/or high-dose zinc. A therapy for resistant cases, requiring vigorous monitoring, is cyclosporine (4–5 mg/kg per day). Anti–TNF-α agents, such as infliximab, adalimumab, and etanercept, have been used with good responses, but these are expensive and do not have Food and Drug Administration (FDA) indication approval.[13] Invariably, severe HS characterized by multiple interconnected tracts, sinuses, and scarring requires surgical removal to achieve long-term relief. Even with surgery, it is essential that concurrent medical therapy be used for prophylaxis.

INFECTIONS/INFESTATIONS

Vulvar infections (yeast, viral, and bacterial) and parasitic infestations have varying presentations, such as edema, erythema, and ulceration.

Vulvovaginal Candidiasis

VVC often causes intense pruritus. Severe VVC is characterized by extensive vulvar edema, erythema (**Fig. 4**), excoriation, and fissure formation. VVC is a common infection and an estimated 75% of women have at least one episode of VVC. Forty percent have two or more episodes. The majority (approximately 70%) of VVC are the result of *Candida albicans*.[14] Symptoms include pruritus, vaginal soreness, vulvar burning, dyspareunia, and dysuria. Fissuring in the interlabial sulci occurring with severe VVC could be confused with herpetic infection. The diagnosis of VVC can be made in a symptomatic woman with either a fungal

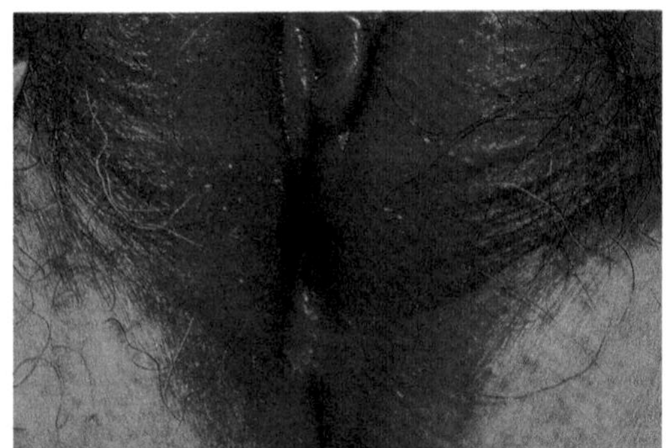

Fig. 4. VVC: diffuse vulvar erythema and mild edema are present.

preparation (10% potassium hydroxide) or Gram stain of vaginal discharge demonstrating yeasts or pseudohyphae. Cultures yield a positive result for a yeast species missed on the wet preparation. *Candida* vaginitis is associated with a normal vaginal pH (≤4.5). The use of 10% potassium hydroxide in wet preparations can improve the visualization of yeast and mycelia by disrupting cellular material that might obscure the yeast or pseudohyphae. RVVC is defined as four or more episodes of symptomatic VVC each year,[15] occurring in less than 5% of women. The pathogenesis of RVVC is unclear. The majority of women with RVVC have no specific underlying conditions. Vaginal cultures are required to confirm the clinical diagnosis in these patients with RVVC and also to identify atypical species, including nonalbicans species. Nonalbicans *Candida* are usually asymptomatic, and do not cause edema. These nonalbicans *Candida* organisms do not form pseudohyphae or hyphae and are difficult to identify on microscopy. *C glabrata* and other nonalbicans *Candida* species are found in up to 30% of patients with RVVC.[14] The standard antiyeast medications are not as effective against these species as they are against *C albicans*. Complicated VVC refers to RVVC, severe VVC, and nonalbicans candidiasis. It also refers to VVC in women with uncontrolled diabetes, debilitation, immunosuppression, or those who are pregnant.

Oral agents (fluconazole [150 mg single dose]) may be preferable for the treatment of *C albicans* because of ease of administration. Creams tend to be messy, irritating, and possibly skin sensitizing.[16] Short-course topical azole drugs are more effective than nystatin in effectively treating uncomplicated VVC. Symptom relief and negative cultures are noted in 80% to 90% of patients who complete therapy.[15] Butaconazole, clotrimazole, miconazole, and terconazole for intravaginal use are available over the counter. Both oral and topical antifungals are used for treatment. Each episode of RVVC caused by *C albicans* responds well to short duration oral or topical azole therapy. To maintain clinical control, the recommendation is a longer duration of initial therapy (eg, 7 to14 days of topical therapy or a 150-mg, oral dose of fluconazole repeated every 72 hours ×3) to achieve mycologic remission. Maintenance therapy with fluconazole (150 mg weekly) is then initiated. Other options recommended for maintenance regimens include clotrimazole, ketoconazole, and itraconazole. Maintenance regimens may be continued for 6 months or longer. Approximately one in 10,000 to 15,000 persons exposed to ketoconazole develops hepatotoxicity, so fluconzaole is preferable. Patients receiving long-term ketoconazole should be monitored for hepatotoxicity.[15]

The optimal treatment of nonalbicans VVC remains unknown. Longer duration of therapy (7 to 14 days) with a nonfluconazole azole drug is recommended as first-line therapy. Boric acid per vagina (600 mg of boric acid in a gelatin capsule) is recommended, administered vaginally once daily for 2 weeks.[15] With this approach, clinical treatment rates are close to 70%. An alternate option is topical 5-flucytosine. Safety data regarding the long-term use of these regimens are lacking. For recurrences of nonalbicans VVC, a maintenance regimen of 100,000 units of nystatin vaginal suppositories daily has been effective.

Cellulitis

Areas of epithelial disruption from scratching of any pruritic vulvar condition may result in superimposed bacterial infections with resultant inflammation and edema. *Staphylococcus aureus* and *Streptococcus pyogenes* are the most common organisms isolated from vulvar cellulitis. Risk factors for cellulitis include diabetes mellitus, arteriosclerosus, obesity, hypertension, and prior irradiation.[17] Cellulitis is manifested by edema, redness, pain, and fever. Sequelae include variable degrees of deep fibrosis and impaired lymphatic return that can occur, predisposing to future recurrent cellulitis and increasing lymphedema with each episode. Antibiotics are usually curative although they do not prevent recurrence. Also, cellulitis of the genitalia is at risk for necrotizing fasciitis compared with other locations. This deep tissue infection characterized by ischemia and necrosis is identified by deteriorating vital signs and a deep, spreading painful erythema, necrosis, tissue hemorrhage, or bullae should raise concern for necrotizing fasciitis (**Fig. 5**). This rapidly

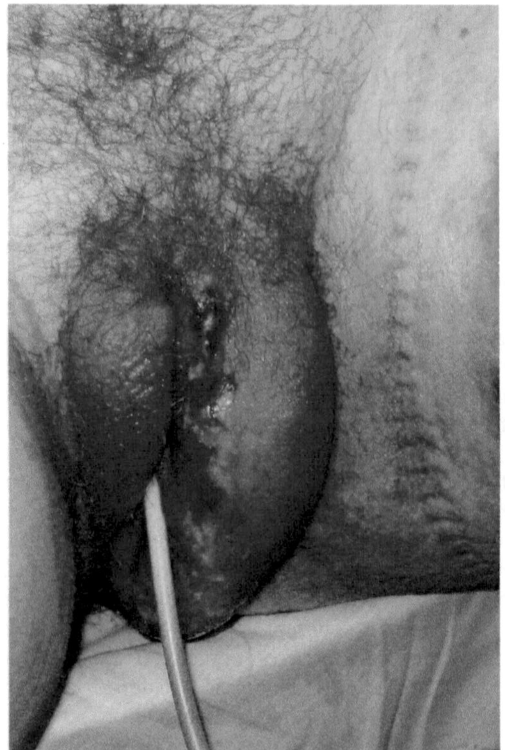

Fig. 5. Necrotizing fasciitis vulvar edema with erosions on the labia majora that were found to have necrosis requiring extensive débridement.

progressive infection is commonly caused by mixed aerobic-anaerobic bacteria. Antibiotic treatment usually proves ineffective. The presence of necrotizing fasciitis is a surgical emergency requiring repeated débridement of the necrotic fascia to prevent septic shock and fatal complications. CT or MRI of the fascial layer in question can effectively diagnose the condition.[18]

Stevens-Johnson Syndrome/Toxic Epidermal Necrolysis

Stevens-Johnson syndrome and toxic epidermal necrolysis, forms of blistering erythema, are hypersensitivity reactions triggered by medication allergy or recurrent HSV infection. These are characterized by a prodrome of malaise and fever, followed by erythematous macules and plaques, generally with cutaneous edema. The skin lesions progress to epidermal necrosis and sloughing. Mucous membranes are affected in 92% to 100% of patients, usually at two or more distinct sites.[19] Stevens-Johnson syndrome and toxic epidermal necrolysis produce erosions, redness, and edema of the mouth, eyes, and genitals as well as inflammation and erosions of the vagina.

Herpes Simplex Virus Infection

Approximately 50 million people in the United States have genital HSV infection. Primary infection of HSV type 1 (HSV-1) or type 2 (HSV-2) presents with multiple, superficial, painful erosions of the lower genital tract. In the primary infection, tender inguinal lymphadenopathy, fever, and malaise may coexist with ulceration. The typical painful multiple vesicular or ulcerative lesions (**Fig. 6**) are absent in a significant number of infected people. HSV-1 is the predominant cause of first episode genital herpes infections although many recurrent genital herpes infections are caused by HSV-2. Approximately 50% of first-episode cases of genital herpes infections are caused by HSV-1.[20] Recurrences and subclinical shedding are much less frequent for genital HSV-1 infection than genital HSV-2 infection.[21,22] Because the specific type of genital herpes infections causing the first episode influences prognosis and counseling, the clinical diagnosis of genital herpes infections should be confirmed by laboratory testing.[23] Recurrent lesions are often less severe and less commonly associated with lymphadenopathy. With recurrent lesions, systemic symptoms are rare although instances have been documented. The diagnosis of HSV is obtained from the clinical presentation and virologic and serologic tests. Virologic tests isolating HSV in cell cultures from genital ulcers and other mucocutaneous lesions is the preferred mode of diagnosis. The sensitivity of culture is generally low and is further lowered for recurrent lesions and lesions in the healing phase. Polymerase chain reaction (PCR) assays for HSV DNA are more sensitive and have been used instead of viral culture.[24,25] PCR assays are, however, not FDA cleared for testing of genital specimens. Because viral shedding is intermittent, lack of HSV detection on culture or PCR does not

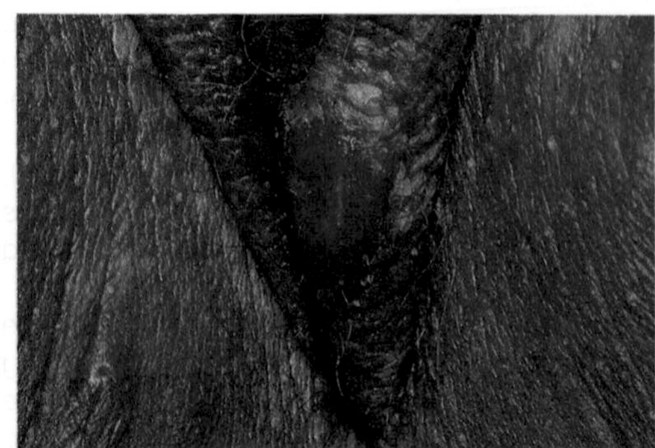

Fig. 6. HSV. Ulceration of the left labium majus with surrounding edema. Note two other lesions of HSV on the right side.

indicate the absence of HSV infection. Antibodies to HSV develop during the first several weeks after infection and persist indefinitely. HSV-specific glycoprotein G2 (HSV-2) and glycoprotein G1 (HSV-1) are identified during type-specific HSV specific tests. Serologic type-specific glycoprotein G–based assays should be specifically requested when serology is performed.[26] The sensitivities of these glycoprotein tests in detecting HSV-2 antibodies approximates 80% to 98%. False-negative results tend to be more common during the early stages of infection. The specificities of these assays are greater than or equal to 96%. False-positive results occur, especially when the likelihood of HSV infection is low. In such cases, repeat or confirmatory testing may be indicated. Three antiviral medications provide clinical benefit for genital herpes infections: acyclovir, valacyclovir, and famciclovir.[27,28] Antiviral drugs partially control the signs and symptoms of herpes episodes either during first clinical outbreaks or recurrent episodes. First-episode herpes may present with mild clinical symptoms but then proceed to later develop severe or prolonged symptoms. Patients with first episode genital herpes infections should, therefore, receive antiviral therapy.[15] Antiviral therapy for recurrent genital herpes infections can be administered either episodically or continuously. Episodic therapy aims to improve symptoms or shorten the duration of lesions whereas continuous suppressive therapy aims to suppress the virus and reduces the frequency of recurrences. For episodic treatment of recurrent herpes to be effective, therapy should be initiated within a day of onset of the lesions or during the prodrome suggesting an impending outbreak. A prescription for the antiviral medication should be given to patients with instructions to start treatment at the earliest sign of a prodrome or lesions. Episodic treatment regimens vary considerably; to give a few examples: Acyclovir 800 mg orally twice a day for 5 days, famciclovir (1000 mg orally twice daily for 1 day), or valacyclovir (1 g orally once a day for 5 days). Suppressive therapy (acyclovir [400 mg orally twice a day], famiciclovir [250 mg orally twice a day], or valacyclovir [500 mg orally once a day]) has the additional advantage of decreasing the risk of genital HSV-2 transmission to susceptible partners.[29] These drugs neither eradicate latent virus nor affect the risk, frequency, or severity of recurrences after the drug is discontinued.

Lymphogranuloma Venereum

LGV is an infection produced by *C trachomatis* serovars L1, L2, or L3.[15,30] This classic cause of vulvar edema is rare in industrialized Western societies.

LGV presents as unilateral tender inguinal and/or femoral lymphadenopathy. The genital ulcer or papule that occurs at the site of inoculation is often self-limited and may have resolved by the time patients seek care. Proctocolitis results from rectal exposure, especially in men having sex with men. The presentation varies from a mucoid and rectal discharge with or without bleeding to fever, constipation, and tenesmus. If LGV is not treated early, it progresses to an invasive, systemic infection. LGV proctocolitis can lead to chronic colorectal fistulas and strictures. Genital and colorectal LGV lesions might also be co-infected with other sexually transmitted pathogens. In addition, secondary bacterial infection of LGV lesions in female patients may produce inflammation and edema of the vulva.

Diagnosis is based on clinical suspicion and the exclusion of other causes (of proctocolitis, inguinal lymphadenopathy, or genital or rectal ulcers) along with *C trachomatis* testing, if available. Genital lesion swabs and aspiration of lymph node specimens (bubo aspirate) may be tested for *C trachomatis* by culture. Immunofluorescent tests and nucleic acid detection have also been used. Nucleic acid amplification tests for *C trachomatis*, however, are not FDA approved for testing rectal specimens. Specialized genotype testing is required for differentiating between *C trachomatis* causing LGV and non-LGV types. These specialized tests are not widely available. Chlamydia serology (complement fixation titers >1:64) may help with diagnosis when the clinical suspicion is high. The interpretation of serologic tests in the setting of proctatitis is neither standardized nor validated. Patients with a clinical picture of LGV presenting with either genital ulcer disease with lymphadenopathy or proctocolitis should be treated for LGV. Treatment aims at curing the infection and preventing ongoing tissue damage and scarring. Buboes might require aspiration or incision and drainage to prevent the formation of inguinal ulcers. The preferred treatment mode of treatment is doxycycline (100 mg orally twice daily for 21 days). Alternately, erythromycin (base 500 mg orally 4 times daily for 21 days) can be used.

Granuloma Inguinale

Granuloma inguinale is a genital ulcerative disease caused by the gram-negative bacterium *Klebsiella granulomatis*, formerly called *Calymmatobacterium granulomatis*. This is a rare disease in North America but is endemic in some tropical and developing countries. It presents as a painless, progressive ulcerative lesions without regional lymphadenopathy. The lesions are highly vascular and bleed easily on contact. The clinical presentation, however, also can include hypertrophic, necrotic, or sclerotic variants, with late lymphedema. The lesions also can develop secondary bacterial infection with surrounding edema. Diagnosis requires visualization of dark-staining Donovan bodies on biopsy or tissue crush preparation. Treatment is with doxycycline (100 mg orally twice daily for a minimum of 21 days) and until all lesions have completely healed. Alternative regimens include azithromycin, ciprofloxacin, erythromycin base, and trimethoprim-sulfamethoxazole.[15]

Chancroid

Chancroid, also uncommon in industrialized countries, is characterized by painful genital ulcers and tender suppurative inguinal adenopathy. It is caused by infection with *Haemophilus ducreyi* and occurs in isolated outbreaks. Vulvar edema may result from surrounding inflammation and bacterial superinfection. Chancroid is a cofactor for HIV transmission. The definitive diagnosis of chancroid requires the identification of *H ducreyi* on special culture media, which is not readily available. The sensitivity of these culture media is less than 80%; thus, the clinical presentation in the absence of positive HSV and syphilis tests supports this diagnosis. There are several options for treatment, including azithromycin (1 g orally in a single dose) or ceftriaxone (250 mg intramuscularly in a single dose). Oral ciprofloxacin or erythromycin base may also be used in the treatment of chancroid.[15] Fluctuant lymphadenopathy tends to require a longer time for resolution in comparison to ulcers and is sometimes managed with needle aspiration, incision, and drainage.

Epstein-Barr Virus

There have been reports of Epstein-Barr virus causing vulvar ulcerations, particularly in adolescents. Symptoms of fever, sore throat, cervical lymphadenopathy, and genital ulcerations and edema may occur during an acute episode of infectious mononucleosis, an Epstein-Barr virus infection.[31,32]

Parvovirus Infection

Parvovirus infection in rare instances can cause vulvar edema. Butler and colleagues[33] described a 7-year-old girl who presented with acute vulvar erythema and pustules. These were associated with a petechial eruption in her flexures and over her feet. There was a mild prodromal illness, no fever, and minimal symptoms associated with the rash. Skin and throat swabs were negative and blood examination showed mild neutrophilia and lymphopenia. Parvovirus B19 IgM was detected on serology and cutaneous features resolved within 4 days. This was a case of parvovirus B19 infection presenting as a bathing trunk exanthem with unique dermatologic features, including the presence of pustules and distant petechiae.

Filariasis

Parasitic infestation of the groin lymph nodes with *Wichereria bancrofti* (filariasis) can cause massive lower-limb and vulvar edema in developing, tropical/subtropical countries.

TRAUMA

Vulvar trauma resulting from various mechanisms might result in massive hematomas and edema. Straddle injuries are the most reported especially in the pediatric and adolescent age groups.

Vulvar Hematoma

Hematomas and impressive edema related to perineal trauma surrounding vaginal deliveries are not unusual. There are reports of hematomas occurring after both consensual sexual intercourse as well as sexual assault in adolescents.[34] Management is conservative and aimed at relief of pain with cool gel packs and narcotics. An indwelling Foley catheter is sometimes required if edema is sufficient to produce obstruction. It is important to assess for hemodynamic stability. In cases with elevated white blood cell counts, antibiotics are started to prevent an infected hematoma. The swelling and associated discoloration (**Fig. 7**) often take several weeks to resolve.

Tourniquet Syndrome

The tourniquet syndrome has been described.[35] It occurs mostly in infants and young children

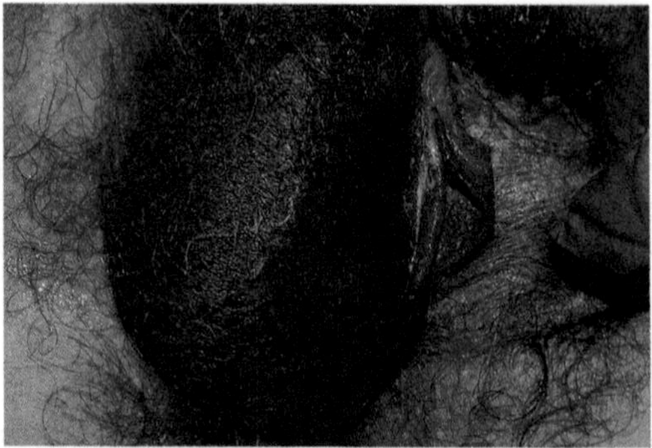

Fig. 7. Vulvar hematoma—large vulvar hematoma with edema and bluish skin discoloration.

whereby there is circumferential strangulation of one or more appendage by single or multiple human hair or fibers. The distal venous and lymphatic drainage is compromised and may result in local edema and inflammation. A circumferential band with distal edema and erythema of finger, toe, penis, or clitoris is typical. Early diagnosis and prompt release of the strangulation are essential to prevent autoamputation of the appendage.

GENERAL MEDICAL CONDITIONS

Vulvar edema may occur as part of anasarca secondary to a generalized medical condition. In renal and cardiac failure, the increased intravascular hydrostastic pressure leads to the formation of edema. Reduced plasma oncotic pressure in severe malnutrition and hepatic failure is another mechanism for generalized edema. Treatment of the underlying condition ultimately resolves the associated vulvar edema.

Iatrogenic

Diagnostic and therapeutic medical/surgical procedures may result in vulvar edema. Levavi and colleagues[36] describe a patient presenting with bilateral severe labial edema 2 days after vaginal and vulvar CO_2 laser treatment for widespread genital condyloma. This finding was attributed to transient local lymphatic drainage obstruction caused by thermal damage from the laser. Vulvar edema has been reported after lower abdominal paracentesis,[37,38] operative laparoscopy,[39,40] vaginal tape procedure complicated by bladder perforation,[41] and intraperitoneal Hyskon administration with fluid shifts.[42] Attempts have been made to explain the underlying pathologic mechanisms in these cases. One cited possibility is the escape of solution through a lower trocar site, with tracking along the subcutaneous planes into a dependent body region (vulvar). In cases of unilateral vulvar edema, another possibility is fluid leakage through a patent canal of Nuck. Lymphedema of the vulva may occur from obstruction of lower-limb lymphatic drainage. Malignancy, surgery, and radiation involving the inguinofemoral group of lymph nodes may impair lymphatic drainage, resulting in edema.

Pregnancy Related

Vulvar edema has been described in association with pregnancy.[43,44] It can occur in preeclampsia as part of generalized edema. There have been reports of vulvar edema with the use of a birthing chair[45] and also after a prolonged second stage. Intravenous tocolytic therapy has been documented to cause edema.[46,47]

Local Vulvar Tumors/Neoplasms

There are a variety of vulvar masses, both benign and malignant, which may be associated with edema or resemble edema clinically. These should be considered differential diagnoses in cases of vulvar edema resistant to the appropriate therapy.

Lipomas

Lipomas of the vulvar are rare benign tumors that consist of mature fat cells often interspersed with strands of fibrous connective tissue. They arise from the vulvar fatty pads and present as soft, multilobulated subcutaneous neoplasms, which can become pedunculated. Although they do not generally produce edema, they often are mistaken for edema. Histologic examination reveals a thin capsule surrounding a lobular proliferation of lipocytes. Lipomas are removed when they are symptomatic, cause cosmetic concerns, or for evaluation their histology when liposarcomas must be ruled out.

Bartholin gland duct cyst

Bartholin cysts are formed when a Bartholin duct is blocked, causing a fluid-filled cyst to develop. A Bartholin cyst can grow from the size of a pea to the size of an egg, or even larger at times. This enlarged cyst can be mistaken for edema. A Bartholin cyst is caused by physical blockage of the Bartholin duct. Or, inflammation or infection of a Bartholin gland duct cyst can produce inflammatory edema. Treatment of Bartholin cysts/abscesses consists of Word catheter placement, marsupialization, or, if recurrent cysts/abscesses, removal of the lesion. Word catheters can be uncomfortable to patients and often do not remain in place for an adequate time. Many providers prefer to go straight to marsupialization rather than use a Word catheter.

Lymphangioma circumscriptum

Lymphangioma circumscriptum (LC) is a rare, benign disorder of lymphatic channels that protrude above the surface of the skin, resembling blisters. It can occur as either a congenital abnormality as a developmental defect of lymphatics in deep and subcutaneous layers, or it can occur as a result of lymphatic obstruction of any cause, including chronic edema, tumor, radiation therapy, and surgery.[48] Lymphangioma circumscriptum may cause symptoms of itching, pain, and oozing of serous fluid. There is a risk of infection, psychosexual dysfunction, and cosmetic disfigurement.[48] The clinical presentation is characterized by localized eruption of grouped thick-walled vesicles filled with clear lymphatic fluid ranging in diameter from 1 to 5 mm (**Fig. 8**).[49] Vesicles may appear pink/purple or black when filled with blood. They may arise over pre-existing papules and in a setting of edema. They may be associated with hyperkeratosis giving verrucous appearance.[50]

The congenital form of LC has been attributed to a hamartomatous malformation of localized, sequestrated lymphatic cisterns lying in deep dermis. These lesions of congenital origin may be large and have deep lymphatic cavernous involvement. The acquired form of LC results from treatment-related obstruction of lymphatics as in pelvic lymphadenectomy.[50] These acquired lesions are generally small and well circumscribed. Treatment for both congenital and acquired vulvar LC ranges from conservative therapy with palliative CO_2 and YAG laser ablation to radical surgery. Surgical removal of the lesion is generally in the form of simple or radical vulvectomy.[51–53] Recurrence is not unusual.

Aggressive angiomyxoma

Aggressive angiomyxoma usually presents as a nonpainful cystlike or polypoid lesion or as an ill-defined swelling of the vulva or pelvic region. The tumor grows and extends locally into soft tissues, displacing the pelvic viscera. Aggressive angiomyxomas occur predominantly in premenopausal women and are often positive for estrogen and/or progesterone receptors. This implies that hormones are potentially important in stimulating growth of the tumor. Complete surgical excision with wide margins seems to be the mainstay of therapy for most patients with aggressive angiomyxoma; however, there is a tendency for recurrence. Gonadotropin-releasing hormone agonist therapy[54] seems to have a significant beneficial role, especially as an adjuvant to surgery or when surgery is not possible. There are a variety of other mesenchymal lesions, such as myofibroblastoma, cellular angiofibroma, and angiomyofibroblastoma, that may mimic aggressive angiomyxoma. McCluggage and colleagues[55] described two cases of massive edema presenting as bilateral vulvar swelling, one in an immobilized patient who was wheelchair bound and the other in an obese woman. These closely mimic aggressive angiomyxoma. Before their report, there had been only a single report of vulva edema presenting as a mass that had undergone surgical resection. This may be a more common condition than is realized in obese and immobile patients. It may be clinically recognized as edema and is managed conservatively with surgical removal only rarely undertaken.

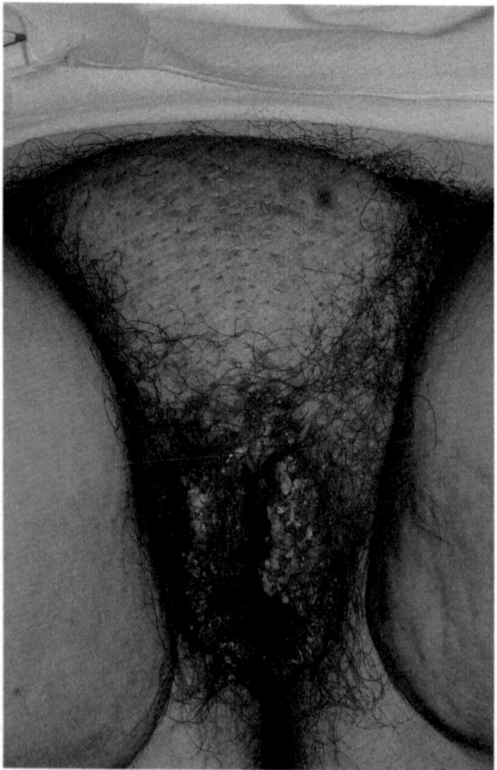

Fig. 8. Lymphangioma circumscriptum: severe edema of the mons pubis. Labia majora bilaterally consist of numerous vesicles containing lymphatic fluid.

Lymphoma

Lymphomas of the vulva are rare, with the majority being non-Hodgkin lymphomas. The most common subtypes of vulvar lymphoma reported are diffuse large B-cell lymphoma and follicular lymphoma. Perianal Hodgkin's lymphoma is also rare. It has been reported in association with HIV infection, Epstein-Barr virus infection, and Crohn disease. Winnicki and colleagues[56] reported a case of Hodgkin's lymphoma of the vulva with involvement of the perianal area. The patient presented with a long history of vulvar swelling, redness, itching, and burning in the setting of a longstanding history of Crohn disease. The patient was subsequently diagnosed as having stage IV disseminated Hodgkin lymphoma with bulky disease of the vulva. She received eight cycles of chemotherapy with doxorubicin, bleomycin, vinblastine, and dacarbazine at the end of which a 50% reduction in the size of the vulvar mass was noted. This is the second reported case of Hodgkin lymphoma of the vulva and the second case of Hodgkin lymphoma involving the perianal area in a female patient. There is currently no evidence that Crohn disease is associated with an increased risk of Hodgkin lymphoma.

TREATMENT OF VULVAR EDEMA

First-line treatment of vulvar edema is guided by the cause. There also are management strategies, however, in addition to treating underlying causes. When vulva edema occurs as part of lower-extremity lymphedema, management includes the treatment of the lymphedema. Complete decongestive therapy is one of the main modalities in lymphedema management. It consists of manual manipulation of the lymphatic ducts, use of compression bandages, therapeutic exercises, and skin care. Intermittent sequential gradient pumps are sometimes used before manual lymphatic drainage. Compression pump technology uses a multichambered pneumatic sleeve. This aims at moving the lymphatic fluid and breaking up fibrotic tissue. Manual lymphatic drainage consists of manipulation of the lymphatic ducts. It consists of gentle skin massage to stimulate the flow of lymph and its return to the blood circulation system. Complete decongestive therapy is generally effective on nonfibrotic lymphedema. It has, however, been shown to help break up fibrotic tissue. Elastic compression garments and nonelastic directional flow foam garments are used for maintenance care once the lymphedema is reduced.

SUMMARY

Vulvar edema has a wide range of causative factors and mechanisms. It is essential that the underlying and associated medical conditions be identified for successful management. In cases that seem resistant to conventional therapy, the rare connective tissue tumors and neoplasms should be considered.

REFERENCES

1. Haeger E, Girton S, Kennedy C. Contact dermatitis of the vulvar. Postgraduate Obstetrics & Gynecology 2007;27:1–6.
2. Shah S, Ormerod A. Pigmented purpuric clothing dermatitis due to disperse dyes. Contact Dermatitis 2000;43:360.
3. Bauer A, Rödiger C, Greif C, et al. Vulvar dermatoses: irritant and allergic contact dermatitis of the vulva. Dermatology 2005;210:143–9.
4. Tavarela VF. Review article: skin complications associated with inflammatory bowel disease. Aliment Pharmacol Ther 2004;20(Suppl 4):50–3.
5. Feller ER, et al. Gynecologic aspects of crohn's disease. Am Fam Physician 2001;64:1725–8.
6. Patton LW, Elgart ML, Williams CM. Vulvar erythema and induration. Extraintestinal crohn's disease of thevulva. Arch Dermatol 1990;126: 1351–2.
7. Vettraino IM, Merritt DF. Crohn's disease of the vulva (review). Am J Dermatopathol 1995;17:410–3.
8. Duhra P, Paula CJ. Metastatic crohn's disease responding to metronodazole. Br J Dermatol 1988; 119(1):87–91.
9. Fitzsimmons JS, Gilbert G. A family study of hidradenitis suppurativa. J Med Genet 1985;22:367–73.
10. Church JM, Fazio VW, Lavery IC. The differential diagnosis and comorbidity of hidradenitis suppurativa and perianal crohn's disease. Int J Colorectal Dis 1993;8:117–9.
11. Jemec GB. Medical treatment of hidradenitis suppurativa. Expert Opin Pharmacother 2004;5(8):1767–70.
12. Brocard A, Knol AC, Khammari A. Hidradenitis suppurativa and zinc: a new therapeutic approach. A pilot study. Dermatology 2007;214(4):325–7.
13. Fardet L, Dupuy A, Kerob B. Infliximab for severe hidradenitis suppurativa: transient clinical efficacy in 7 consecutive patients. J Am Acad Dermatol 2007;56: 624–8.
14. Richter SS, Galask RP, Messer SA, et al. Antifungal susceptibilities of Candida species causing vulvovaginitis and epidemiology of recurrent cases. J Clin Microbiol 2005;43:2155–62.
15. 2006 CDC Std Treatment Guidelines.http://www.cdc.gov/std/treatment/2006/toc.htm. Accessed March 2, 2010.
16. Nwokolo NC, Boag FC. Chronic vaginal candidiasis. Management in the postmenopausal patient (review). Drugs Aging 2000;16:335–9.
17. Adelson MD, Joret DM, Gordon LP, et al. Recurrent necrotizing fasciitis of the vulva. a case report. J Reprod Med 1991;36:818–22.
18. Brothers TE, Tagge DU, Stutley JE, et al. Magnetic resonance imaging differentiates between necrotizing and non-necrotizing fasciitis of the lower extremity. J Am Coll Surg 1998;187:416–21.
19. Letko E, Papaliodis DN, Papaliodis GN, et al. Stevens-Johnson syndrome and toxic epidermal necrolysis: a review of the literature. Ann Allergy Asthma Immunol 2005;94:419–36.
20. Roberts CM, Pfister JR, Spear SJ. Increasing proportion of herpes simplex virus type 1 as a cause of genital herpes infection in college students. Sex Transm Dis 2003;30:801–2.
21. Benedetti JK, Corey L, Ashley R. Recurrence rates in genital herpes after symptomatic first-episode infection. Ann Intern Med 1994;121:847–54.
22. Engelberg R, Carrell D, Krantz E, et al. Natural history of genital herpes simplex virus type 1 infection. Sex Transm Dis 2003;30:174–7.
23. Scoular A. Using the evidence base on genital herpes: optimising the use of diagnostic tests

and information provision. Sex Transm Infect 2002; 78:160–5.
24. Scoular A, Gillespie G, Carman WF. Polymerase chain reaction for diagnosis of genital herpes in a genitourinary medicine clinic. Sex Transm Infect 2002;78:21–5.
25. Wald A, Huang M-L, Carrell D, et al. Polymerase chain reaction for detection of herpes simplex virus (HSV) DNA on mucosal services: comparison with HSV isolation in cell culture. J Infect Dis 2003;188: 1345–51.
26. Song B, Dwyer DE, Mindel A. HSV type specific serology in sexual health clinics: use, benefits, and who gets tested. Sex Transm Infect 2004;80: 113–7.
27. Leone PA, Trottier S, Miller JM. Valacyclovir for episodic treatment of genital herpes: a shorter 3-day treatment course compared with 5-day treatment. Clin Infect Dis 2002;34:958–62.
28. Chosidow O, Drouault Y, Leconte-Veyriac F, et al. Famciclovir vs. aciclovir in immunocompetent patients with recurrent genital herpes infections: a parallel-groups, randomized, double-blind clinical trial. Br J Dermatol 2001;144:818–24.
29. Romanowski B. Valtrex HS230017 Study Group, Marina RB, Roberts JN. Patients' preference of valacyclovir once-daily suppressive therapy versus twice-daily episodic therapy for recurrent genital herpes: a randomized study. Sex Transm Dis 2003; 30:226–31.
30. O'Farrell N. Donovanosis. Sex Transm Infect 2002; 78:452–7.
31. Halvorsen JA, Brevig T, Aas T, et al. Genital ulcers as initial manifestation of Epstein–Barr virus infection: two new cases and a review of the literature. Acta Derm Venereol 2006;86: 439–42.
32. Cheng SX, Chapman MS, Margesson LJ, et al. Genital ulcers caused by Epstein–Barr virus. J Am Acad Dermatol 2004;51:824–6.
33. Butler GJ, Mendelsohn S, Franks A. Parvovirus B19 infection presenting as 'bathing trunk' erythema with pustules. Australas J Dermatol 2006;47(4): 286–8.
34. Jones JS, Rossman L, Hartman M, et al. Anogenital injuries in adolescents after consensual sexual intercourse. Acad Emerg Med 2003;10(12): 1378–83.
35. Serour F, Gorenstein A, Dan M. Tourniquet syndrome of the clitoris in a 4-year-old girl. J Emerg Med 2007; 33(3):283–4.
36. Levavi H, Perez-Davidi Y, Sabah G. Labial edema following treatment of condyloma acuminata with co2 laser in an adolescent: a case report and literature review. J Pediatr Adolesc Gynecol 2006;19:105–7.
37. Luxman D, Cohen JR, Gordon D, et al. Unilateral vulvar edema associated with paracentesis in patients with severe ovarian hyperstimulation syndrome. A report of nine cases. J Reprod Med 1996;41:771.
38. Vavilis D, Tzitzimikas S, Agorastos T, et al. Postparacentesis bilateral massive vulvar edema in a patient with severe ovarian hyperstimulation syndrome. Fertil Steril 2002;77:841.
39. Pados G, Vavilis D, Pantazis K, et al. Unilateral vulvar edema after operative laparoscopy: a case report and literature review. Fertil Steril 2005;83:471.
40. Guven S, Guven ES, Ayhan A. Vulvar edema as a rare complication of laparoscopy. J Am Assoc Gynecol Laparosc 2004;11:429.
41. Tseng LH, Lo TS, Wang AC, et al. Bladder perforation presenting as vulvar edema after the tension-free vaginal tape procedure. A case report. J Reprod Med 2003;48:824.
42. Sauer M, Rodi I, Bustillo M. Unilateral vulvar edema after intraperitoneal Hyskon administration. Fertil Steril 1985;44:546.
43. Deren O, Bildirici I, Al A. Massive vulvar edema complicating a diabetic pregnancy. Eur J Obstet Gynecol Reprod Biol 2000;93:209.
44. Tam KS, Woods ML, Hill D. Staphylococcus septicaemia and massive vulvar oedema in pregnancy. Aust N Z J Obstet Gynaecol 2002;42:554.
45. Goodlin RC, Frederick IB. Postpartum vulvar edema associated with birthing chair. Am J Obstet Gynecol 1983;146:334.
46. Brittain C, Carlson JW, Gehlbach DL, et al. A case report of massive vulvar edema during tocolysis of preterm labor. Am J Obstet Gynecol 1991;165:420.
47. Trice L, Bennert H, Stubblefield PG. Massive vulvar edema complicating tocolysis in a patient with twins. A case report. J Reprod Med 1996;41:121.
48. Roy KK, Agarwal R, Agarwal S, et al. Recurrent vulval congenital lymphangioma circumscriptum—a case report and literature review. Int J Gynecol Cancer 2006;16:930–4.
49. Whimster IW. The pathology of lymphangioma circumscriptum. Br J Dermatol 1976;94:473–86.
50. Tulasi NR, John A, Chauhan I, et al. Lymphangioma circumscriptum. Int J Gynecol Cancer 2004;14: 564–6.
51. Ochsendorf FR, Kaufmann R, Runne U. YAG laser ablation of acquired vulval lymphangioma. Br J Dermatol 2001;144:442–4.
52. Vlastos AT, Malpica A, Follen M. Lymphangioma circumscriptum of the vulva; a review of literature. Obstet Gynecol 2003;101:946–54.
53. Horn LC, Kühndel K, Pawlowitsch T, et al. Acquired lymphangioma circumscriptum of the vulva

mimicking genital warts. Eur J Obstet Gynecol Reprod Biol 2005;123:117–24.

54. Sereda D, Sauthier P, Rachid Hadjeres R, et al. J Low Genit Tract Dis 2009;13(1):46–50.
55. McCluggage WG, Nielsen GP, Young RH. Massive vulval edema secondary to obesity and Immobilization: a potential mimic of aggressive angiomyxoma. Int J Gynecol Pathol 2008;27(3):447–52.
56. Winnicki M, Gariepy G, Sauthier PG, et al. Hodgkin lymphoma presenting as a vulvar mass in a patient with crohn disease: a case report and literature review. J Low Genit Tract Dis 2009;13(2):110–4.

Hidradenitis Suppurativa

F. William Danby, MD, FRCPC[a,b,*], Lynette J. Margesson, MD, FRCPC[a,b]

KEYWORDS

- Hidradenitis suppurativa • Acne inversus
- Follicular hyperkeratosis • Diet • Treatment

Hidradenitis suppurativa (HS) is a chronic, inflammatory, scarring condition involving the intertriginous skin of the axillary, inguinal, inframammary, genital, and perineal areas of the body. It is also referred to as acne inversa and, in the old literature, as Verneuil disease.[1]

HS has been linked to the apocrine sweat (hidros) glands (aden) that were first described in 1921. This link became merely historical in 1990, when Yu and Cook[2] showed follicular occlusion to be the primary event in HS. It is now accepted that the first pathogenetic change is in the pilosebaceous follicular ducts, like acne, and so there has been a move to rename this disorder acne inversa.[3] Despite the legitimate argument that HS is a misnomer, the term has become generally accepted.[4]

DEFINITION

HS is defined clinically by its various features and by its chronicity. It is a recurrent disease, classically, but not exclusively, in the apocrine gland–bearing areas of the skin, manifesting as painful, recurrent, deep-seated, inflamed nodules that can result in abscesses, sinuses, and varying degrees of chronic draining sinus tracts with scarring, disfigurement, and disability.

The Second International HS Research Symposium (San Francisco, March 2009) adopted the following consensus definition[5]: "HS is a chronic, inflammatory, recurrent, debilitating, skin follicular disease that usually presents after puberty with painful deep seated, inflamed lesions in the apocrine gland-bearing areas of the body, most commonly the axilla, inguinal and anogenital region."[6]

HS is frequently misdiagnosed as boils. This results in delayed diagnosis, fragmented care, and progression to a chronic, disabling condition that has a profoundly negative effect on quality of life.

DIAGNOSTIC CRITERIA

The Second International HS Research Symposium also adopted the following diagnostic criteria:

1. Typical lesions: either deep-seated painful nodules (blind boils) in early primary lesions or abscesses, draining sinuses, bridged scars, and tombstone open comedones in secondary lesions
2. Typical topography: axillae, groin, genitals, perineal, and perianal region, buttocks, infra- and intermammary folds
3. Chronicity and recurrences.

These 3 criteria must be met to establish the diagnosis.[6]

HS is recognized by the characteristic skin lesions appearing in the typical locations. The pattern in one area of recurrent boils that do not respond to standard antibiotics is a good clue. Normal boils caused by bacteria respond well to antibiotics and seldom recur after treatment. Normal boils point vertically to, and discharge onto, the surface, unlike typical HS lesions, which are rounded and tend not to burst. HS is characterized by deep, painful, subcutaneous nodules that rupture horizontally under the skin and then tend to track subcutaneously. HS is chronic; 90% of patients in one study had the disease for an average of 19 years.[7]

[a] Dartmouth Medical School, Hanover, NH, USA
[b] Danby & Margesson, 721 Chestnut Street, Manchester, NH 03104, USA
* Corresponding author. Danby & Margesson, 721 Chestnut Street, Manchester, NH 03104.
E-mail address: billd860@gmail.com

Dermatol Clin 28 (2010) 779–793
doi:10.1016/j.det.2010.07.003

There are questions that can help diagnose HS and differentiate it from other disorders (**Box 1**).

DIFFERENTIAL DIAGNOSIS

HS has an extensive differential diagnosis (**Box 2**).[8] The appearance, age of onset, typical locations, poor response to antibiotics, and lack of signs of systemic sepsis can all help distinguish this condition, so the diagnosis should be obvious. There are few conditions that cause recurrent abscesses and sinus tract formation in the intertriginous skin areas, such as Crohn disease, ulcerative colitis, and granuloma inguinale. The most common differential diagnoses are the follicular pyodermas: folliculitis, furuncles, and carbuncles. Infected Bartholin glands and epidermal cysts can also present with HS-like lesions. Atypical infections from any organism, from deep fungi to mycobacteria, can mimic HS, although this is rare. Tumors such as epidermoid cysts, even steatocystoma multiplex, can be confused with HS. The swelling and lymphedema of Crohn disease can cause confusion. Acne produces many lesions similar to HS but the distribution is different.

Because the sites of involvement of HS are so varied and the lesions are sometimes nonspecific, patients present the problem to many specialists. They may see surgeons, gynecologists, urologists, plastic surgeons, dermatologists, infectious disease specialists, proctologists, and even gastroenterologists. Patients seen in emergency departments are often treated with simple incision and drainage. Too often, a short course of antibiotic is given or the lesions are just incised and drained. This treatment is generally ineffective in controlling the disorder and is discouraging for patients. Delay in diagnosis is common, averaging about 7 years, and can be decades.

Box 1
Questions to help diagnosis HS

1. Does anyone in your family have the same symptoms?
2. Do the boils recur in the same spots?
3. Do you smoke or use tobacco products?
4. Do your boils flare before your menstrual period?
5. Have the treatments received been helpful?
6. Do you get a fever with these boils?
7. Do you have infections elsewhere?

Patients with HS normally respond "Yes" to questions 1 to 4 and "No" to 5 to 7.

Data from Poli F, Jemec GB, Revuz J. Clinical presentation. In: Jemec GB, Revuz J, Leyden J, editors. Hidradenitis suppurativa. Berlin: Springer; 2006. p. 22.

Box 2
Differential diagnosis of HS

- Infections
  - Bacterial
    - Carbuncles, furuncles, abscesses, ischiorectal/perirectal abscess, Bartholin duct abscess, erysipelas
    - Mycobacteria: tuberculous abscess
    - Sexually transmitted infections: granuloma inguinale, lymphogranuloma venereum, noduloulcerative syphilis
  - Deep fungi: blastomyces, nocardia
- Tumors
  - Cysts: epidermoid, Bartholin, pilonidal
    - Other: steatocystoma multiplex
  - Trichoepithelioma
- Miscellaneous
  - Crohn disease
  - Anal or vulvovaginal fistulae

PREVALENCE AND EPIDEMIOLOGY

HS is a common, forgotten, and orphaned disease. It is often not recognized by physicians, even dermatologists, and the results are devastating for patients. HS is mistakenly referred to as a rare disease. The global prevalence has been reported as between 1% and 4%, depending on the definitions used.[9] Jemec[10] reported a prevalence of 4% in a series of self-reported cases, with a high prevalence in young adults that was confirmed in another study.[11] Revuz reported the prevalence in persons 55 years and older as 0.5% in contrast to 1.4% for younger people. There may be an increased incidence in black people but most investigators report no racial differences.[5,7,12,13] It is more common in women than men, at a ratio of 3.3:1.14. HS affects the genders differently, being more common found under the breasts (22%) and in the groin (93%) in women and on the buttocks (40%) and perianal area (51%) in men.[11] The average age of onset is 23 years, with a range of 11 to 50 years. It rarely occurs before puberty,[14] occurs earlier in those with a family history of HS,[15] and is unusual after menopause.[12] In men, HS can continue into old age,[16] it can be more severe, and associated squamous cell carcinoma, although infrequent, is more common in men.[5]

ETIOLOGY

Several factors are related to the development of HS.

Genetic Factors

Patients with HS have a 35% to 40% positive family history. An autosomal dominant inheritance pattern has been noted. Studies on 4 generations in a Chinese family indicate linkage to a locus at chromosome 1p21.1 to 1q25.3 but no specific gene was defined.[17] Despite the dominant inheritance pattern, a positive history is usually found in fewer than 50% of family members, probably because of lack of adequate family reporting, poor recognition or hiding of HS, or development of HS in family members after the survey. These findings were supported by von der Werth and Williams[7] who also suggested that HS is most likely a heterogeneous disease, probably with several genes involved. Revuz[5] pointed out that patients with a family history of HS usually have milder disease with earlier onset. More genetic studies are needed.

Infection

Bacteria have long been considered in the pathogenesis of HS. Various strains have been cultured but all are considered to be secondary invaders. It is generally agreed that bacteria do not have a major direct role in the cause of HS but may share in the pathogenesis of the chronic relapsing lesions of deep Hurley stage III, in which they may be responsible for some of the destructive processes that are seen.[18]

Hormonal Factors

Although there has been controversy for years about the role of androgens in HS, there is a strong relationship between sex hormones and HS. It has been suggested that the preponderance in women argues against the role of androgens, a suggestion that ignores the greater sensitivity of women to androgens. HS is more common in women; it occurs around menarche, flares premenstrually, improves with pregnancy, fades after menopause, and does not occur in eunuchs or eunuchoids. Even the studies of HS in children are associated with premature adrenarche or early puberty, when androgens are dominant. As in acne, there are no increases in serum androgens in most patients with HS[19] and the effect is assumed to be caused by end organ sensitivity. The ultimate support for the role of androgens is the effectiveness of antiandrogen therapy, as discussed later.[20–22]

Immune Factors

Even in its most aggressive Hurley stage III form, the disease does not usually produce acute systemic inflammatory effects. There is no fever, no lymphadenopathy, no septicemia, no local cellulitis, cultures are often sterile, and, if the offending material beneath the surface is removed, the disease heals without further difficulty and without antibiotics, which is strongly suggestive of inflammation mediated on the local level by the innate immune system. The simple model of the disorder is the inflammatory reaction around a simple ingrown hair; flick out the foreign hair so it is no longer in contact with dermal toll-like receptors (as an unproven example) and the inflammation fades immediately. Adaptive immunity therefore seems to play no significant part in the cause of HS.

Other Factors

HS can be triggered by, or flared because of, lithium,[23] which can enhance neutrophil migration, increase epithelial cell proliferation, and cause follicular plugging by a direct effect on follicular keratinocytes, as in acne. Sirolimus has been related to the new onset of HS,[24] and medroxyprogesterone acetate acting as an androgen has precipitated or aggravated HS in personal cases. Although HS can be found in both obese and thin patients, shearing forces and hormone-related factors in the obese can worsen HS,[18] and obesity seems to result in more severe disease.[25] Smoking is common in patients with HS, 70% to 89% of patients with HS have been smokers, and nicotine has been shown to activate nonneuronal acetylcholine receptors causing increased keratinization of the pilosebaceous duct, suggesting a role for nicotine in the cause of HS.[25–27]

Pathogenesis

The pathogenesis of the disease consists of follicular plugging, ductal rupture, and secondary inflammation leading to numerous downstream changes. HS is subject to genetic, mechanical, hormonal, and other influences.[28] The sequential story is likely as follows, although some links remain to be proven.

When hormonal overstimulation of the production of ductal keratinocytes results in failure of terminal differentiation of the keratinocytes lining the ducts, they fail to separate from each other, leading to the accumulation of keratinocytes known as a comedo. The comedo causes a tight plug in the acroinfundibulum of the duct. It seems that a genetic weakness or deficiency of the PAS-positive glassy membrane glycoprotein material that supports the duct (Danby FW. The glassy membrane in hidradenitis suppurativa, unpublished work, 2009) under the centrifugal pressure of a bulging follicular canal, permits the wall of the duct to lose its structural integrity. Molecule-sized follicular contents leak out, stimulating the innate immune system, leading to the rupture of the congenitally weak wall of the duct. Healing processes attempt to repair the normal anatomy of the pilosebaceous unit, and sometimes succeed, but the failure of the inflammatory contents to simply discharge to the surface and then heal is what differentiates HS from acne, folliculitis, or a simple boil. After rupturing beneath the surface, the follicular fragments and their growth cause the extensive lateral spread and the characteristic inflammatory reaction.[29]

The epithelial material caught in the dermis is not simply sitting there as isolated, benign pieces of damaged tissue, waiting to dissolve. These fragments are alive and are still exposed to the hormones and growth factors that nourished the initial overproduction of keratinocytes. Continuous growth of these hormonally stimulated remnants beneath the surface produces the communicating sinuses (**Fig. 1**) and provides increasing volumes of irritating material, some almost certainly derived from the pluripotential stem cells in the bulge area of the exploded follicle. This aberrant epithelial repair response drives the inflammation in the dermis and subcutis.[30]

The innate immune system is the prime mover in HS (–discussed earlier), just as in acne vulgaris and even acne rosacea. The ongoing reaction to an enlarging and extending mass of epithelial and ductal elements produces continuous and increasing amounts of innate inflammatory reaction, which explains the relentless course of the disorder. This mass of interactive material forms the central core of HS, and the disorder will not settle until this active mass is eliminated. These and numerous other pathogenetic considerations were recently discussed by a panel of experts.[28]

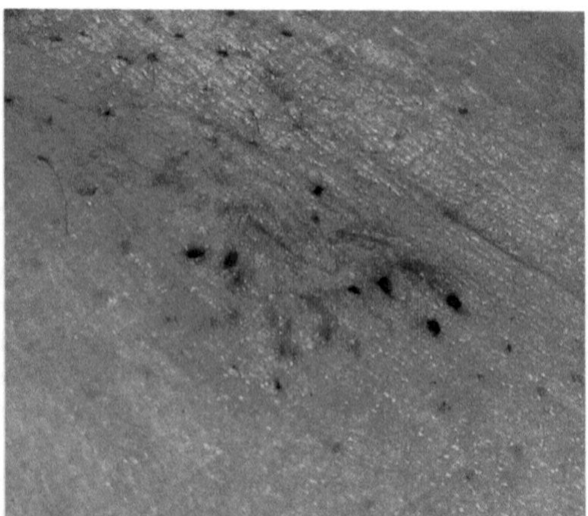

Fig. 1. Classic multiheaded comedones over a sinus track in HS.

CLINICAL DESCRIPTION

HS classically occurs in the early 20s. The onset can be insidious, with apparently random small lesions that develop as a red, indurated papule, pustule, or nodule that may resolve without leaving any mark (**Box 3**). The lesions may develop in only 1 area, or several areas over weeks or months. The discomfort varies from vague itching to mild to moderate pain. In some cases, the onset can be severe, even frightening, with large, deep, painful lesions that result in restriction of activities. Too often they are diagnosed as recurrent boils or furunculosis. Lesions are generally intertriginous and involve, in order of frequency, the axillae, inguinal areas, inner thigh, perianal and perineal areas, mammary and inframammary area, buttocks, pubic region, scrotum, vulva, chest, scalp, and retroauricular region. Women typically

Box 3
Clinical description

HS Lesions

Primary lesions

Recurrent or persistent/painful

- Red papules less than 1 cm in diameter
- Red nodules larger than 1 cm in diameter
- Pustules or abscesses

Secondary lesions

Persistent red, painful, draining sinus(es)

Ulcerations with or without granulation tissue

Tertiary lesions

Scars

- Pitted or cribriform
- Dense fibrotic plaques or linear, ropelike scars

Epidermoid cysts

Single or multiple tombstone comedones

Lymphedema with or without lymphangiectasia

have involvement in the groin, axilla, and under the breasts. In men, it is found in the axillae and groin and is more common perianally than in women.[7] Involvement of the perineal and perianal areas is more debilitating than axillary involvement because of frequent recurrence.[31]

Primary lesions of HS are individual, painful nodules, 0.5 to 2 cm in diameter that persist for weeks or months with a varying degree of inflammation. The diagnosis is frequently delayed. These lesions can be deep and patients complain of pain although all that is visible is redness with barely any swelling, despite major discomfort. A prodrome has been reported in 50% of all patients, consisting of burning, stinging, pain, and pruritus, with or without hyperhidrosis, occurring 12 to 48 hours before the onset of nodules.[5] The first lesion may be a small (<1 cm), red papule that may resolve and recur or rupture with purulent drainage. Deep, red, round, painful nodules (>1 cm) are typical. They may be individual or coalesce into groups. The HS nodules do not point centrally but are deep, round, red, and sore, without the spontaneous drainage seen in furunculosis. Nodules can last from 7 to 15 days. They then may progress to resolution, or persist, or drain. With more severe disease, and more time, there is eventual drainage with spontaneous resolution of the pain. Patients often squeeze or pinch these lesions to get relief (some even attempt home surgery to open lesions). Lesions may be grouped or come and go in various areas, depending on the individual. Sheets of small folliculopapules and folliculopustules and acneform lesions may be scattered over the buttocks, mons pubis, and around the breasts. These lesions occur both in early and late HS and may occur in an area separate from the main HS activity. Patients may present, for example, active papules, nodules, and draining sinuses in one area (the groin) and sheets of perifollicular papule pustules elsewhere (around the breasts or buttocks). All these lesions wax and wane.

Secondary lesions develop as a result of persistence of the process in an area. The subcutaneous coalescence of several neighboring cysts, or the lateral extension of actively proliferating pilosebaceous material with rupture to the surface, results in formation of chronic interlinked sinuses. Drainage from these lesions may be serous, purulent, bloody, or a mixture, with or without odor. Uncommonly there may be persistent ulcerations and even the formation of red granulation tissue around a sinus opening. With healing, hypertrophic scars develop and eventually dense ropelike linear fibrotic bands develop that may crisscross an area of involvement. Sinus tracts can be single or multiple; they may be hardly visible, with intermittent serous drainage, or they may be swollen, painful, and inflamed with 1 or more draining sinuses forming a honeycombed pattern of draining nodules or tracts.

Tertiary lesions occur as a result of aberrant healing. Small HS lesions typically heal with small, acneform, pitted, and, less commonly, cribriform scars. Occasionally, indolent epidermal cysts of 1 to 6 cm can develop on the face, behind the ears, at the nape of the neck, on the trunk, and in the genital area. These cysts are more common in men than in women.[5,7] Sinus tracks can coalesce forming hypertrophic, fibrous, fistular tracts involving entire zones. These subcutaneous networks of sinuses can form a solid plaque or thick, bridged, ropelike scars. Both can result in contractures and may decrease range of motion so that patients cannot lift arms or separate thighs. Scarring can result in lymphatic obstruction with lymphedema and eventual lymphangiectasia. One of the classic features of HS is the tombstone comedones that form in a burned out area because of permanently dilated pores. They are often associated with multiple small, superficial sinuses and are present in up to 50% of patients.[11]

CLINICAL COURSE

The mean age of onset is 22.1 years and HS lasts about 19 years.[7] It can remit or partially remit with pregnancy and breastfeeding. The course for patients can be variable. It may be intermittent and benign, with mild but chronic painful disease, acute exacerbations, premenstrual flares, and usually resolution after menopause. It may remit for weeks to months, lesions may flare continuously or only intermittently, and marked involvement may occur in only 1 area with a long deep-draining sinus and discharge typical of Hurley stage III. Revuz[5] describes 2 types of severe disease. The first shows typical solid plaques of coalescent nodules, fistulae, and scars with smelly discharge, pain, and debility. The other type shows new lesions; deep, painful, separate nodules, and draining lesions, continually appearing and each lasting 10 to 30 days. Patients do not necessarily progress from mild to moderate to severe disease but may instead present with a certain degree of severity and remain in that range. Those with severe disease may have marked severity from the beginning and the lesions often develop rapidly, sometimes with the predictive prodrome of itch, pain, and/or malaise.

Patients have varied difficulty with mobility, ranging from minor soreness and discomfort to being unable to walk or sit without pain. With large draining areas, odor may be significant. Patients may need to wear diapers for the drainage. With such pain, debility, and disruption in their daily lives it is common for patients with HS to withdraw and become depressed and, eventually, dysfunctional.

The severity of HS can be classified using Hurley clinical staging and this can also be used to help direct future management.[32]

HURLEY STAGES

In the recent report by Canoui-Poitrine and colleagues,[16] 68.2% of patients are Hurley stage I, 27.6% Hurley stage II, and 3.9% Hurley stage III (**Box 4**). To more accurately assess outcome variables related to HS treatment, the Sartorius score has been developed to monitor patients. It is to act as a complimentary system to the Hurley classification, and is presently undergoing evaluation as a research tool.[33]

MORBIDITY/QUALITY OF LIFE

It is usual for patients with severe disease to be unemployable and socially isolated because of the painful, draining, and malodorous lesions.[34] HS has a profoundly negative effect on patients, not only at a physical level but socially and economically. von der Werth and Jemec[35] studied 144 patients with HS with a dermatology life quality *index* and found a higher morbidity index than in mild to moderate psoriasis or alopecia. The high score was related to pain, malodorous discharge, intimate sites of eruptions, and lack of medical care because of incorrect diagnosis.

In a study of the quality of life of 61 patients with HS, impairment was higher than that for urticaria, neurofibromatosis, psoriasis, and atopic dermatitis.[36] The effect on quality of life is correlated with the number of active lesions and, in particular, severity of pain. Pain is the most limiting factor. Long, continuous duration, and pelvic area involvement, especially with a malodorous discharge, are other major factors.[37]

Patients with HS lose an average of 2 to 7 days of work per year, and this number tends to be greater in women.[13] They are often unemployed, poor, socially isolated, or reclusive.[38,39]

Box 4
Hurley stages

Stage I: abscess formation, single or multiple without sinus tracts and cicatrization

Stage II: recurrent abscesses with tract formation and cicatrization, single or multiple widely separated lesions

Stage III: diffuse or near-diffuse involvement, or multiple interconnecting tracts and abscesses across entire area

ASSOCIATED DISEASES

HS has been associated with severe acne (acne conglobata), dissecting cellulitis of the scalp, and pilonidal cysts (**Box 5**).[40,41] Pilonidal cysts have been associated with HS in up to 30% of cases. Acne vulgaris is only found with HS in about 10% of women and 30% of men but a history of long-lasting, scarring acne was found in 23% of women and 44% of men. Dissecting cellulitis of the scalp is rare (1%); Revuz[5] has never seen the follicular triad in 500 patients he has followed.

KERATITIS-ICHTHYOSIS-DEAFNESS SYNDROME

Two rare pigmentary disorders have been associated with HS. Dowling-Degos disease is a genetic condition with flexural pigmented macules in the axilla, neck, and groin. Kitamura disease has reticulate acropigmentation on hands and feet. The association of these conditions with HS is soft.[9]

Box 5
Associated diseases

- Follicular occlusive diseases (follicular tetrad)
  - Acne vulgaris
  - Acne conglobata
  - Dissecting cellulitis of the scalp
  - Pilonidal cysts/sinus
- Pigmentary disorders
  - Dowling-Degos disease
  - Kitamura disease
- Rheumatologic diseases
  - Arthritis
  - Synovitis, acne, pustulosis, hyperostosis, and osteitis (SAPHO) syndrome
- Miscellaneous
  - Fox-Fordyce disease
  - Steatocystoma multiplex
  - Pityriasis rubra pilaris
  - Human immunodeficiency virus (HIV)–associated pityriasis rubra pilaris
  - Pyoderma gangrenosum

There are many reports of rheumatologic associations or complications of HS, especially in African American men. This seems to be related to chronic inflammation.[42–45] SAPHO syndrome has been associated with HS.[46,47]

Crohn disease may be either associated with HS or in the differential diagnosis, because it can mimic the appearance of advanced, scarred HS with lymphedema and draining sinuses in the genital and perianal areas. There are a few series and case reports of HS and Crohn disease, but this may be a coincidence, so it needs to be further studied.[48] It has been postulated that both diseases have a related pathogenesis caused by an abnormal host-microbial interaction.[49] There are reports of associations with several other conditions, as listed in **Box 5**. Some of these conditions may be related to structural or functional abnormalities in the follicle.[15,50,51] Pyoderma gangrenosum has 15 reported cases associated with HS.[52] Keratitis-ichthyosis-deafness syndrome has a tenuous link.[53]

COMPLICATIONS

HS is associated with several complications, especially in long-term untreated disease (**Box 6**). Fistulae are rare and associated with long-standing disease.[8] The most common complications are anal and perianal fistulae, and it is speculated that these occur because of repeated or persistent abscess formation in the anal glands between the internal and external sphincter.[54] Arthropathy can be associated with or can complicate HS (see earlier discussion). In late disease in the genital and perianal areas, significant lymphedema can occur, which can progress to lymphangiectasia with draining lesions and recurrent cellulitis. Secondary infection from clinically open skin areas results rarely in repeated cellulitis, very rarely in septicemia, and exceptionally in epidural abscesses and sacral osteomyelitis.[55] Incapacitating cases of massive scrotal and vulvar edema have been reported. As with any long-term inflammatory condition, metabolic complications may occur, with anemia, hypoproteinemia, and, rarely, amyloidosis.[8,55]

Squamous cell carcinoma is a late and uncommon complication of HS. Almost two-thirds of cases affect the buttocks and perineum, mostly in men in a ratio of 4:1 to women. The poor prognosis may reflect the likelihood of delayed or missed diagnosis.[55,56] Almost 50% of patients die within 2 years of developing a squamous cell carcinoma, which in turn usually develops after about 25 years.[55–57]

Other skin and visceral cancers have also been associated with HS.[55,58] In one study, patients with HS were found to have a 50% increase in incidence of malignancy including buccal cancer and primary liver cancer. This increase may be explained by smoking and alcohol.[55,58]

The thick plaques and ropelike scars can bind and limit limb movement, especially in axillae and, less often, the groin. Scarring in the perineal area can cause anal, urethral, and rectal strictures.[59] Patients severely affected with HS are withdrawn, frequently depressed, and suicide is a serious risk.

Box 6
Complications of HS

Fistulae into urethra, bladder, rectum (rare)

Arthropathy

Infections

- Cellulitis
- Lumbosacral epidural abscess
- Sacral bacterial osteomyelitis

Lymphatic obstruction with lymphedema

Complications from chronic inflammatory disease

- Anemia, hypoproteinemia, amyloidosis

Squamous cell carcinoma

Contractures and limb mobility limitations

Malaise, depression, suicide

TREATMENT

There is no single effective treatment or cure for HS. The only permanent cure has been reported for very severe HS (Hurley III) with wide surgery. Most patients with HS require a combination of medical and surgical strategies, beginning with gentle atraumatic care.

General care for HS is based on clinical experience:

- Gentle local hygiene. Washing with a mild nonsoap cleansing bar is all that is necessary. If there is odor then an antiseptic cleanser with triclosan could be used. Washing should be with hands only (no washcloths) to prevent further friction and irritation.
- Reducing trauma to the involved areas is important. This involves reduction in heat, humidity, sweating, and friction. The aim is to stop any follicular trauma and maceration that could promote more inflammation,

plugging, and rupture of the follicles. Friction must be avoided. Clothing must be loose and ventilated, specifically avoiding tight synthetic garments. Patients must not pinch or squeeze the lesions. Weight loss to ideal weight is desirable. Tampon use may be preferable to sanitary pads.
- Stopping smoking and avoiding all tobacco and nicotine-replacement products is recommended.

There have been no large, well-controlled studies of HS treatment, so most recommendations are from small series and case reports. Treatment depends on the stage of HS (see Hurley classification), frequency of flares, and the goals of the patient **Box 7**.[5] The goal of treatment is to reduced the extent and progression of the disease and bring the disease activity down to the mildest stage possible.

Surgical Management

Standard surgical management of HS has for decades consisted of wide excision. The margins are estimated before surgery; width and depth vary case by case. Primary closure, flaps or grafts, or healing by secondary intention follows. This treatment is usually limited to Hurley stage III disease in which HS has progressed beyond successful medical management.[60]

Unroofing

Unroofing is another simple technique. It is not well described in the literature and not generally taught, but it is useful for the lesions occupying the middle ground between the early hot nodules of Hurley stage I and the advancing branching lesions of stage III. Elimination of the deep, epithelialized, subcutaneous sinus tracts of HS is invaluable, but is not a new technique; it that has been ignored for years.[61] It requires only sturdy scissors and a malleable probe, although a variation of the technique with laser has been described.[62] It is far more effective than prolonged antibiotics and anti-inflammatory therapy, which do not address the pathogenesis of the disorder.

Unroofing is not technically difficult. It can be performed in the office setting under local anesthesia and so is easily adapted to the emergency room. It requires simple postoperative dressing care, and postoperative pain is remarkably, indeed surprisingly easy to manage.

Lidocaine anesthesia with epinephrine is used. Controlled volumes are injected peripherally, avoiding leakage from sinuses. Time for adequate vasoconstriction reduces pain and minimizes blood loss.

A fluctuant mass is best initially incised and drained by digital pressure. The central linear incision is extended to the edge of the loose overlying tissue that covers the original fluctuant area and the incision is extended through 360 degrees at the edge of the redundant overlying tissue, beveling the edges if possible. The base of the wound is then debrided using simple scrubbing with coarse gauze. Excision of fat at the base of the wound is unnecessary and compromises both the speed of healing and the cosmetic result. All depths and margins are explored digitally, visually, and with appropriate instruments. Any linear fibrous tissue is suspect as a possible sinus track and is best removed. Communicating sinuses are discovered and removed. Draining sinuses and all sinus tracks and openings must be explored because they can be surprisingly extensive. They must be totally unroofed, but only tissue that is involved with active disease, or is devitalized, or, if left behind, would interfere with healing should be removed. The wound base is dried and sealed with simple chemical hemostasis, preferably ferric chloride. Small bleeders also respond to this simple chemical cauterant; electrodesiccation or electrocautery are rarely needed. The scars are normally soft, contract to a size much smaller than the unroofed area, and are acceptable to the patients (**Figs. 2–4**).

A single lesion being managed on an emergency basis for pain relief requires only unroofing (not incision and drainage) and ferric chloride.

After the operation, the wound is dressed with a thick coat of simple petrolatum. No antibacterial soaps and no washcloths are used. Thick layers of petrolatum on cotton or soft gauze are reapplied once or twice daily or as needed. Patients (and wound care staff) must be instructed to avoid debriding the wound. Healing by secondary intent and epithelialization will proceed only if the fresh epidermis is allowed to cover the wound and is not debrided away. HS is not an infection; the inflammation was caused by the material removed by this procedure, so antibiotics are rarely necessary and are best avoided.[28] This minimizes the risk of encouraging the overgrowth of yeast and resistant bacteria.

Unroofing eliminates the risk and costs of hospital or ambulatory surgical center care, laser, anesthesia, graft donor sites, dehiscence, infection, the burying of residual inflammatory foci, postoperative antibiotics, time lost from work, and the need for travel to major centers.[63] Most importantly, when performed correctly it stops forever the progression of the treated lesion.

In severely involved patients, several visits may be required to clear all areas. An unroofed area is

Box 7
General therapy

Education and support

Improve environment:

- Reduce heat, sweating, obesity, friction in the area
- Loose clothing, boxer-type underwear
- Tampon use, if appropriate (avoid pads)

Antiseptic wash (Triclosan cleanser)

Consider antiandrogen treatment

Stop all dairy foods

Stop smoking

Hurley stage I

Aim: reduce duration of flares

Clindamycin 1% lotion morning and evening

Short courses of antibiotics 7 to 10 days:

- Tetracylines (doxycycline, minocycline)
- Amoxicillin+clavulanic acid
- Clindamycin

Zinc gluconate

Intralesional triamcinolone

Stage I: only a few flares yearly

If more than 1 flare/mo or severe flares, treatment as stage II

Hurley stage II

Aim: reduce to stage I

Medical treatment

- Control acute inflammation
- Prepare for surgery

For little scarring and severe inflammation:

Clindamycin+rifampicin for 3 months, or dapsone

Intralesional triamcinolone

Maintenance: tetracyclines or dapsone

Zinc orally

Scarring/sinus tracts:

- Surgical treatment: early local unroofing
- Wide excision reserved for Hurley III

Good control:

- Treatment as stage I (therapy for flares only)

Hurley stage III

Medical treatment:

- Antiinflammatory antibiotics
  - Clindamycin+rifampin
  - Prednisone, triamcinolone, or cyclosporine
- Tumor necrosis factor α (TNFα) inhibitors and other biologicals
  - Infliximab, adalimumab, etanercept

Surgery:

- Extensive surgery with special nursing and wound care

Medical treatment is short term, preparatory for surgery, or palliative

a deactivated area. Patients learn and appreciate this. The chronic patients' tendency to hide from life gradually yields to an enthusiasm for final clearance.

Medical Management

Medical treatments include antibiotics, antiandrogens and other immunosuppressives (eg, corticosteroids, cyclosporine, TNFα inhibitors), combined with diet and metabolic management. Isotretinoin, although controversial, in low dose and used as a systemic comedolytic, is worth considering in early cases as gentle concurrent prophylactic therapy.[64] Prohibit smoking totally.[5] Nicotine in any form must cease if failure is to be avoided.

Antibiotics

Antibiotics are used extensively for HS despite few studies on efficacy.[65] They treat only the epiphenomena of HS, not the cause, and are used topically and systemically for their antiinflammatory

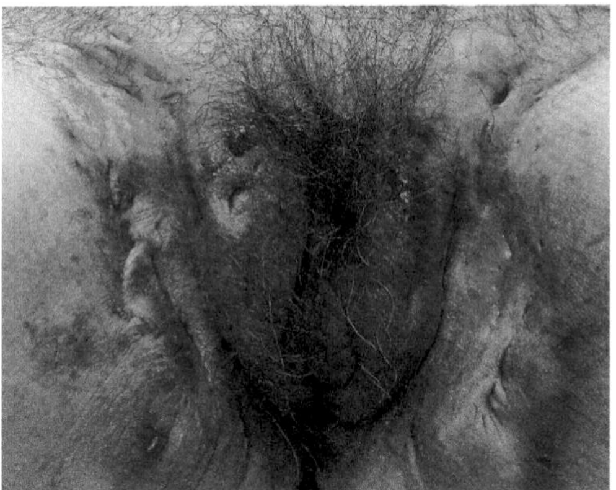

Fig. 2. Hurley stage III with extensive interconnecting, draining sinuses involving inguinal and labiocrural folds, and labia majora with pitted scars. Chronic granulation tissue is seen at the opening of the sinus tract on the right upper labium majus.

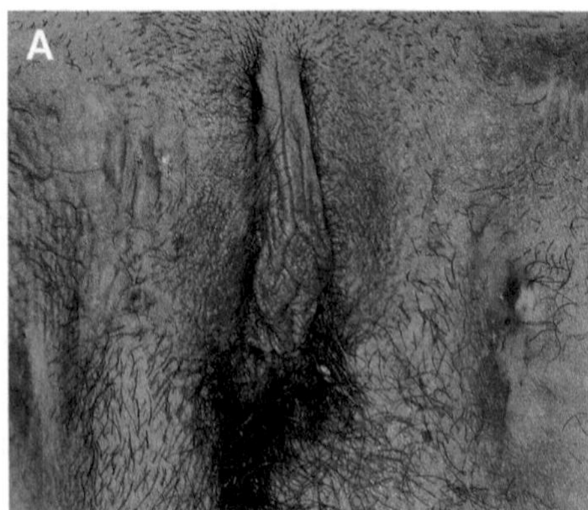
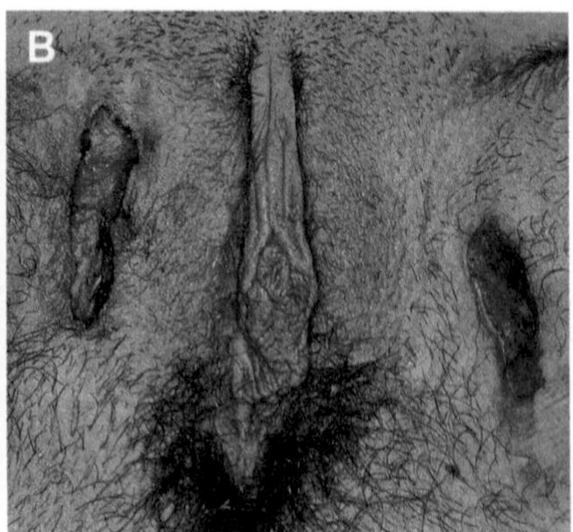

Fig. 3. (*A*) Preoperative Hurley stage II, showing 2 areas of interconnecting chronic sinuses in the labiocrural folds. (*B*) Postoperative Hurley stage II, showing the unroofed sinuses with clean bases and no bleeding.

actions. Antibiotics may also decrease odor and reduce pain but the natural history of HS is not altered by antibiotic therapy.[66,67]

Topical clindamycin 1% solution twice a day in a randomized placebo-controlled study for 12 weeks reduced abscesses and pustules but not the inflammatory nodules.[68] In another 3-month study, 1% clindamycin solution was found to be as effective as oral tetracycline (500 mg twice daily).[69]

Oral antibiotics (doxycycline, minocycline, erythromycin, amoxicillin plus clavulanic acid, and cephalosporins) have been recommended for short and long courses. Amoxicillin plus clavulinic acid may be most useful for acute HS flares.[69] Oral clindamycin (600 mg daily) with rifampin (600 mg daily) in a small study of 14 patients after 10 weeks resulted in significant remission in 8 out of 14. The 2 patients who had diarrhea from the clindamycin were successfully switched to minocycline.[70] Dapsone has been used successfully in a small study of 5 patients. Responses were seen after 4 to 12 weeks. Patients were kept on maintenance therapy (50 to 150 mg daily) with a medium follow-up of 24 months.[71] Revuz[5] counsels caution if using dapsone.

Antiandrogens

There are now a few studies on the use of antiandrogens. Two address cyproterone acetate and 3 concern finasteride. Cyproterone acetate 50 mg/ethinyl estradiol 50 μg was compared in a crossover trial with norgestrel 500 μg/ethinyl estradiol 50 μg for 6 months. Women in both groups improved; 7 out of 24 cleared and remained clear for 19 months.[72] The second report used a fairly high dose of cyproterone acetate, 100 mg daily, in 4 patients with control and good results.[73] Cyproterone acetate is not available in the United States. Finasteride 5 mg, usually used for prostate cancer, has been successfully used in 3 reports. Kraft and Searles[20] showed the superiority of finasteride to oral antibiotics in 64 patients. Searles[21] reported on 41 women who failed antibiotics, retinoids, and surgery, but showed 75% improved after 2 to 10 months of therapy, including 59% asymptomatic. Side effects were minor with some swelling and menstrual

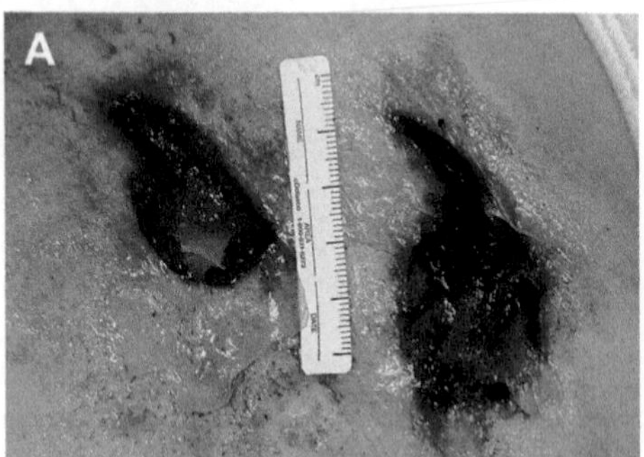
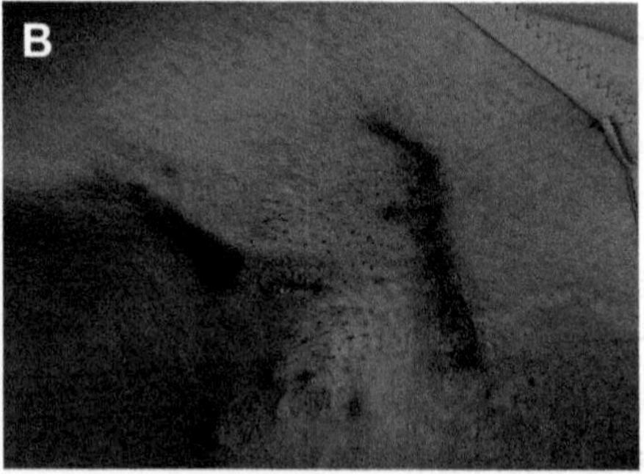

Fig. 4. (*A*) Hurley stage II in the left axilla with unroofed sinuses, postoperatively, showing clean bases. The wounds are coated with petrolatum. (*B*) Hurley stage II 8 weeks after operating, showing the final healing of the surgery.

irregularities. Dutasteride has helped clear both men and women in several anecdotal personal cases. Finasteride and dutasteride must be used with caution because they are teratogenic. If oral contraceptives are considered, those containing ethinyl estradiol and drospirenone are preferred, combined with the antiandrogen spironolactone, 50 to 100 mg, when possible.[20,21,74]

Dietary and metabolic management

Hormonal stimulation of the genetically susceptible pilosebaceous population by dairy hormones and high glycemic load diets, as in acne, has recently been recognized. This stimulation is likely caused by the presence in all dairy products of androgens and their precursors, numerous growth factors, and unknown factors that promote hyperinsulinemia and higher levels of insulinlike growth factor 1, all leading to a greater exposure of the pilosebaceous unit to androgens.[75] The link to obesity is documented[33] and the use of metformin in maximally tolerated doses to help drive weight loss is part of our HS strategy.[76] Personal and additional reported cases (Bibb R. Dairy elimination clears hidradenitis suppurativa 97%, personal communication, 2009) illustrating successful clearing with dietary control are being collected for publication.

Recognition of this link imposes an obligation on dermatologists to discuss restrictive dietary management with patients with HS, and offer assistance and advice with zero dairy intake and low glycemic load diets. For further information, kindly review and refer patients to www.hs-foundation.org, www.acnemilk.com, www.thepaleodiet.com, www.godairyfree.org, and www.glycemicindex.com.

Immunosuppressives

Patients with HS have significant inflammation and display altered immune responses.[77] Whether these variations actually contribute to the cause or are merely a reflection of the pathogenesis, immunosuppressants are sometimes used to modify these responses. They are usually ineffective when used alone, so are best combined with other medications and surgery. There are only a few case reports to support their use, although more studies on the use of the biologic group are now available (see later discussion).

Corticosteroids have been used successfully intralesionally and systemically, mainly for symptomatic care.[59,78–80] High doses of systemic steroids, rapidly tapered, can be effective in aborting an acute HS lesion, quickly reducing pain and inflammation. Intralesional steroids (a small amount of triamcinolone acetonide 5–10 mg/mL) injected into an acute lesion can effect rapid resolution.[5] Cyclosporine (4–5 mg/kg/d) has been reported to help in a few cases.[81–84] Methotrexate orally has been used unsuccessfully.[84]

Retinoids

Isotretinoin has not been found to be consistently effective, in contrast to its use in acne. Nevertheless, in one study of 68 cases, 23.5% completely cleared and 11 maintained improvement in follow-up, but 29 did not finish the study because of lack of effect, side effects, or both.[64] Isotretinoin in low doses, although controversial, has been useful for long-term prophylaxis in several personal cases, but can cause flaring in usual doses.

TNFα inhibitors

Crohn and HS sometimes coexist, and infliximab used to treat the Crohn may dramatically improve both conditions.[85] More than 50 patients with HS have now been reported for this off-label use and more trials are ongoing. So far only 1 double-blind, placebo-controlled crossover trial for moderate to severe HS has been reported, with improvement but not cure.[86] With infliximab there is often dramatic improvement, especially for quality of life.[87] In one study of 7 cases, there was a short-term response in severe HS for 2 of the cases, but severe side effects in 3.[88] There are now more than 10 cases reported for the use of adalimumab and almost 30 for the use of etanercept, which has the advantage of subcutaneous injections instead of the intravenous infusions of infliximab. In a prospective study of 15 patients treated with etanercept, only 3 responded.[89] Adalimumab has also been used after infliximab failed because of antibody-induced resistance. Like etanercept, it has the advantage of subcutaneous administration. A series of 6 cases of resistant HS were reported by Blanco and colleagues,[90] all treated with adalimumab; all responded and the medication was well tolerated. Like infliximab, it can induce dramatic and rapid control.[91] These medications can make unroofing and wide excisional surgery easier by decreasing the preoperative swelling, inflammation, and discharge but do not affect the chronic sinus tracts, so they are not a cure. There is improvement but it cannot be considered permanent.

The risk/benefit ratio of these drugs remains to be determined and their role as the purported ultimate alternative needs to be defined.[92] Significant side effects have been reported, ranging from lupuslike reactions, neuropathy, and hypersensitivity to reactivation of tuberculosis and other serious infections. Efficacy and safety studies, cost-effectiveness, and a head-to-head comparison with other standard HS treatments for effectiveness are needed.

Miscellaneous: experimental therapies

Zinc Zinc salts have been found to be antiinflammatory and have been used for mild to moderate acne. Zinc is also antiandrogenic, acting through inhibition of both isoenzymes of 5α-reductase. Two clinical trials showed improvement at 30 to 60 mg per day. Zinc gluconate was found to be only 15% less effective than minocycline in a randomized trial.[93,94] In a study of 22 patients using 90 mg of zinc gluconate, there were 8 complete and 14 partial remissions. The side effects include gastrointestinal upset and potential blocking of copper metabolism resulting in anemia.

Photodynamic therapy 5-Aminolevulinic acid has been used with exposure to various wavelengths of laser, visible light, and intense pulsed light. There have been mixed results, with reports ranging from 75% to 100% improvement to no improvement.[95,96] No cures are reported.

Botulinum toxin There are 2 reports of treatment, 1 with a single injection session followed by more than 10 months improvement.[97] The suggested mechanism, a decrease in apocrine output and so less stress against the plugged orifice, represents a prolonged response to botulinum toxin.

Radiotherapy Radiation treatment was extensively used in the past, with variable response. It was believed to be helpful for early lesions.[98]

Unresolved questions Despite recent advances on a molecular level, several questions need to be resolved before this disease can be fully understood, prevented, and controlled (**Box 8**).

THE FUTURE

Extensive information is available from the Hidradenitis Suppurativa Foundation at www.HS-foundation.org and the International Society for the Study of Vulvovaginal Disease at its educational site www.issvd.org, and the subject is regularly updated at www.UpToDate.com.

Patients with HS (and their physicians, surgeons, and dieticians) need to understand this disease to develop realistic expectations and to work with each other for the best outcome. They need to know that HS is not contagious and is not caused by poor hygiene; that diet may prove more valuable than surgery; that hormone control is more valuable than antibiotics; that surgery should be undertaken as early as possible; and that surgery need not be mutilating, expensive, or painful. HS is an orphan disease that is ready to be adopted, now that the causes are becoming understood and logical, scientific therapies are being brought to the patient. HS is not easy to manage, but it is becoming manageable, and, for an increasing number of patients, the word cure is no longer out of reach.

Box 8
Unresolved HS questions

Pathophysiology

Usefulness of infliximab and its role in therapy

Relation to Crohn disease

Role of diet and metabolic control in prevention and therapy

Usefulness of medical therapies and how best to combine with unroofing or excision

Long-term most effective modalities

REFERENCES

1. Verneuil A. Etudes sur les tumeurs de la peau; de quelques maladies des grandes sudoripares. Archives Generales de Medicine 1854;4:447–68.
2. Yu CC, Cook MG. Hidradenitis suppurativa: a disease of follicular epithelium, rather than apocrine glands. Br J Dermatol 1990;122(6):763–9.
3. Sellheyer K, Krahl D. "Hidradenitis suppurativa" is acne inversa! An appeal to (finally) abandon a misnomer. Int J Dermatol 2005;44(7):535–40.
4. Jansen T, Plewig G. What's new in acne inversa (alias hidradenitis suppurativa)? J Eur Acad Dermatol Venereol 2000;14(5):342–3.
5. Revuz J. Hidradenitis suppurativa. J Eur Acad Dermatol Venereol 2009;23(9):985–98.
6. Diagnostic Criteria. In: Second International HS Research Symposium 2009.
7. von der Werth JM, Williams HC. The natural history of hidradenitis suppurativa. J Eur Acad Dermatol Venereol 2000;14(5):389–92.
8. Alikhan A, Lynch PJ, Eisen DB. Hidradenitis suppurativa: a comprehensive review. J Am Acad Dermatol 2009;60(4):539–61.
9. Naldi L. Epidemiology. In: Jemec G, Revuz J, Leyden J, editors. Hidradenitis suppurativa. Berlin: Springer; 2006. p. 58–64.
10. Jemec GB. The symptomatology of hidradenitis suppurativa in women. Br J Dermatol 1988;119(3):345–50.
11. Jemec GB, Heidenheim M, Nielsen NH. The prevalence of hidradenitis suppurativa and its potential precursor lesions. J Am Acad Dermatol 1996;35(2 Pt 1):191–4.

12. Parks RW, Parks TG. Pathogenesis, clinical features and management of hidradenitis suppurativa. Ann R Coll Surg Engl 1997;79(2):83–9.
13. Jemec GB, Heidenheim M, Nielsen NH. Hidradenitis suppurativa–characteristics and consequences. Clin Exp Dermatol 1996;21(6):419–23.
14. Weber-LaShore A, Huppert J. Hidradenitis suppurativa in a pre-pubertal female. J Pediatr Adolesc Gynecol 2009;22(2):e53.
15. Mengesha YM, Holcombe TC, Hansen RC. Prepubertal hidradenitis suppurativa: two case reports and review of the literature. Pediatr Dermatol 1999; 16(4):292–6.
16. Canoui-Poitrine F, Revuz JE, Wolkenstein P, et al. Clinical characteristics of a series of 302 French patients with hidradenitis suppurativa, with an analysis of factors associated with disease severity. J Am Acad Dermatol 2009;61(1):51–7.
17. Gao M, Wang PG, Cui Y, et al. Inversa acne (hidradenitis suppurativa): a case report and identification of the locus at chromosome 1p21.1-1q25.3. J Invest Dermatol 2006;126(6):1302–6.
18. Slade DE, Powell BW, Mortimer PS. Hidradenitis suppurativa: pathogenesis and management. Br J Plast Surg 2003;56(5):451–61.
19. Barth JH, Layton AM, Cunliffe WJ. Endocrine factors in pre- and postmenopausal women with hidradenitis suppurativa. Br J Dermatol 1996;134(6):1057–9.
20. Kraft JN, Searles GE. Hidradenitis suppurativa in 64 female patients: retrospective study comparing oral antibiotics and antiandrogen therapy. J Cutan Med Surg 2007;11(4):125–31.
21. Searles GE. Daily oral finasteride 5mg for hidradenitis suppurativa. Annual Meeting, Canadian Dermatology Association. Vancouver, BC (Canada), July 1–5, 2009.
22. Mortimer PS, Dawber RP, Gales MA, et al. Mediation of hidradenitis suppurativa by androgens. Br Med J (Clin Res Ed) 1986;292(6515):245–8.
23. Gupta AK, Knowles SR, Gupta MA, et al. Lithium therapy associated with hidradenitis suppurativa: case report and a review of the dermatologic side effects of lithium. J Am Acad Dermatol 1995;32(2 Pt 2):382–6.
24. Mahe E, Morelon E, Lechaton S, et al. Cutaneous adverse events in renal transplant recipients receiving sirolimus-based therapy. Transplantation 2005;79(4):476–82.
25. Revuz J. HS patients' frequently asked questions. In: Jemec G, Revuz J, Leyden J, editors. Hidradenitis suppurativa. Berlin: Springer; 2006. p. 191.
26. Hana A, Booken D, Henrich C, et al. Functional significance of non-neuronal acetylcholine in skin epithelia. Life Sci 2007;80(24–25):2214–20.
27. Konig A, Lehmann C, Rompel R, et al. Cigarette smoking as a triggering factor of hidradenitis suppurativa. Dermatology 1999;198(3):261–4.
28. Kurzen H, Kurokawa I, Jemec GB, et al. What causes hidradenitis suppurativa? Exp Dermatol 2008;17(5):455–6.
29. Schauber J, Gallo RL. Expanding the roles of antimicrobial peptides in skin: alarming and arming keratinocytes. J Invest Dermatol 2007;127(3):510–2.
30. Gniadecki R, Jemec GBE. Lipid raft-enriched stem cell-like keratinocytes in the epidermis, hair follicles and sinus tracts in hidradenitis suppurativa. Exp Dermatol 2004;13:361–3 [electronic citation].
31. Williams ST, Busby RC, DeMuth RJ, et al. Perineal hidradenitis suppurativa: presentation of two unusual complications and a review. Ann Plast Surg 1991; 26(5):456–62.
32. Hurley HE. Axillary hyperhidrosis, apocrine bromhidrosis, hidradenitis suppurativa, and familial benign pemphigus: surgical approach. In: Roenigk RK, Roenigk RH, editors. Dermatologic surgery. New York: Marcel Dekker; 1989. p. 729–39.
33. Sartorius K, Emtestam L, Jemec GB, et al. Objective scoring of hidradenitis suppurativa reflecting the role of tobacco smoking and obesity. Br J Dermatol 2009;161(4):831–9.
34. Ramasastry SS, Conklin WT, Granick MS, et al. Surgical management of massive perianal hidradenitis suppurativa. Ann Plast Surg 1985;15(3): 218–23.
35. von der Werth JM, Jemec GB. Morbidity in patients with hidradenitis suppurativa. Br J Dermatol 2001; 144(4):809–13.
36. Wolkenstein P, Loundou A, Barrau K, et al. Quality of life impairment in hidradenitis suppurativa: a study of 61 cases. J Am Acad Dermatol 2007;56(4):621–3.
37. Wolkenstein P. Quality of life in hidradenitis suppurativa. In: Jemec G, Revuz J, Leyden J, editors. Hidradenitis suppurativa. Berlin: Springer; 2006. p. 116–9.
38. Anderson BB, Cadogan CA, Gangadharam D. Hidradenitis suppurativa of the perineum, scrotum, and gluteal area: presentation, complications, and treatment. J Natl Med Assoc 1982;74(10): 999–1003.
39. Anderson DK, Perry AW. Axillary hidradenitis. Arch Surg 1975;110(1):69–72.
40. Scheinfeld NS. A case of dissecting cellulitis and a review of the literature. Dermatol Online J 2003; 9(1):8.
41. Chicarilli ZN. Follicular occlusion triad: hidradenitis suppurativa, acne conglobata, and dissecting cellulitis of the scalp. Ann Plast Surg 1987;18(3):230–7.
42. Rosner IA, Richter DE, Huettner TL, et al. Spondyloarthropathy associated with hidradenitis suppurative and acne conglobata. Ann Intern Med 1982;97(4):520–5.
43. Bhalla R, Sequeira W. Arthritis associated with hidradenitis suppurativa. Ann Rheum Dis 1994;53(1): 64–6.

44. Libow LF, Friar DA. Arthropathy associated with cystic acne, hidradenitis suppurativa, and perifolliculitis capitis abscedens et suffodiens: treatment with isotretinoin. Cutis 1999;64(2):87–90.
45. Thein M, Hogarth MB, Acland K. Seronegative arthritis associated with the follicular occlusion triad. Clin Exp Dermatol 2004;29(5):550–2.
46. Kahn MF, Bouvier M, Palazzo E, et al. Sternoclavicular pustulotic osteitis (SAPHO). 20-year interval between skin and bone lesions. J Rheumatol 1991; 18(7):1104–8.
47. Kahn MF, Chamot AM. SAPHO syndrome. Rheum Dis Clin North Am 1992;18(1):225–46.
48. Church JM, Fazio VW, Lavery IC, et al. The differential diagnosis and comorbidity of hidradenitis suppurativa and perianal Crohn's disease. Int J Colorectal Dis 1993;8(3):117–9.
49. Cario E, Podolsky DK. Differential alteration in intestinal epithelial cell expression of toll-like receptor 3 (TLR3) and TLR4 in inflammatory bowel disease. Infect Immun 2000;68(12):7010–7.
50. Misery I, Faure M, Claidy A. Pityriasis rubra pilaris and human immunodeficiency virus infection–type 6 pityriasis rubra pilaris? Br J Dermatol 1996;135(6):1008–9.
51. Gonzalez-Lopez A, Velasco E, Pozo T, et al. HIV-associated pityriasis rubra pilaris responsive to triple antiretroviral therapy. Br J Dermatol 1999;140(5): 931–4.
52. Ah-Weng A, Langtry JA, Velangi S, et al. Pyoderma gangrenosum associated with hidradenitis suppurativa. Clin Exp Dermatol 2005;30(6):669–71.
53. Maintz L, Betz RC, Allam JP, et al. Keratitis-ichthyosis-deafness syndrome in association with follicular occlusion triad. Eur J Dermatol 2005;15(5):347–52.
54. Endo Y, Tamura A, Ishikawa O, et al. Perianal hidradenitis suppurativa: early surgical treatment gives good results in chronic or recurrent cases. Br J Dermatol 1998;139(5):906–10.
55. Russ E, Castillo M. Lumbosacral epidural abscess due to hidradenitis suppurativa. AJR Am J Roentgenol 2002;178(3):770–1.
56. Maalouf E, Faye O, Poli F, et al. [Fatal epidermoid carcinoma in hidradenitis suppurativa following treatment with infliximab]. Ann Dermatol Venereol 2006;133(5 Pt 1):473–4 [in French].
57. Maclean GM, Coleman DJ. Three fatal cases of squamous cell carcinoma arising in chronic perineal hidradenitis suppurativa. Ann R Coll Surg Engl 2007; 89(7):709–12.
58. Lapins J, Ye W, Nyren O, et al. Incidence of cancer among patients with hidradenitis suppurativa. Arch Dermatol 2001;137(6):730–4.
59. Wiseman MC. Hidradenitis suppurativa: a review. Dermatol Ther 2004;17(1):50–4.
60. Rhode JM, Burke WM, Cederna PS, et al. Outcomes of surgical management of stage III vulvar hidradenitis suppurativa. J Reprod Med 2008;53(6):420–8.
61. Barron J. The surgical treatment of perianal hidradenitis suppurativa. Dis Colon Rectum 1970;13(6): 441–3.
62. Madan V, Hindle E, Hussain W, et al. Outcomes of treatment of nine cases of recalcitrant severe hidradenitis suppurativa with carbon dioxide laser. Br J Dermatol 2008;159(6):1309–14.
63. Danby FW. Surgical unroofing for hidradenitis suppurativa, why and how? J Am Acad Dermatol 2010;63:481.e1–3.
64. Boer J, van Gemert MJ. Long-term results of isotretinoin in the treatment of 68 patients with hidradenitis suppurativa. J Am Acad Dermatol 1999;40(1): 73–6.
65. Lee RA, Yoon A, Kist J. Hidradenitis suppurativa: an update. Adv Dermatol 2007;23289–306.
66. Brown TJ, Rosen T, Orengo IF. Hidradenitis suppurativa. South Med J 1998;91(12):1107–14.
67. Harrison BJ, Mudge M, Hughes LE. Recurrence after surgical treatment of hidradenitis suppurativa. Br Med J (Clin Res Ed) 1987;294(6570):487–9.
68. Clemmensen OJ. Topical treatment of hidradenitis suppurativa with clindamycin. Int J Dermatol 1983; 22(5):325–8.
69. Jemec GB, Wendelboe P. Topical clindamycin versus systemic tetracycline in the treatment of hidradenitis suppurativa. J Am Acad Dermatol 1998; 39(6):971–4.
70. Mendonca CO, Griffiths CE. Clindamycin and rifampicin combination therapy for hidradenitis suppurativa. Br J Dermatol 2006;154(5):977–8.
71. Kaur MR, Lewis HM. Hidradenitis suppurativa treated with dapsone: A case series of five patients. J Dermatolog Treat 2006;17(4):211–3.
72. Mortimer PS, Dawber RP, Gales MA, et al. A double-blind controlled cross-over trial of cyproterone acetate in females with hidradenitis suppurativa. Br J Dermatol 1986;115(3):263–8.
73. Sawers RS, Randall VA, Ebling FJ. Control of hidradenitis suppurativa in women using combined anti-androgen (cyproterone acetate) and oestrogen therapy. Br J Dermatol 1986;115(3):269–74.
74. Stewart EG, Margesson LJ, Danby FW. Treatment of hidradenitis suppurativa. In: Berman RS, Dellavalle RP, editors. Boston: UpToDate Online; 2009. 17.3. 11-22-2009.
75. Kurokawa I, Danby FW, Ju Q, et al. New developments in our understanding of acne pathogenesis and treatment. Exp Dermatol 2009;18(10):821–32.
76. Golay A. Metformin and body weight. Int J Obes (Lond) 2008;32(1):61–72.
77. Giamarellos-Bourboulis EJ, Antonopoulou A, Petropoulou C, et al. Altered innate and adaptive immune responses in patients with hidradenitis suppurativa. Br J Dermatol 2007;156(1):51–6.

78. Auerbach R. Treatment of hidradenitis suppurativa. JAMA 1973;223(5):556–7.
79. Kipping HF. How I treat hidradenitis suppurativa. Postgrad Med 1970;48(3):291–2.
80. Camisa C, Sexton C, Friedman C. Treatment of hidradenitis suppurativa with combination hypothalamic-pituitary-ovarian and adrenal suppression. A case report. J Reprod Med 1989;34(8):543–6.
81. Gupta AK, Ellis CN, Nickoloff BJ, et al. Oral cyclosporine in the treatment of inflammatory and noninflammatory dermatoses. A clinical and immunopathologic analysis. Arch Dermatol 1990; 126(3):339–50.
82. Buckley DA, Rogers S. Cyclosporin-responsive hidradenitis suppurativa. J R Soc Med 1995;88(5): 289P–90P.
83. Rose RF, Goodfield MJ, Clark SM. Treatment of recalcitrant hidradenitis suppurativa with oral ciclosporin. Clin Exp Dermatol 2006;31(1):154–5.
84. Jemec GB. Methotrexate is of limited value in the treatment of hidradenitis suppurativa. Clin Exp Dermatol 2002;27(6):528–9.
85. Martinez F, Nos P, Benlloch S, et al. Hidradenitis suppurativa and Crohn's disease: response to treatment with infliximab. Inflamm Bowel Dis 2001;7(4): 323–6.
86. Grant A, Gonzalez F, Kerdel FA. Long-term efficacy and safety results (52 weeks of a double blind, placebo controlled, cross over trial of infliximab for patients with moderate to severe HS. In: Second International HS Research Symposium. San Francisco (CA), March 5, 2009.
87. Thielen AM, Barde C, Saurat JH. Long-term infliximab for severe hidradenitis suppurativa. Br J Dermatol 2006;155(5):1105–7.
88. Fardet L, Dupuy A, Kerob D, et al. Infliximab for severe hidradenitis suppurativa: transient clinical efficacy in 7 consecutive patients. J Am Acad Dermatol 2007;56(4):624–8.
89. Lee RA, Dommasch E, Treat J, et al. A prospective clinical trial of open-label etanercept for the treatment of hidradenitis suppurativa. J Am Acad Dermatol 2009;60(4):565–73.
90. Blanco R, Martinez-Taboada VM, Villa I, et al. Long-term successful adalimumab therapy in severe hidradenitis suppurativa. Arch Dermatol 2009;145(5):580–4.
91. Alexis AF, Strober BE. Off-label dermatologic uses of anti-TNF-a therapies. J Cutan Med Surg 2005;9(6): 296–302.
92. Brunasso AM, Delfino C, Massone C. Hidradenitis suppurativa: are tumour necrosis factor-alpha blockers the ultimate alternative? Br J Dermatol 2008;159(3):761–3.
93. Dreno B, Moyse D, Alirezai M, et al. Multicenter randomized comparative double-blind controlled clinical trial of the safety and efficacy of zinc gluconate versus minocycline hydrochloride in the treatment of inflammatory acne vulgaris. Dermatology 2001;203(2):135–40.
94. Brocard A, Knol AC, Khammari A, et al. Hidradenitis suppurativa and zinc: a new therapeutic approach. A pilot study. Dermatology 2007;214(4): 325–7.
95. Gold M, Bridges TM, Bradshaw VL, et al. ALA-PDT and blue light therapy for hidradenitis suppurativa. J Drugs Dermatol 2004;3(Suppl 1):S32–5.
96. Strauss RM, Pollock B, Stables GI, et al. Photodynamic therapy using aminolaevulinic acid does not lead to clinical improvement in hidradenitis suppurativa. Br J Dermatol 2005;152(4): 803–4.
97. O'Reilly DJ, Pleat JM, Richards AM. Treatment of hidradenitis suppurativa with botulinum toxin A. Plast Reconstr Surg 2005;116(5):1575–6.
98. Schenck SG. Hidradenitis suppurativa axillaris; an analysis of 54 cases treated with roentgen rays. Radiology 1950;54(1):74–7 [illust].

Pigmented Lesions of the Vulva

Aruna Venkatesan, MD

KEYWORDS

- Melanoma • Vulva • Nevus • Pigmented lesion
- Melanosis • Management

Roughly 1 of every 10 women will have a pigmented vulvar lesion in her lifetime.[1,2] Given the risk associated with melanomas and vulvar intraepithelial neoplasia (VIN, squamous cell carcinoma in situ), careful evaluation is critical. In contrast to melanocytic lesions on fully keratinized skin, pigmented lesions on the vulva can appear quite different, both grossly and histologically. Pigmented lesions encompass lesions containing melanin as well as lesions that appear pigmented, but do not contain melanin, such as purpura, vascular lesions, and debris-filled comedones.

This review article outlines an approach to the undifferentiated pigmented vulvar lesion and includes descriptions of the most clinically significant pigmented lesions of the vulva.

EVALUATING THE PIGMENTED VULVAR LESION

Relevant History

Women rarely examine the vulva, so history is of minimal importance. A lesion should be evaluated on its appearance and, when atypical, a biopsy taken, rather than the patient's report of duration and change.

Relevant Clinical Features

Clinical morphology is the primary, initial indicator of risk and abnormality. In addition, some pigmented lesions are more likely to be single, whereas others are more likely to be multifocal.

Diagnostic Tools

As with keratinized skin, skin biopsies are sometimes essential to distinguish benign from malignant growths. Because pigmented lesions on genital skin are less typical morphologically than on extragenital skin, the threshold to biopsy a genital pigmented lesion should be lower. A punch or excisional biopsy, rather than a shave biopsy, should be performed for any potential melanoma, to facilitate diagnosis and measurement of thickness. Borderline histologic results may require consultation with other dermatopathologists with an expertise in the diagnosis of melanocytic lesions.

Dermoscopy can be a useful diagnostic tool in the evaluation of pigmented lesions on nonmodified mucous membranes, but this is a tool not available to nondermatologists, and also this is not used routinely in many dermatology practices. This can be useful for vulvar lesions as well and is discussed in context with the relevant diseases.

DIFFERENTIAL DIAGNOSIS

Physiologic Hyperpigmentation

Different skin types show different degrees of pigmentation on the vulva. Physiologic hyperpigmentation in the vulvar region sometimes is concerning for a disease process when it is outside the range of normal for that skin type (**Fig. 1**). Physiologic hyperpigmentation is normal hyperpigmentation that is most common in individuals who are darkly complexioned; this is accentuated at the posterior introitus, the tips of the labia minora, and the perianal skin. Often there is hyperpigmentation of the hair-bearing labia majora as well. The proximal, medial thighs sometimes exhibit uniform hyperpigmentation that fades to the color of the nonmodified mucous membrane. These lesions are macular and symmetric, with

Department of Dermatology, Stanford Hospital and Clinics, 450 Broadway Street, Pavilion C, Redwood City, CA 94063, USA
E-mail address: arunavenk@gmail.com

Dermatol Clin 28 (2010) 795–805
doi:10.1016/j.det.2010.08.007

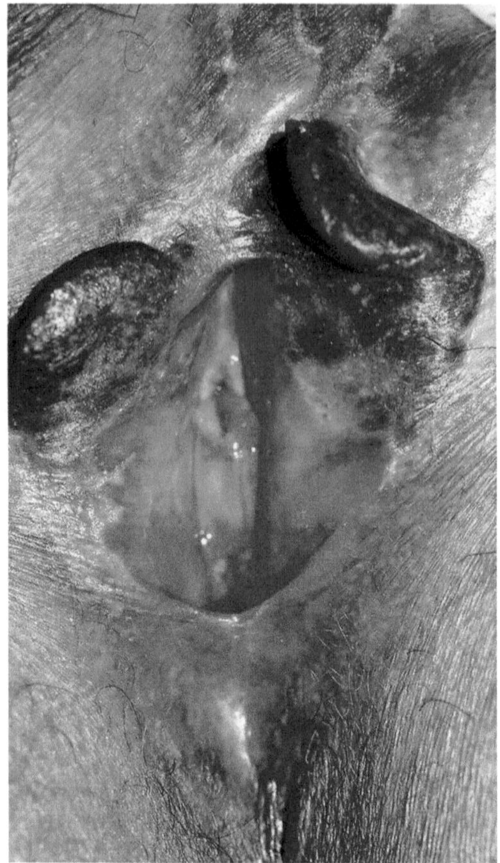

Fig. 1. Physiologic hyperpigmentation occurs most often in darkly pigmented individuals and it is characterized by macular, symmetric hyperpigmentation, often most marked on the labia minora, but sometimes also in the introitus, and perianally. (*Courtesy of* Libby Edwards, MD, Charlotte, NC.)

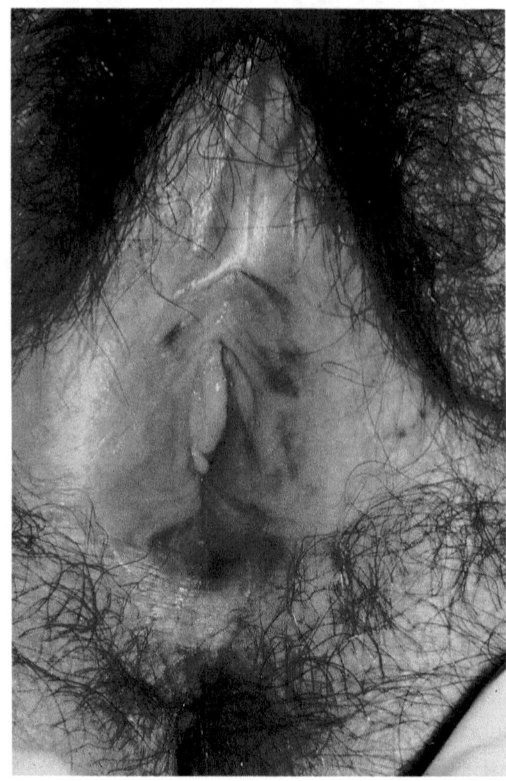

Fig. 2. Postinflammatory hyperpigmentation consists of macular hyperpigmentation occurring in the distribution of a previous inflammatory condition, as has occurred in this woman with lichen sclerosus. (*Courtesy of* Libby Edwards, MD, Charlotte, NC.)

no scale or change in texture from normal skin, and this is asymptomatic. Genital tissue has a higher density of melanocytes than the rest of the body, magnifying the effect of physiologic hyperpigmentation.[3] The degree of hyperpigmentation can change with different hormonal stages, such as adolescence and menopause, as well as pregnancy and contraceptive use. If a biopsy is performed, the melanin content and number of melanosomes of the melanocytes and keratinocytes of the basal layer is higher than normal.[4] Congenital adrenal hyperplasia, Addison's disease, or Cushing's disease can result in hyperpigmentation that is similar in appearance.[4]

Postinflammatory hyperpigmentation

Postinflammatory hyperpigmentation (PIH) occurs in patients of all skin types, including on the vulva, but this is most striking in patients of color (**Fig. 2**). This presents as macules and patches of varying shades of brown, which are usually less symmetric than physiologic hyperpigmentation, and occur most often in a distribution of previous injury or dermatosis. The postinflammatory pigment change in and of itself is asymptomatic, but pruritus can be present with concomitant active inflammation from an underlying skin disease. Causes of PIH include inflammatory skin disease, trauma, dermatologic treatments, and fixed drug eruption.[4]

Signs of associated inflammatory conditions may be, but are not always, present. Lichen sclerosus and lichen planus are relatively common inflammatory dermatoses that sometimes produce striking postinflammatory hyperpigmentation. The basement membrane disruption of these diseases, as well as of fixed drug eruptions and erythema multiforme, are especially likely to create postinflammatory hyperpigmentation because of the characteristic basement membrane damage that allows melanin release into the dermis.[4] If the pattern of the hyperpigmentation is atypical, the diagnosis should be confirmed by biopsy, especially because there may be an association of lichen sclerosus with melanoma. Patients with darker skin types sometimes exhibit dark color not only from postinflammatory hyperpigmentation, but also from active inflammation that appears pigmented only because of their skin type. Treatment of any underlying active inflammation minimizes patient discomfort and further worsening of postinflammatory hyperpigmentation. PIH is usually not treated. Hydroquinone can be tried, but it removes epidermal pigment rather than dermal pigment and it can be irritating to genital skin. The hyperpigmentation of lichen sclerosus and lichen planus resolves slowly if at all.

Acanthosis nigricans

Practitioners are familiar with acanthosis nigricans on the folds of the neck, axilla, and groin. Acanthosis nigricans can also be found on the vulva and consists of the same velvety, leathery, wrinkly texture with a darkened appearance as on other parts of the body, and is often associated with skin tags within skin folds (**Fig. 3**). Acanthosis nigricans is most commonly associated with diabetes mellitus, obesity, and some medications such as niacin and prednisone. Rarely, this is a marker of cancer, most commonly adenocarcinoma.[4,5] In the latter case, this is most likely in thin patients with marked changes of acanthosis nigricans, and can occur in atypical areas rather than skin folds. Histologically, acanthosis nigricans is papillomatous, producing its thickened and darkened appearance clinically. In a cross-sectional study of nondiabetic women being evaluated for hirsutism with documented hyperandrogenism at a university teaching hospital, 56% of the women were found to have acanthosis nigricans. Although different body sites were found to be involved, such as the axilla, nape of neck, breasts, and inner thighs, interestingly, vulvar acanthosis nigricans was always present in the women who displayed at least one lesion.[6] Acanthosis nigricans can usually be distinguished from physiologic hyperpigmentation by its velvety texture and usual sparing of mucous membranes and modified mucous membranes.

Seborrheic keratoses

Seborrheic keratoses (SKs) are common benign tumors of epidermal cells that are most prevalent in older adults and found on all keratinized skin surfaces, although there is no predisposition for the genitalia (**Fig. 4**). They are a proliferation of keratinocytes of unknown cause, occurring in all white patients older than 40 years, with a familial predilection for large numbers. These can be seen in other races and in younger patients as well. Typical SKs are keratotic, flat-topped, sharply demarcated, brown lesions with a stuck-on appearance, showing keratotic and follicular plugging, uniform color and shape, and a slightly verrucous surface. They can lose their coloration and uniformity when irritated, and the moisture and heat of the genital area can make vulvar seborrheic keratoses appear less keratotic. These lesions often mimic nevi, pigmented condylomata acuminata, and vulvar intraepithelial neoplasia (VIN, squamous cell carcinoma in situ, Bowenoid papulosis) and, less often, melanoma or dysplastic nevi. These atypical lesions should be biopsied. In general, HPV (human papillomavirus)-related lesions tend to be multiple, whereas SKs are more likely to be single within this area. SKs are unlikely to occur on the vulva if there are not typical SKs noted on other skin surfaces.

Atypical-appearing SKs may benefit from the use of dermoscopy.[7] At least one melanomalike SK was analyzed with dermoscopy and found to

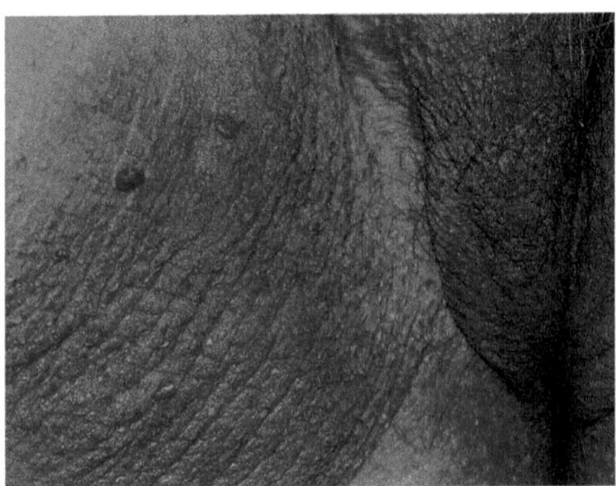

Fig. 3. Thickened-appearing, velvety, brown plaques in skin folds, usually of overweight individuals, is characteristic of acanthosis nigricans. (*Courtesy of* Libby Edwards, MD, Charlotte, NC.)

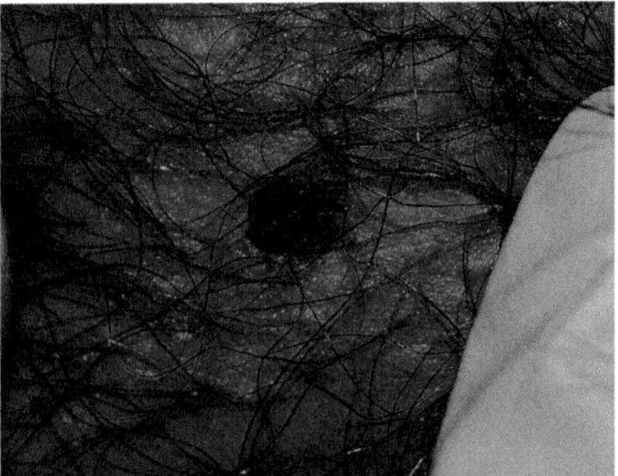

Fig. 4. Seborrheic keratoses classically are warty, brown, flat-topped papules indistinguishable from pigmented warts. (*Courtesy* of Libby Edwards, MD, Charlotte, NC.)

demonstrate numerous milialike cysts, a "pseudonetwork" of numerous gland openings, and an absence of pigment network, globules, and streaks. The comedolike openings (ie, keratin-filled invaginations in the epidermis) appreciated in cutaneous SKs are not seen in the vulva, possibly because of friction preventing their formation.

In difficult-to-diagnose, suspected SKs, biopsy is recommended, as roughly 0.5% may be melanomas.[8]

SKs are usually not removed. If the diagnosis is in doubt, they should be removed and submitted for histology. Typical but symptomatic lesions can be removed by cryotherapy, curettage, liquid nitrogen, electrocautery, or shave biopsy.

Pigmented condylomata acuminata (anogenital warts)

Condylomata acuminata, or anogenital warts, are HPV-related growths usually found as multiple lesions on the genitalia (**Fig. 5**). They have variable morphology, to include papillomatous, verrucous, fleshy papules, and flat-topped. Although most warts are skin colored, some are hyperpigmented, as regularly occurs in patients of darker skin types.

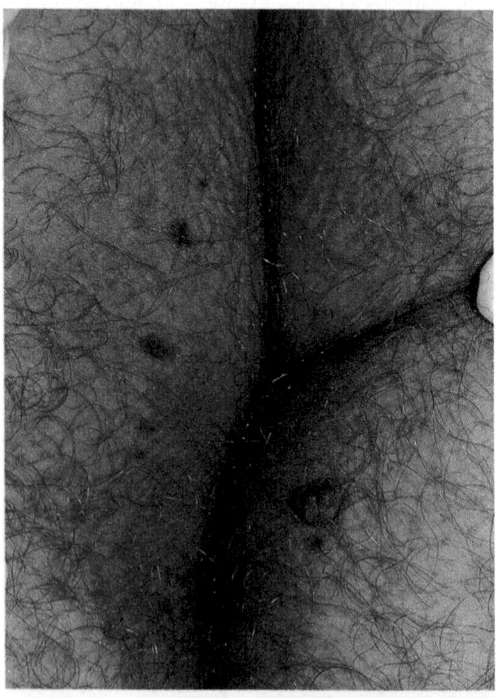

Fig. 5. Brown anogenital warts are usual in patients who are genetically dark complexioned, but in lighter people, hyperpigmented warts are suspicious for dysplasia. (*Courtesy of* Libby Edwards, MD, Charlotte, NC.)

Flat-topped, brown, anogenital warts in individuals of light skin types should be biopsied to evaluate for VIN, also known as squamous cell in situ and Bowenoid papulosis. Anogential warts are often indistinguishable from SKs. Dermoscopically, anogenital warts exhibit exophytic papillary structures with variation in pigment that includes jet-black color (ie, hemorrhage), red dots, and whitish halo (ie, keratinization).[9]

Vulvar melanosis/lentiginosis

Roughly 68% of pigmented vulvar lesions in reproductive-age women are lentigines.[1] Vulvar melanosis or lentiginosis presents as multiple asymptomatic, asymmetric macules that have the following features: tan to black coloration, irregular borders, color variation within single lesions, and are of varying size (**Fig. 6**). Their macular, nontextured nature is an important distinguishing factor from other vulvar lesions. Melanosis can occur throughout the vulva including the labia minora and medial labia majora, introitus, and perineum. Vulvar melanosis can occur as a postinflammatory hyperpigmentation, such as in patients with lichen sclerosus.[10]

Although the diagnosis of vulvar melanosis is largely made by inspection, and biopsy confirmation, dermoscopy may play a role as well. Vulvar melanosis demonstrates different patterns, including structureless, parallel, and reticular-like[11] or ringlike pattern,[12] differing from dermoscopic features of melanoma. More studies are needed to differentiate melanomas from melanosis using these patterns. Features that indicate a diagnosis other than vulvar lentiginosis include the presence of a papular component, erosions,

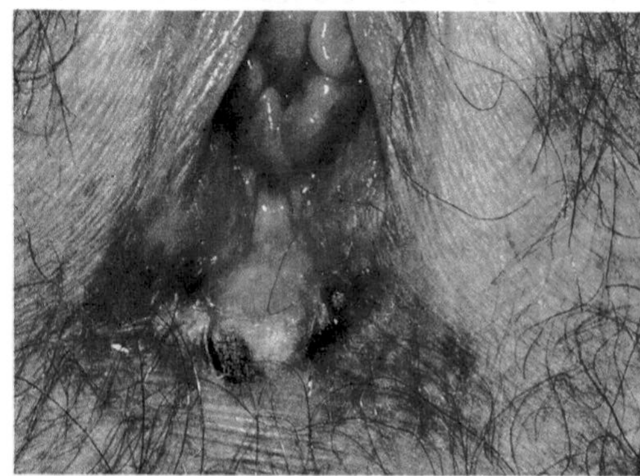

Fig. 6. The macular, irregular hyperpigmentation of melanosis can be extremely black at times, and indistinguishable from melanoma, and virtually always requires a biopsy to rule out dangerous disease of melanoma and pigmented vulvar intraepithelial neoplasia. (*Courtesy of* Libby Edwards, MD, Charlotte, NC.)

or symptoms such as pruritus or pain. A biopsy is nearly always indicated to rule out melanoma and pigmented VIN.

Histologically, these lesions contain melanin pigment confined to the basal layer of squamous epithelium.[13] Lentigines show basal layer hyperpigmentation, mild melanocytic hyperplasia arranged as solitary units at the dermoepidermal junction rather than nests, epithelial hyperplasia, and stromal melanophages without cytologic atypia.[14–17] If biopsies are negative, reassurance and observation is the appropriate management. Removal is solely a cosmetic issue and can be attempted via destructive or excisional modalities. The association of vulvar melanosis with malignancy is unlikely but has not been disproven at this point. Patients with vulvar melanosis appear to have no increase in melanomas or squamous cell carcinomas, although a single case of genital melanosis in a patient with melanoma of the urinary bladder has been reported.[18] Also, vulvar melanosis is associated with lichen sclerosus, and there has been reported a possible association between lichen sclerosus and melanoma. Thus, a reasonable approach would be to follow these patients at some sort of regular interval, especially if they have concomitant lichen sclerosus.

Genodermatoses characterized by lentigines There are several genodermatoses that exhibit genital and, often, extragenital mucosal pigmentation showing histologic changes of lentigines as a characteristic feature. These lentigines generally consist of multiple small, dark macules that variably occur on the mucous membranes, modified mucous membranes, and nearby keratinized skin. Bannayan-Riley-Ruvalcaba syndrome carries autosomal dominant inheritance and involves the triad of macrocephaly, genital lentiginosis, and intestinal polyposis.[19] The genital lentigines have been shown to histologically demonstrate hyperplasia of the epidermis with increased basal layer pigmentation and a slight increase in number of melanocytes compared with normal.[20] LAMB syndrome is a cardiocutaneous syndrome that includes atrial myxomas, black and blue nevi in the skin and genital mucosa, and papules and dermal nodules on the skin and tongue.[21] Laugier-Hunziker syndrome involves acquired hyperpigmentation of the oral and genital mucosa (benign to malignant) that can include longitudinal melanonychia.[22] Beare-Stevenson cutis gyrate syndrome is a rare genetic disorder characterized by craniosynostosis, cutis gyrate (furrowed, wrinkled skin), and acanthosis nigricans that can involve the genital skin. Dowling-Degos disease is a rare inherited disease that is characterized by flexoral reticular hyperpigmentation where pigmented macules may be present on the genitalia.[23] LEOPARD, or multiple lentigines syndrome, is an autosomal dominant trait characterized by hypertelorism, sensoneurial deafness, and cardiac abnormalities. Carney complex or NAME syndrome is characterized by hypercortisolism, mucocutaneous lentigines, and nonendocrine and endocrine tumors such as myxomas. Peutz-Jeghers syndrome is an autosomal dominant disorder characterized by intestinal hamartomatous polyps and mucocutaneous melanocytic macules, with an increased risk of a variety of cancers.

Melanocytic nevi (pigmented nevi, nevocellular nevi, common nevi)

A melanocytic nevus is a benign proliferation of melanocytes. Roughly 23% of pigmented vulvar lesions in reproductive-aged women are melanocytic nevi, and roughly 2% of women have vulvar nevi.[1] Clinically, nevi can be flat (junctional) or domed (compound or intradermal). Common nevi range from tan to dark brown in color; rarely these can be blue because of dermal pigment. Individual nevi are generally symmetric, with sharp and regular borders, even color throughout the lesion, and size smaller than 7 mm (**Fig. 7**). Nevi that stray from this characterization warrant biopsy, and may be dysplastic nevi (atypical moles) whose presence increases an individual's risk of cutaneous melanoma. The gross and microscopic appearance of dysplastic nevi falls between those of common nevi and melanoma. Surgical removal of atypical nevi on the vulva is warranted. Nevi on the vulva can at times be difficult to distinguish

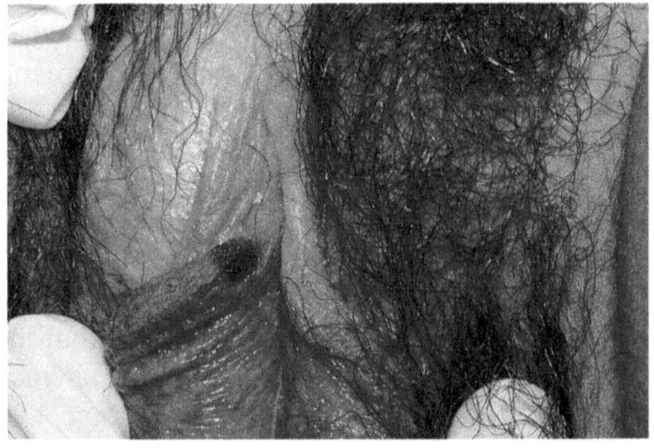

Fig. 7. Although pigmented nevi generally exhibit a predilection for sun-exposed skin, these small, regular, soft or flat, well-demarcated, brown papules also occur on the vulva and can mimic genital warts or pigmented vulvar intraepithelial neoplasia. (*Courtesy of* Libby Edwards, MD, Charlotte, NC.)

from seborrheic keratoses, pigmented warts, and pigmented VIN, for which dermoscopy and/or biopsy can be helpful to differentiate these lesions. Virtually all nevi are acquired, but uncommon congenital nevi can be larger and carry a greater risk of malignancy.[4]

The early medical literature described concern over the premalignant potential of vulvar nevi as compared with nevi on other parts of the body. However, a large majority of vulvar nevi are identical histologically to extragenital nevi, with most being junctional.[24] A minority subgroup of unusual vulvar nevi occurs in premenopausal women, with the distinguishing feature of enlarged junctional melanocytic nests.[24,25] Distinct from dysplastic nevi found on all skin surfaces, these vulvar nevi sometimes demonstrate cytologic atypia, focal pagetoid spread, with a dermal nevus component, adnexal spread, and dense eosinophilic fibrosis in the superficial dermis.[26,27] The Gleason and colleagues study[26] reported recurrence of a single nevus from 45 removed by excision after 3.5 years, and no recurrences after 11.5 years, suggesting that these are not malignant. Such lesions have been termed "nevi with site-related atypia," of which the genitalia is one of these sites,[28] or "atypical melanocytic nevus of the genital type" (AMNGT).[29] It is important to note that these nevi can be misdiagnosed as melanoma even among experienced pathologists.

Some clinicians suggest removal of any nevi found within lichen sclerosus. These nevi can appear histologically similar to melanoma despite being of benign character, with features such as confluence of junctional nests, nests within dermal fibrosis, lymphocytic inflammation, and pagetoid upward spread of melanocytes.[30] Ideally, lichen sclerosus should be controlled before benign-appearing nevi are excised.

Melanoma

Melanoma is a malignancy of the pigment-producing cells of the epidermis. Only about 3% of all melanomas involve the genital tract[31]; however, 8% to 10% of genital malignancies are melanomas,[32] making it the second most common malignancy of the vulva behind squamous cell carcinoma. Patients with lighter skin types are most at risk; however, it should be noted that the incidence ratio of genital melanomas between different ethnicities is less marked than that observed for other cutaneous melanomas. The Surveillance, Epidemiology, and End Results (SEER) database of vulvar and vaginal melanomas from 1992 to 2005 found the overall white-to-black incidence ratio in vulvar melanomas was 3.14 to 1.00 and in vaginal melanomas was 1.02 to 1.00, which is much less than compared with cutaneous, nongenital melanomas (13 to 1 and 17 to 1, respectively).[33] Genetic factors, such as family history of melanoma or inherited dysplastic nevus syndrome, appear to be more important than UV exposure in the development of vulvar melanomas. Vulvar melanomas at time of diagnosis tend to be large, with red, white, blue, or black hues, irregular coloration, asymmetric and indistinct borders, and size larger than 7 mm (**Fig. 8**). They most commonly occur on the labia majora in women of age 50 or older, and can be flat or nodular.[34] At least one quarter of cases in lighter skin types are amelanotic, which distinguishes vulvar melanomas from those on other parts of the body.[34] Because vulvar melanomas usually present at a more advanced stage than melanoma on more visible surfaces, patients are often symptomatic with a palpable mass, pain, pruritus, or bleeding, or they have noticed an enlarging lesion. Most vulvar melanomas are of the mucosal lentiginous subtype on the mucosal surface of the genitalia, but these can also be superficial spreading or nodular, especially on the keratinized surfaces.[34] Vulvar melanomas of the mucosal lentiginous subtype appear to emerge de novo rather than being associated with prior nevi as is often observed in cutaneous, nongenital melanomas.[34]

If melanoma is suspected, an excisional biopsy with 1- to 2-mm margins is ideal, but punch biopsy of a subsection of a large lesion is reasonable. Shave biopsies should not be performed to

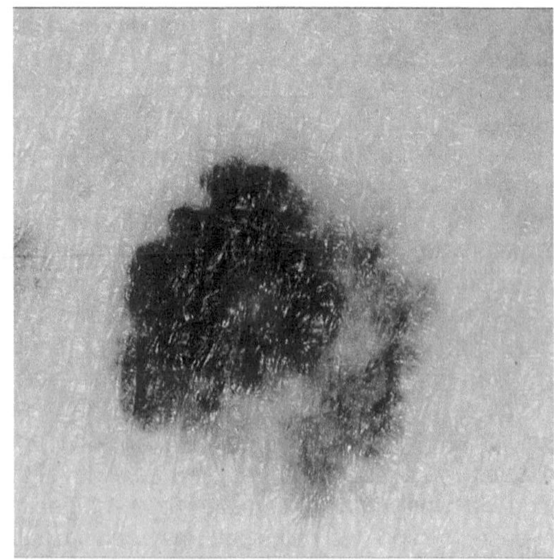

Fig. 8. Melanoma is described as large, irregularly pigmented and shaped brown papules or macules; however, amelanotic melanoma is more common on the vulva than on other areas of the body. (*Courtesy of* Libby Edwards, MD, Charlotte, NC.)

preserve diagnostic and prognostic accuracy. Pathologists experienced in reading large volumes of vulvar pigmented lesions should be consulted when the initial biopsy is inconclusive but identifies atypia. Histologically, melanoma shows a significant increase in the number of atypical melanocytes at all epidermal levels, arranged as solitary units and as nests, with striking dendrites and some melanocytes being mitotic.[17]

Once diagnosed, melanomas are staged with Breslow thickness being the most important predictor of survival.[35,36] Because vulvar melanomas tend to be more advanced on presentation, the typical Breslow thickness at presentation is 2 to 3 mm.[37] Staging is performed using the American Joint Committee on Cancer classification system. In a large review of SEER cases, most vulvar melanomas were found in white women (90%), of which 61% represented localized disease, 9% had nodal metastases, and only 6% had distant disease. Five-year disease-specific survival rates were 75.5% in patients with local disease, 38.7% with regional disease, and 22.1% in distant disease. Younger women and those with fewer positive lymph nodes had the best chance at survival.[38]

Treatment is largely surgical. Local excision with 1- to 2-cm margins carries similar survival as a radical vulvectomy, with groin dissection or sentinel lymph node biopsy performed for tumors thicker than 1 mm.[39] Sentinel lymph node biopsies sometimes have a useful place in practice. A recent small study of patients with vulvar melanoma without palpable groin nodes demonstrated that Breslow thickness alone does not predict the presence of lymph node metastases, and that sentinel lymph node biopsy could be useful to help guide which patients should be recommended radical lymph node dissection.[40] Dacarbazine chemotherapy has been shown to have response rates in the 15% to 25% range[32] and interferon has been used with melanoma in general as an adjuvant therapy. Radiation and chemotherapy are often used for palliation. Routine skin checks should be performed as follow-up in patients with a history of melanoma.

Vulvar intraepithelial neoplasia

There are 2 major clinical types of vulvar intraepithelial neoplasia (VIN): those that are largely multifocal HPV-related disease occurring in younger women, and those that are largely unifocal HPV-unrelated disease occurring in older women. HPV-related VIN is linked to high-risk HPV types, most commonly 16, 18, and 31. Risk factors include smoking, multiple sexual partners, and immunosuppression, such as HIV. Multifocal VIN, or Bowenoid papulosis, is HPV-related and often appears as hyperpigmented, flat-topped papules or plaques with distinct margins (**Fig. 9**). The diagnosis is based clinically with histologic confirmation, as the lesions can grossly be mistaken for banal genital warts, SKs, and melanocytic nevi. They most commonly occur on the vestibule and lateral labia minora.[41] Clinicians should avoid biopsying lesions recently treated with podophyllin, as its effect on the skin may be interpreted histologically as VIN.

VIN generally is treated because of the risk of progression to invasive vulvar carcinoma without treatment. This can be as high as 87.5% in those, usually older, women with untreated unifocal disease often associated with lichen sclerosus or lichen planus.[42] However, a small study of almost completely non-white Pacific Islanders showed spontaneous regression of warty/basaloid VIN in women younger than 30 with multifocal pigmented lesions, many of whom were smokers and symptomatic.[43] Thus, multifocal lesions can sometimes be observed over a 12-month period in woman

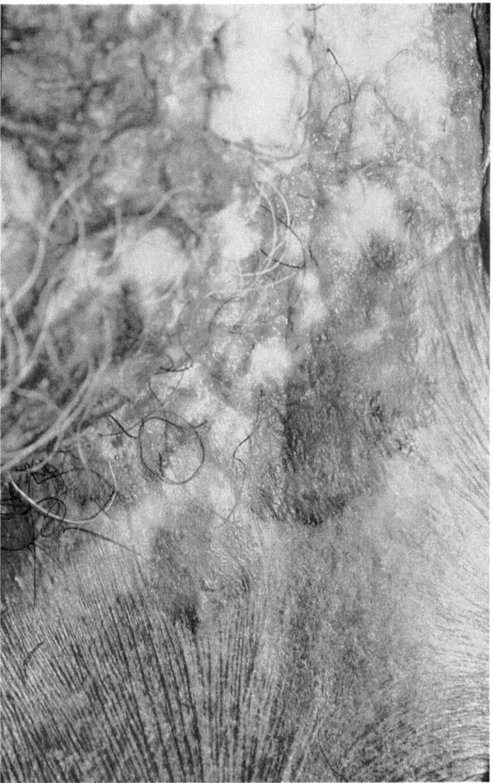

Fig. 9. Pigmented vulvar intraepithelial neoplasia is clinically indistinguishable from brown genital wart infection, particularly when flat. A high index of suspicion is required to make this diagnosis. (*Courtesy of* Libby Edwards, MD, Charlotte, NC.)

younger than 30 before treating them, assuming patients have regular clinical follow-up.

Typical treatment modalities include surgery, cryotherapy, and CO2 laser excision or vaporization. For larger lesions, imiquimod has become an often-used therapy, but this does not have Food and Drug Administration approval. Less often, 5-fluorouracil (5-FU) cream is considered, and topical 5-aminolevulinic acid–based photodynamic therapy is a new modality. It involves application of a photosensitizing compound that collects in neoplastic tissue, followed by nonthermal light of a wavelength matching the photosensitizer's absorption characteristics, thereby producing reactive oxidants than can kill the local cells.[44] It has been studied to treat high-grade VIN, but pigmented and multifocal lesions appear to be less responsive compared with unifocal lesions.[45,46]

Squamous cell carcinoma

Squamous cell carcinoma (SCC) constitutes the great majority of vulvar malignancies.[47] From 1999 to 2004, the rate of vulvar cancer in the United States among all women was 1.7 per 100,000. Cancer rates rose about 3% per year among black women but were stable among other racial and ethnic groups.[48] White women older than 50 carry the highest rates of SCC.[47] Risk factors include long-term inflammation (eg, lichen sclerosus and lichen planus) in older woman and HPV-related disease in younger women. It appears that roughly 60% of vulvar SCC cases are associated with lichen sclerosus,[49,50] and that untreated lichen sclerosus carries a 3% to 5% risk of SCC. Risk factors for HPV-positive SCCs include tobacco and alcohol use and cervical dysplasia.[51] Immunosuppression by virtue of disease or medication significantly increases the risk of invasive SCC in all types of VIN.

At presentation, about half of invasive SCC cases are symptomatic, notably pruritic. Multiple biopsies of lesions of different morphologies increase the yield of detecting SCC.[52] There are 3 main types of SCC. Two are associated with HPV: the classic Bowenoid type, which most often presents as keratotic, verrucous nodules or masses, and verrucous carcinoma (Buschke-Lowenstein tumor), which appears as large, cauliflowerlike lesions that rarely metastasize but are locally invasive. The third type of SCC is the non-HPV–associated keratinizing or differentiated SCC, which appears as crustlike lesions that on biopsy show groups of keratinocytes with cornified material in the lamina propria. This type most often occurs in a setting of long-term inflammation, such as lichen sclerosus or lichen planus.

Staging is dictated by the International Federation of Gynecology and Obstetrics. Five-year survival ranges from 100% for localized, stage I disease, to 20% for stage IVB disease. Unlike melanoma, tumor depth rather than thickness is the primary histologic feature that predicts prognosis and directs therapy.[53] The primary treatment modality is surgery, reserving radical vulvectomies for only advanced cases. Alternatively, chemotherapy and radiation are used in those who are not surgical candidates. Sentinel lymph node biopsy compared with inguinofemoral lymph node dissection for staging carries a reduction in morbidity and has a false negative rate of about 2%[54]; however, both approaches are still used in practice.

Pigmented basal cell carcinoma

Basal cell carcinoma (BCC) is a low-grade neoplasm often classified as an epithelioma rather than a carcinoma because of its very rare metastatic potential. This tumor usually is pink or flesh-colored, with a pearly, translucent sheen; however, it occasionally is pigmented, sometimes exhibiting irregular browns and black. BCC is

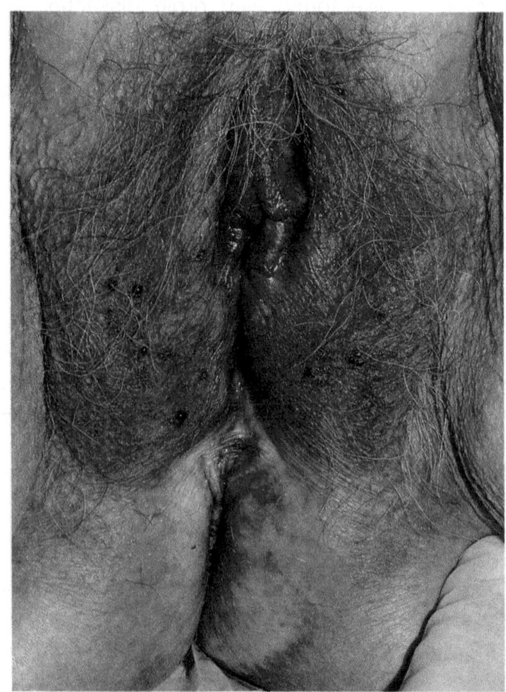

Fig. 10. Angiokeratomas are common vascular growths that usually appear purple. However, at times they can be nearly black and can be confused with true pigmented lesions. (*Courtesy of* Libby Edwards, MD, Charlotte, NC.)

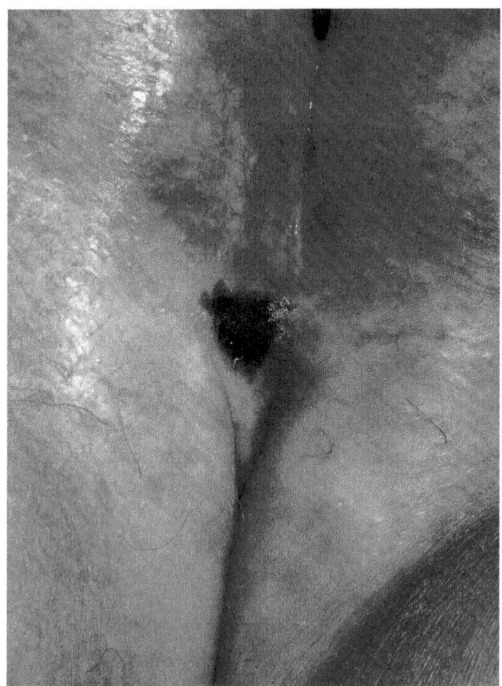

Fig. 11. Like angiokeratomas, purpura can sometimes appear brown or black and raise the specter of more serious disease. (*Courtesy of* Libby Edwards, MD, Charlotte, NC.)

uncommon in the vulva, constituting approximately 5% of primary vulvar cancers.[55] BCCs can appear as nodules, polyps, ulcers, or flat areas of hyperpigmentation or hypopigmentation. These eventually enlarge and ultimately ulcerate. BCCs of the genitalia usually require a biopsy to diagnose. Although metastasis is not a concern, up to 10% recurred in a study of vulvar BCC in the United Kingdom,[55] and were virtually never fatal. Basal cell nevus syndrome is a rare disorder that can also affect the perineum. Thus, patients with this disease are recommended to have routine anogenital examinations.[56,57]

Others

There are a variety of other vulvar lesions that may appear pigmented to the naked eye but do not contain melanin. Using a lens magnifier can help differentiate these from true pigmented lesions.

Angiokeratomas are benign, common hemangiomas that are usually multiple and familial (**Fig. 10**) and present as small, smooth papules usually found on the hair-bearing vulvar skin, increasing with age.[4] They vary in color from red to purple that is so dark as to appear black, and, when solitary, these can mimic nodular melanoma, thus warranting biopsy. Treatment is cosmetic. Electrocautery can be done, but new lesions occur.

Like hemangiomas, Kaposi's sarcoma on the genitalia can appear violaceous or black owing to vascular channels or hemosiderin, especially in patients of African background; however, it is virtually always reported in homosexual males with HIV rather than in women.[58]

Purpura, or cutaneous hemorrhage, presents as well-demarcated dark red or purple patches that are nonblanching (**Fig. 11**). Isolated vulvar purpura is overwhelmingly most common within active, fragile vulvar lichen sclerosus.

SUMMARY

Brown vulvar lesions are quite common in the general population. Although the great majority of these lesions are benign, those that cannot be definitively diagnosed clinically should be biopsied. Reviewing difficult cases with colleagues who specialize in vulvar lesions is highly recommended, given that in the vulva some lesions that grossly, dermoscopically, and microscopically appear atypical can actually be normal variants and thus are not associated with risk of malignancy. The benefit of careful, experienced evaluation is significant for the patient's physical and emotional well-being, preserving the skin when possible, but this must be balanced against the potential risk of invasive, life-threatening malignancy.

REFERENCES

1. Rock B, Hood AF, Rock JA. Prospective study of vulvar nevi. J Am Acad Dermatol 1990;22(1):104–6.
2. Friedrich E, Burch K, Bahr J. The vulvar clinic: an eight-year appraisal. Am J Obstet Gynecol 1979; 135:1036–40.
3. Lynch PJ. Pigmented disorders. In: Edwards L, Lynch PJ, editors. Genital dermatology atlas. 2nd edition. Philadelphia: Lippincott Williams & Wilkins; 2010. p. 170–85.
4. Wiseman MC, Klemperer E. Brown lesions. In: Edwards L, editor. Genital dermatology atlas. 1st edition. Philadelphia: Lippincott Williams & Wilkins; 2004. p. 170–85.
5. Pipkin C, Lio P. Cutaneous manifestations of internal malignancies: an overview. Dermatol Clin 2008;26: 1–15.
6. Grasinger C, Wild R, Parker I. Vulvar acanthosis nigricans: a marker for insulin resistance in hirsute women. Fertil Steril 1993 Mar;59(3):583–6.
7. de Giorgi V, Massi D, Salvini C, et al. Pigmented seborrheic keratoses of the vulva clinically mimicking a malignant melanoma: a clinical, dermoscopic-pathologic case study. Clin Exp Dermatol 2005;30 (1):17–9.

8. Izikson L, Sober AJ, Mihm MC Jr, et al. Prevalence of melanoma clinically resembling seborrheic keratosis: analysis of 9204 cases. Arch Dermatol 2002; 138:1562–6.
9. Ozdemir F, Kilinc-Karaarslan I, Akalin T. A pigmented, hemorrhagic genital wart: clinical, dermoscopic, and histopathologic features. Arch Dermatol 2008;144(8):1072–3.
10. El Shabrawi-Caelen L, Soyer HP, Schaepp H, et al. Genital lentigines and melanocytic nevi with superimposed lichen sclerosus: a diagnostic challenge. J Am Acad Dermatol 2004;50:690–4.
11. Mannone F, De Giorgi V, Cattaneo A, et al. Dermoscopic features of mucosal melanosis. Dermatol Surg 2004;30(8):1118–23.
12. Ferrari A, Buccini P, Covello R, et al. The ringlike pattern in vulvar melanosis: a new dermoscopic clue for diagnosis. Arch Dermatol 2008;144(8):1030–4.
13. Karney MY, Cassidy MS, Zahn CM, et al. Melanosis of the vagina. A case report. J Reprod Med 2001;46 (4):389–91.
14. Barnhill RL, Albert LS, Shama SK, et al. Genital lentiginosis: a clinical and histopathologic study. J Am Acad Dermatol 1990;22(3):453–60.
15. Jih DM, Elder DE, Elenitsas R. A histopathologic evaluation of vulvar melanosis. Arch Dermatol 1999;135(7):857–8.
16. Rudolph RI. Vulvar melanosis. J Am Acad Dermatol 1990 Nov;23(5 Pt 2):982–4.
17. Sison-Torre EQ, Ackerman AB. Melanosis of the vulva. A clinical simulator of malignant melanoma. Am J Dermatopathol 1985;7(Suppl):51–60.
18. Kerley SW, Blute ML, Keeney GL. Multifocal malignant melanoma arising in vesicovaginal melanosis. Arch Pathol Lab Med 1991;115(9):950–2.
19. Erkek E, Hizel S, Sanlý C, et al. Clinical and histopathological findings in Bannayan-Riley-Ruvalcaba syndrome. J Am Acad Dermatol 2005;53(4): 639–43.
20. Fargnoli MC, Orlow SJ, Semel-Concepcion J, et al. Clinicopathologic findings in the Bannayan-Riley-Ruvalcaba syndrome. Arch Dermatol 1996;132(10): 1214–8.
21. Rhodes AR, Silverman RA, Harris TJ, et al. Mucocutaneous lentigines, cardiomucocutaneous myxomas, and multiple blue nevi: the "LAMB" syndrome. J Am Acad Dermatol 1984;10(1):72–82.
22. Gencoglan G, Gerceker-Turk B, Kilinc-Karaarslan I, et al. Dermoscopic findings in Laugier-Hunziker syndrome. Arch Dermatol 2007;143(5):631–3.
23. Wu YH, Lin YC. Generalized Dowling-Degos disease. J Am Acad Dermatol 2007;57(2):327–34.
24. Christensen WN, Friedman KJ, Woodruff JD, et al. Histologic characteristics of vulvar nevocellular nevi. J Cutan Pathol 1987;14(2):87–91.
25. Friedman RJ, Ackerman AB. Difficulties in the histologic diagnosis of melanocytic nevi on the vulvae of premenopausal women. In: Ackerman AB, editor. Pathology of malignant melanoma. New York: Masson; 1981. p. 119.
26. Gleason BC, Hirsch MS, Nucci MR, et al. Atypical genital nevi. A clinicopathologic analysis of 56 cases. Am J Surg Pathol 2008;32(1):51–7.
27. Ribé A. Melanocytic lesions of the genital area with attention given to atypical genital nevi. J Cutan Pathol 2008;35(Suppl 2):24–7.
28. Hosler GA, Moresi JM, Barrett TL. Nevi with site-related atypia: a review of melanocytic nevi with atypical histologic features based on anatomic site. J Cutan Pathol 2008;35(10):889–98.
29. Clark WH Jr, Hood AF, Tucker MA, et al. Atypical melanocytic nevi of the genital type with a discussion of reciprocal parenchymal-stromal interactions in the biology of neoplasia. Hum Pathol 1998; 29(1 Suppl 1):S1–24.
30. Carlson JA, Mu XC, Slominski A, et al. Melanocytic proliferations associated with lichen sclerosus. Arch Dermatol 2002;138(1):77–87.
31. Gungor T, Altinkaya SO, Ozat M, et al. Primary malignant melanoma of the female genital tract. Taiwan J Obstet Gynecol 2009;48(2):169–75.
32. Irvin WP Jr, Legallo RL, Stoler MH, et al. Vulvar melanoma: a retrospective analysis and literature review. Gynecol Oncol 2001;83:457–65.
33. Hu DN, Yu GP, McCormick SA. Population-based incidence of vulvar and vaginal melanoma in various races and ethnic groups with comparisons to other site-specific melanomas. Melanoma Res 2010;20: 153–8.
34. Ragnarsson-Olding BK, Kanter-Lewensohn LR, Lagerlöf B, et al. Malignant melanoma of the vulva in a nationwide, 25-year study of 219 Swedish females: clinical observations and histopathologic features. Cancer 1999;86(7):1273–84.
35. Piura B. Management of primary melanoma of the female urogenital tract. Lancet Oncol 2008;9:973–81.
36. Ragnarsson-Olding BK, Nilsson BR, Kanter-Lewensohn LR, et al. Malignant melanoma of the vulva in a nationwide, 25-year study of 219 Swedish females: predictors of survival. Cancer 1999;86: 1285–93.
37. Wechter ME, Gruber SB, Haefner HK, et al. Vulvar melanoma: a report of 20 cases and review of the literature. J Am Acad Dermatol 2004;50:554–62.
38. Sugiyama VE, Chan JK, Shin JY, et al. Vulvar melanoma: A multivariable analysis of 644 patients. Obstet Gynecol 2007;110:296–301.
39. Trimble EL, Lewis JL Jr, Williams LL, et al. Management of vulvar melanoma. Gynecol Oncol 1992;45: 254–8.
40. Trifirò G, Travaini LL, Sanvito F, et al. Sentinel node detection by lymphoscintigraphy and sentinel lymph node biopsy in vulvar melanoma. Eur J Nucl Med Mol Imaging 2010;37(4):736–41.

41. Pelisse M, Edwards L. Red plaques and patches. In: Edwards L, editor. Genital dermatology atlas. 1st edition. Philadelphia: Lippincott Williams & Wilkins; 2004. p. 18–44.
42. Jones RW, Rowan DM. Vulvar intraepithelial neoplasia III: a clinical study of the outcome in 113 cases with relation to the later development of invasive vulvar carcinoma. Obstet Gynecol 1994;84:741–5.
43. Jones RW, Rowan DM. Spontaneous regression of vulvar intraepithelial neoplasia 2-3. Obstet Gynecol 2000;96(3):470–2.
44. Peng Q, Berg K, Moan J, et al. 5-aminolevulinic acid-based photodynamic therapy: principles and experimental research. Photochem Photobiol 1997; 65:235–51.
45. Abdel-Hady ES, Martin-Hirsch P, Duggan-Keen M, et al. Immunological and viral factors associated with the response of vulval intraepithelial neoplasia to photodynamic therapy. Cancer Res 2001;61(1):192–6.
46. Hillemanns P, Untch M, Dannecker C, et al. Photodynamic therapy of vulvar intraepithelial neoplasia using 5-aminolevulinic acid. Int J Cancer 2000 Mar 1;85(5):649–53.
47. Saraiya M, Watson M, Wu X, et al. Incidence of in situ and invasive vulvar cancer in the US, 1998-2003. Cancer 2008;113(Suppl 10):2865–72.
48. Watson M, Saraiya M, Wu X. Update of HPV-associated female genital cancers in the United States, 1999-2004. J Womens Health (Larchmt) 2009;18(11):1731–8.
49. Leibowitch M, Neill S, Pelisse M, et al. The epithelial changes associated with squamous cell carcinoma of the vulva: a review of the clinical, histological and viral findings in 78 women. Br J Obstet Gynaecol 1990;97(12):1135–9.
50. Carli P, Cattaneo A, De Magnis A, et al. Squamous cell carcinoma arising in vulval lichen sclerosus: a longitudinal cohort study. Eur J Cancer Prev 1995;4(6):491–5.
51. Madsen BS, Jensen HL, van den Brule AJ, et al. Risk factors for invasive squamous cell carcinoma of the vulva and vagina—population-based case-control study in Denmark. Int J Cancer. 2008;122(12): 2827–34.
52. Tyring SK. Vulvar squamous cell carcinoma: guidelines for early diagnosis and treatment. Am J Obstet Gynecol 2003;189(Suppl 3):S17–23.
53. Yoder BJ, Rufforny I, Massoll NA, et al. Stage IA vulvar squamous cell carcinoma: an analysis of tumor invasive characteristics and risk. Am J Surg Pathol 2008;32(5):765–72.
54. Johann S, Klaeser B, Krause T, et al. Comparison of outcome and recurrence-free survival after sentinel lymph node biopsy and lymphadenectomy in vulvar cancer. Gynecol Oncol 2008;110(3): 324–8.
55. Feakins RM, Lowe DG. Basal cell carcinoma of the vulva: a clinicopathologic study of 45 cases. Int J Gynecol Pathol 1997;16(4):319–24.
56. Wang SQ, Goldberg LH. Multiple polypoid basal cell carcinomas on the perineum of a patient with basal cell nevus syndrome. J Am Acad Dermatol 2007;57 (Suppl 2):S36–7.
57. Chen KT. Pigmented apocrine hamartoma of the vulva: a report of two cases. Int J Gynecol Pathol 2005;24(1):85–7.
58. Helton JL. Genital dermatology in the immunosuppressed patient. In: Edwards L, editor. Genital dermatology atlas. 1st edition. Philadelphia: Lippincott Williams & Wilkins; 2004. p. 186–201.

Extramammary Paget's Disease: Summary of Current Knowledge

Christina Lam, MD[a,b], Deana Funaro, MD, FRCPC[c,*]

KEYWORDS

- Extramammary Paget's disease • Vulva • Vulvar neoplasia
- Genital disease

Extramammary Paget's disease (EMPD) is a rare cutaneous malignancy accounting for approximately 1% to 2% of vulvar cancers.[1] Its pathogenesis has been debated, but most cases are thought to arise as a primary intraepidermal neoplasm of glandular origin. A minority seems to represent intraepithelial spread of an underlying dermal adnexal malignancy or a regional neoplasm with contiguous epithelium.[2,3]

The rarity of this disease has caused difficulties in its characterization. Controversies exist in the literature regarding the prevalence of concurrent underlying adenocarcinoma or invasive EMPD, associated malignancies, and optimal treatment. Drawing conclusions has been difficult due to the limited number of case series, usually involving a small number of patients, which have used not only widely differing investigative approaches but also showed significantly variable results.[4–6] This inconsistency can be explained in part by retrospective reviews combining multiple institutions and multiple surgeons, and the lack of uniformity in the immunohistochemical analysis of specimens. One of the largest multi-institutional series of vulvar EMPD cases to date provided retrospective data on 100 patients with this condition, but immunohistochemical analysis was not performed.[6]

This article aims to summarize what is known about EMPD to date in the literature. In addition, based on current knowledge, an approach to diagnosis and treatment is elaborated to aid clinicians faced with patients presenting this disease.

EPIDEMIOLOGY

EMPD is a rare condition with only a few hundred cases reported in the world medical literature. Precise incidence is unknown. EMPD represents 6.5% of all cutaneous Paget's disease and affects predominantly patients between 50 to 80 years of age, with a peak age of 65.[3,7] Women and Caucasians are more commonly affected,[3,5] although a male predominance seems to exist in Asia.[1,7] The vulva remains the most frequently involved site with 65% of EMPD located in this area.[8] Familial occurrence is rare, with six reports in the Japanese literature and one in the British literature.[7]

PATHOLOGY

In EMPD, the proliferative neoplastic cell is the Paget cell (PC). Characteristically, histopathologic examination with hematoxylin and eosin stain will

Financial disclosure obligations: The authors do not have any relationship with a commercial company that has a direct financial interest in the subject matter or materials discussed in this article or with a company making a competing product.

[a] Department of Dermatology, CHUM, University of Montreal, Quebec, Canada
[b] Dermatology Clinic, St-Luc Hospital, 7th floor, Édouard-Asselin pav, 264 René-Lévesque, Montreal, Quebec, H2X 1P1, Canada
[c] Vulvar Disease Division, Department of Dermatology, CHUM, University of Montreal, Quebec, Canada
* Corresponding author. Department of Dermatology, Notre-Dame Hospital, CHUM, 1560, Sherbrooke Street East, Montreal, Quebec H2L 4M1, Canada.
E-mail address: rouleaufunaro@videotron.ca

Dermatol Clin 28 (2010) 807–826
doi:10.1016/j.det.2010.08.002
0733-8635/10/$ – see front matter

reveal an intraepithelial proliferation of large round cells with abundant, pale-staining, basophilic cytoplasm and large, centrally situated nuclei, sometimes with a prominent nucleolus. Some have referred to this as the classic type (or type A).[9] These cells are most often found concentrated in the lower epidermis, but may scatter higher. They can be distributed singly or in groups forming clusters, nests, or glandular structures within the epidermis and epithelium of adnexal structures. Hyperkeratosis, acanthosis, and parakeratosis may be seen. A dense dermal inflammatory infiltrate composed of small round cells and plasma cells can also be found in the upper dermis.[2,3,7]

Immunohistochemical staining is being used to identify PCs and to help differentiate between primary and secondary forms of EMPD. The unique histopathological pattern produced by the intraepidermal infiltration of PCs has led to the recognition of the pagetoid spread pattern in other pathologic conditions. Differential diagnoses to be considered with this particular pattern include malignant melanoma, Bowen's disease, Langerhans cell histiocytosis, mycosis fungoides, sebaceous carcinoma, and Merkel cell carcinoma.[2,10]

As PCs contain intracytoplasmic sialomucin, positive staining with periodic acid-Schiff, mucicarmine, alcian blue, and colloidal iron often aids in diagnosis, especially with EMPD demonstrating more mucin than mammary Paget's disease (MPD).[7,10] When large mucin droplets are present, the nucleus can be displaced to the periphery, creating signet ring PCs (or type B).[9] As well, differential staining patterns of mucin core proteins (MUC) may help in the confirmation of disease. PCs in both MPD and EMPD frequently express MUC1. MUC5A2 appears to be associated much more commonly with EMPD (particularly of vulvar or male genitalia location) than MPD and its loss may signify a more invasive disease.[11–13] Finally, Kuan and colleagues[12] found MUC2 expression in all three perianal EMPD cases associated with an underlying rectal adenocarcinoma.

Adding cytokeratins (CK), carcinoembryonic antigen (CEA), and gross cystic disease fluid protein-15 (GCDFP-15) to the immunohistochemical panel also helps narrow the diagnosis and may point to an underlying malignancy. High-molecular-weight CKs stain the surrounding epidermis but not the PC, whereas low-molecular-weight CKs (such as Cam 5.2) demonstrate the reverse.[2,11,14] As well, CK7 seems to have very good sensitivity, for PC in both MPD and EMPD, ranging from 86% to 100% depending on the study, whereas CK20 may be more specific for EMPD.[15–17] In addition, a particular pattern has been observed in patients with perianal Paget's disease in which CK20+/GCDFP-15- was more frequently associated with an underlying rectal adenocarcinoma, whereas CK20-/GCDFP-15+ was not.[9,18,67] This may also hold true for vulvar cases, but both merit further study.[19] As for CEA, positive staining is quite sensitive for EMPD and a negative result seems to be associated more frequently with underlying carcinomas.[15,20,21] An initial approach to biopsy specimens is outlined in **Fig. 1**.

Various other immunohistochemical markers have been described in the literature, attempting to identify prognostic indicators, pathogenetic

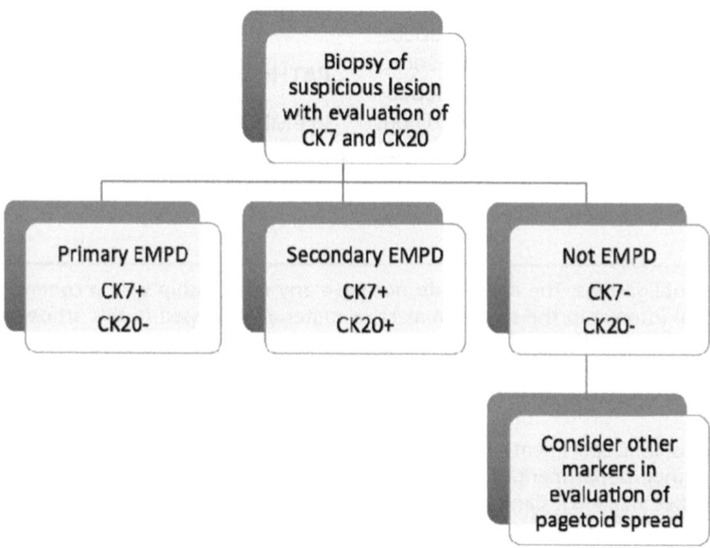

Fig. 1. Approach to initial histologic evaluation.

mechanisms, or possible targeted-therapy. Among the hormonal receptors studied, there appears to be a frequent lack of positivity for both estrogen and progesterone receptors, whereas androgen receptors are found more than 50% of the time.[22,23] Significance of this finding remains unclear. In addition HER-2 protein overexpression, as can be frequently found in MPD, may be detected in 30% to 50% of EMPD cases[23–25] and may be associated with a more aggressive, recurrent disease.[26] Expression of tumor proliferation markers have also been examined, showing that combination high expressivity of Ki-67 and cyclin D1 may be highly associated with invasiveness in EMPD lesions,[27] whereas Ki-67 alone seems to have no prognostic role.[28] As well, presence of the tumor suppressor protein p53 might predict invasive[28,29] and secondary EMPD.[30] Interestingly, Yamada and colleagues[31] evaluated the use of immunostain D2-40 for lymphatic endothelium and found a positive correlation between dermal invasion greater than 1 mm, lymphatic invasion as demonstrated by the D2-40 stain, and nodal metastasis. The investigators suggested using a combination of D2-40 immunostain as a predictor of lymphatic invasion and depth of dermal invasion greater than 1 mm as a predictor for nodal metastasis. Finally, the demonstration of uroplakin-III (a transmembrane protein on urothelial cells found to be highly specific for urothelial carcinoma) in vulvar EMPD lesions may be useful in characterizing secondary EMPD as being of urothelial origin.[32]

PATHOGENESIS

The precise pathogenesis of EMPD is still the subject of great debate. Cell origin remains controversial because this condition, although mostly found on apocrine gland-bearing skin, can also be diagnosed on apocrine-poor sites.[3,7] Though immunohistochemical staining show the epithelial-glandular nature of these cells, a precise origin remains unclear.[2,7] Many theories have been brought forward as PCs have been associated with skin adnexae (both apocrine and eccrine glands), pluripotent keratinocyte stem cells within the epidermis, and, more recently, Toker cells, which are present in both mammary and vulvar tissue.[2,33]

EMPD is considered to be a heterogenous condition encompassing two distinct pathogenetic mechanisms. In primary EMPD (or intraepidermal EMPD), PCs are thought to originate in the epidermis at the sweat gland level or from primitive epidermal basal cells. This form is not associated with an underlying adenocarcinoma, though it can become invasive, infiltrate the dermis, and even metastasize to local lymph nodes and distant sites. By contrast, secondary EMPD arises from epidermotropic spread of malignant cells from an underlying adenocarcinoma in a dermal adnexal gland or within a contiguous epithelium, usually of the genitourinary (GU) or gastrointestinal (GI) tract.[2,3]

Finally, it has also been suggested that EMPD can result from a multicentric oncogenic stimulus, inducing intraepidermal, adnexal, and distant adenocarcinoma—a theory supported by the occasional association between EMPD and MPD.[7]

CLINICAL FINDINGS

The lesions in EMPD are nonspecific and multiple topical therapies are often tried before the diagnosis is made. A median delay of 2 years has been reported.[4] The primary lesion is an erythematous and scaly plaque (**Fig. 2**), usually well delineated, and may demonstrate crusting, weepy erosions (**Fig. 3**), and even ulcerations (**Fig. 4**). Infiltrated nodules, vegetative lesions, and regional lymphadenopathy may be present. Pigmentary changes may also be noted, more often hypo- rather than hyperpigmentation.[4,34] Lesions are often solitary, but may be multiple, in which cases the plaques seem to be separated by areas of normal skin.[7] With such a presentation, the

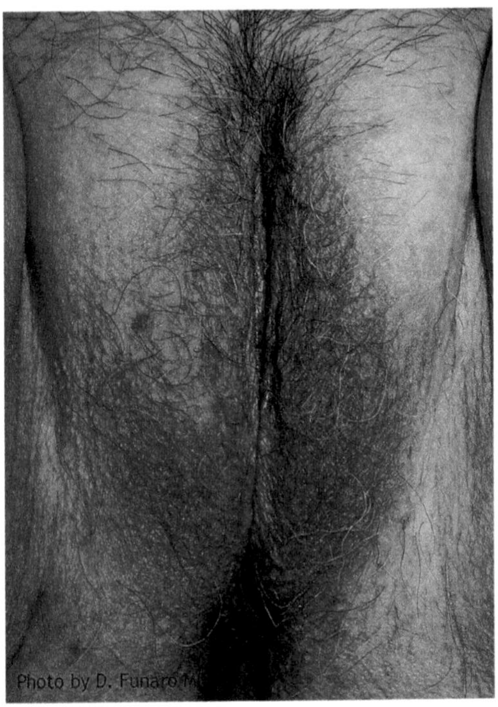

Fig. 2. Discrete EMPD of the right labium majora.

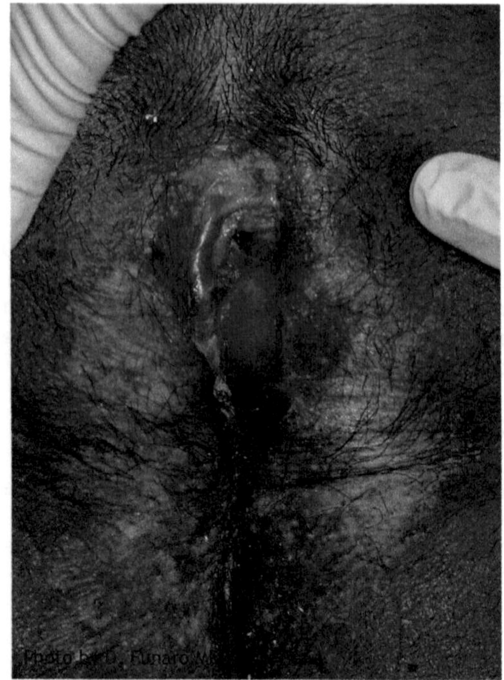

Fig. 3. Extensive EMPD involving vulva, buttocks, and perianal area.

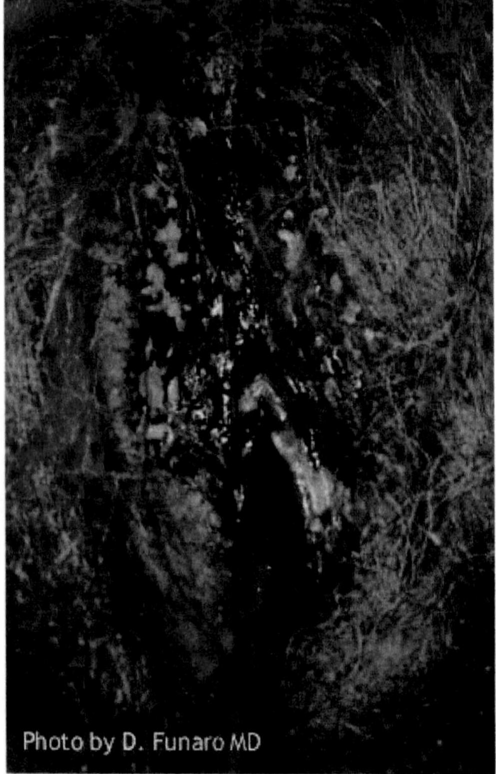

Fig. 4. Erosive EMPD with adenocarcinoma.

diagnoses most frequently considered are those of superficial fungal infections, psoriasis, and various eczematous dermatitides, prompting initial treatment with topical corticosteroids or antifungals.[10] EMPD affects typically apocrine-rich areas of the body (axillae, groin), but cases of "ectopic EMPD" have been described, in particular the cheek,[35,36] abdomen,[37] and external ear.[38] The most commonly involved area is the vulva (up to 65% of EMPD cases), but the perianal area (20%) and male genitalia (14%), that is, scrotum or penis, are also quite frequent.[7,8] Patients often complain of pruritus (up to 60%–72%), but burning, tenderness, and edema may be experienced as well.[39,40] Up to 39% of patients may have associated lymphadenopathy, either unilateral or bilateral.[4]

ASSOCIATION WITH INTERNAL MALIGNANCY

As stated previously, reports in the literature are unclear regarding exact incidence of underlying malignancy and which investigations to do under specific circumstances. Various factors contribute to the difficult interpretation of results and include: (1) disparate definitions of the term "underlying malignancy," ranging from underlying adnexal carcinoma to locoregional malignancy of contiguous epithelium to distant neoplasm; (2) lack of precise chronology from diagnosis of internal malignancy to that of EMPD, shedding doubt on a veritable association; (3) unknown evolution of the internal malignancy relative to that of EMPD; (4) lack of rigor or nonuniform methods used to investigate for possibility of internal malignancy; (5) incomplete data and bias stemming from retrospective studies and large tertiary-care institutions; and (6) lack of correlation between the prevalence of various internal malignancies associated with EMPD relative to that seen by age group independent of EMPD. Despite these difficulties, certain topographic locations of EMPD may be associated more frequently with specific neoplasms, in which case a directed search could be undertaken based on clinical presentation.[7] As demonstrated by Chanda[8] in a large review of 197 cases of EMPD in which 29% of them were associated with an internal malignancy (12% of them within a year of diagnosis), certain parallels can be drawn between the location of the primary lesion of EMPD and the anatomic site of the associated neoplasm. In particular, the study found that all 4 of the male GU system malignancies had presented with male genitalia EMPD; that 8 out of 9 GI tract neoplasms were associated with perianal EMPD; and that 27 out of 31 female GU tract cancers had been seen with vulvar EMPD.

In addition, all reported malignancies were carcinomas. To add to this list, certain series have shown an increased association with breast cancer,[39,41] but whether this is due primarily to its high incidence in the general female population rather than a real association with EMPD has yet to be fully explored. As well, the possibility of an oncogenic stimulus provoking multifocal lesions in anatomically noncontiguous sites exists. In recent years, others have tried to revisit the issue with widely differing results (the risk often quoted as 15%–30%), a summary of which is detailed in **Tables 1–4**. As well, a tendency for a higher percentage of perianal EMPD to be associated with underlying neoplasia has been alluded to in the past,[9,42] but may in part reflect referral bias at large institutions.[48,49] As for underlying adnexal carcinomas, prevalence usually ranges from 15% to 35%,[8,39,41,55,56] with the one of the largest multicenter reviews to date showing 4%.[6]

COURSE AND PROGNOSIS

As most of the research relating to EMPD has come from retrospective analyses, this question has not been formally evaluated in a prospective study. However, information can be gleaned from various larger case series and reviews on the subject.

Patients with localized and intraepithelial EMPD seem to experience a favorable prognosis.[41,56] In a series of 33 patients with EMPD (57% of which had invasive growth on histopathology, although depth was not specified) and negative clinical lymph nodes, no patient died of EMPD during a median follow-up of 68 months and the standard mortality rate was not significantly different from that of the general matched population.[5] An analysis of 46 patients with intraepithelial vulvar disease showed no death from EMPD during a mean follow-up of 6.89 years.[39] As well, there have been a few documented cases of progressive dermal invasion from initial purely intraepithelial vulvar disease over an extended follow-up period of greater than 10 years, with subsequent lymphatic metastases[19,41]; thus showing that primary disease has the potential to become disseminated.

Several factors may portend a greater risk of death, such as: presence of dermal invasion, elevated CEA levels, clinical presence of nodules in the primary lesion, and bilateral lymph node metastases. Of these, presence of dermal invasion may be the most significant factor.[4] In addition, certain studies have shown that it may be possible to risk-stratify patients with dermal invasion based on depth. Minimally invasive EMPD, defined by some as up to 1 mm of PC invasion below the basement membrane,[19,41] has been found in some studies to be associated with a similar prognosis to that of intraepithelial disease.[19,68] Alternatively, others have classified minimally (or micro-) invasive as up to the level of the papillary dermis and shown variable outcomes. A study of 22 patients with minimally invasive disease demonstrated a 5-year survival rate of 88%,[4] whereas another reported no death from disease in 9 similar patients,[56] thus expounding the difficulty in interpreting data. Another interesting association appears to be the serum CEA level, possibly predictive of systemic metastases from EMPD with a sensitivity of 70% and specificity of 94%.[4] If elevated initially, it may parallel disease course in patients with metastases.[68] Overall mortality rates in certain series, from metastatic EMPD or from associated internal malignancy, have been reported as elevated as 26% and appear greater in those with an associated underlying adnexal carcinoma (46% vs 18%).[8] As well, recurrence rates appear high despite conventional surgical treatment, from 8% to 44%,[4,5,40] likely due to the multifocal nature of the disease and ill-defined margins.[54] Interestingly, recurrences up to 12 years after initial treatment have been reported.[19]

INVESTIGATIONS

As mentioned previously, intraepithelial or minimally invasive EMPD is associated with a good prognosis. At the other end of the spectrum, patients presenting with metastatic disease, particularly to draining lymph nodes, suffer a much poorer outcome, with a reported mortality of up to 66%.[4,39] In addition, a lymph node staging system has been proposed by Hatta and colleagues,[4] where N0 implies no lymph node involvement; N1, unilateral involvement; and N2 bilateral or distant-site disease. The Kaplan-Meier overall survival curve figured in this study clearly depicts decreasing survival with increasing lymph node status. Thus, a clinical quandary arises when faced with managing a patient with histologically proven EMPD and negative clinical lymphadenopathy. Can prognosis be improved by determining possibility of lymphatic invasion in invasive disease? This issue has been broached recently in the literature, specifically relating to two surgical aspects: the value of sentinel lymph node biopsy (SLNB) with or without complete lymph node dissection (CLND) and the pertinence of elective lymph node dissection (ELND) in managing invasive EMPD. The principle from which these procedures stem is based on the notion that metastases first pass through the

Table 1
Reported series or cases of underlying malignancy with perianal EMPD

Studies	Total No. of Patients	No. of Patients Affected (%)	Malignancy	Chronology with EMPD Diagnosis
Williams et al,[42] 1978	7	5 (71%)	3 perianal adenocarcinoma 1 sweat gland carcinoma	Synchronous
			1 perianal gland adenocarcinoma + sigmoid villous adenoma + SCC of neck (in same patient)	SCC diagnosed after, others synchronous
Chanda,[8] 1985	24	6 (25%)	4 rectal adenocarcinoma 2 anaplastic (cloacogenic) carcinoma	Within 1 y
		3 (17%)	2 rectal adenocarcinoma 1 other	>1 y before or after
Beck & Fazio,[43] 1987	10	3 (30%)	1 SCC of anus 1 rectal cancer 1 prostate cancer	10 y after 4 y after Unclear
Berardi et al,[44] 1988	86	34 (39%)	14 carcinoma of anus 13 carcinoma of rectum 5 carcinomas (skin, prostate, nasopharynx, neck) 1 "3 separate carcinomas" 1 sigmoid carcinoma in situ	NA
Armitage et al,[45] 1989	8	3 (37%)	2 mucinous adenocarcinoma	1 at presentation 1 at 3 y after
			1 poorly differentiated adenocarcinoma	10 y after
Goldman et al,[46] 1992	5	4 (80%)	2 anorectal adenocarcinoma 1 sweat gland adenocarcinoma	Synchronous
			1 anorectal jct adenocarcinoma	4 y after
Marchesa et al,[47] 1997	14	4 (28%)	1 SCC of anus 2 rectal adenocarcinoma 1 apocrine carcinoma	56 mo after NA
Sarmiento et al,[48] 1997	13	4 (31%)	1 anal adenocarcinoma 2 prostate adenocarcinoma 1 rectal adenocarcinoma	Previous to diagnosis Synchronous
Goldblum & Hart,[9] 1998	11	5 (45%)	5 rectal adenocarcinoma	4 synchronous 1 metachronous (30 mo after)
Zollo & Zeitouni,[40] 2000	2	0	—	—
McCarter et al,[49] 2003	27	9 (33%)	4 anal carcinoma 3 rectal carcinoma 1 prostate cancer 1 SCC of skin	NA
Pierie et al,[5] 2003	8	NA	2 colorectal carcinoma 1 BCC	Synchronous
Tulchinsky et al,[50] 2003	5	1 (20%)	1 breast carcinoma	20 y previous
Minicozzi et al,[51] 2009	6	1 (17%)	1 rectal adenocarcinoma + history of prostatic cancer	Synchronous

Abbreviations: BCC, basal cell carcinoma; NA, not applicable; SCC, squamous cell carcinoma.

lymphatic system before disseminating systemically and that, by interrupting this passage, it may be possible to prevent widespread disease.[69]

Tsutsumida and colleagues[64] studied 34 patients with genital EMPD to specifically determine indications for ELND. Intentional procedural evaluation of lymph nodes was undertaken only if clinical or histologic (as seen on the initial biopsy specimen) evidence of lymph node involvement was found. No intervention was necessary for the 22 patients with in situ and papillary dermis invasion; however, 4 of the 6 patients with reticular dermis invasion underwent ELND and 3 had histologic evidence of lymphatic disease, whereas all 6 of the patients with invasion to the subcutaneous tissues had nodal metastases with a significant increase in mortality rate. Details pertaining to specific correlations between clinical and histologic evidence of lymphadenopathy were not provided. Based on their results, the investigators strongly recommended ELND for all patients with EMPD invasion into the reticular dermis and beyond, even in the absence of clinical lymphadenopathy. Kodama and colleagues[56] reviewed 30 cases of vulvar EMPD and reported no death from disease in 10 patients with intraepithelial and 9 with minimally invasive (depth not specified) disease, of which 12 had had a bilateral groin node dissection with negative histologic evaluation. Clinical status of lymph nodes was not mentioned and no specific recommendations regarding nodal dissection were given. At the other end of the spectrum, Fanning and colleagues,[6] in a large retrospective review of 100 patients with vulvar EMPD, provided data for 12 patients with invasive lesions, 7 of which were microinvasive (depth not specified) and 5 deeply invasive. None of these patients underwent lymphadenectomy or died from disease, although 3 recurred after surgical excision (1 of them invasively, within a median follow-up time of 7 years). Despite their results, the investigators' guidelines recommended performing a modified radical vulvectomy with inguinal lymphadenectomy (unilateral for ipsilateral lesions and bilateral for central lesions) in patients with underlying adenocarcinoma or intraepithelial EMPD. The reason for including intraepithelial disease was referenced to a sole case report of a patient with microinvasive (<1 mm of invasion) vulvar EMPD who rapidly developed clinical lymphadenopathy with bilateral histologically positive nodes.[70] This approach does not seem to be standard in the literature and does not reflect the practice at the authors' institution.

In the early 1990s, Morton and colleagues[71] reported their initial experience with intraoperative lymphatic mapping and sentinel lymphadenectomy relative to melanoma. In essence, the technique uses the injection of dye and lymphoscintigraphy to map the lymphatic drainage pathway of the primary lesion and thus identify the first draining lymph node (or sentinel node), the underlying concept being that this node represents the status of all nodes in the draining basin. The sentinel node is then excised and examined by permanent section for evidence of disease. If disease is demonstrated, the surgeon can then perform a CLND.[69,71] The technique's utility lies in that it is a minimally invasive procedure and a more morbid surgery (ie, a CLND) can be prevented if the node is negative for disease.

Hatta and colleagues[72] performed, in one of the largest series to date, SLNB in 13 patients with primary genital EMPD. Clinical evidence of lymphadenopathy before the procedure was unclear. Of 4 patients with a positive SLNB, 3 had reticular dermal invasion and 1 had microinvasive disease to the papillary dermis. The 3 patients with deep dermal invasion underwent total lymphadenectomy and interestingly, 2 had no additional nodes but 1 died of visceral metastases 3 months later, whereas the one with additional nodes had bone metastases. No patient with intraepithelial disease had a positive sentinel node and all 9 node-negative patients were free from disease during the 3 to 50 month follow-up period. Based on their findings, the investigators concluded that SLNB was warranted for all EMPD patients except in those with strictly intraepithelial disease and that its positivity correlated well with poorer prognosis and need for additional therapy.

Other smaller case series have reported on SNLB in invasive EMPD, but these have all been limited by the short follow-up period and lack of a control group. Ewing and colleagues[73] described three cases of vulvar microinvasive (<1 mm in depth) EMPD in which one patient had a unilaterally positive sentinel node and underwent bilateral CLND with resultant negative histopathology. The other two had negative sentinel nodes and all three cases had no recurrence of invasive or metastatic disease with a maximum follow-up of 26 months (one case was not specified). Baron and colleagues[74] reported two cases of vulvar EMPD, of which one was microinvasive (<1 mm) and one was unclear, both of which had negative SLNB and no recurrence up to 4 years post intervention. Two case reports very briefly detail negative SLNBs in intraepithelial EMPD and clinically normal nodes.[75,76]

Despite the attraction of performing SLNB in invasive disease to minimize risks of chronic lymphedema, pain and infection from nodal dissection, the technique remains to be standardized

Table 2
Reported series or cases of underlying malignancy with vulvar EMPD

Studies	Total No. of Patients	No. of Patients Affected (%)	Malignancy	Chronology with EMPD Diagnosis
Taylor et al,[52] 1975	18	3 (17%)	1 breast adenocarcinoma 1 ovary adenocarcinoma 1 SCC cervix	39 y previous 3 y previous Synchronous
Breen et al,[53] 1978	13	5 (38%)	1 breast carcinoma 1 cervical carcinoma 1 SCC of vulva 1 BCC of face 1 uterine adenocarcinoma	10 y previous 5 y previous 12 y previous Recurrent 8 mo previous
Gunn & Gallager,[54] 1980	4	1 (25%)	1 breast carcinoma	NA
Chanda[8] 1985	109	10 (9%)	3 cervical squamous carcinoma 3 cervical adenocarcinoma 2 breast carcinoma 1 Bartholin gland adenocarcinoma 1 gall bladder adenocarcinoma	Within 1 y
		21 (19%)	9 breast carcinoma 3 uterine carcinoma 3 vaginal carcinoma 3 bladder carcinoma 1 ovarian carcinoma 2 others	>1 y before or after
Feuer et al,[41] 1990	19	6 (31%)	1 carcinoma in situ of cervix + breast carcinoma 1 BCC 1 cervical carcinoma 1 ovarian carcinoma 1 esophageal carcinoma 1 breast carcinoma	NA
		1 (5%)	1 adenocarcinoma of periurethral gland	NA
Fishman et al,[55] 1995	14	9 (64%)	2 breast carcinoma 1 endometrial carcinoma 1 bladder carcinoma 1 skin cancer 1 vulvar carcinoma 1 colon carcinoma	Metachronous
			2 focally invasive adenocarcinoma	Synchronous
Kodama et al,[56] 1995	27	11 (41%)	Carcinoma of skin appendage 2 carcinoma in situ	NA
Goldblum & Hart,[19] 1997	19	2 (10%)	1 breast carcinoma 1 bladder TCC	Metasynchronous 9 mo after
Fanning et al,[6] 1999	100	20 (20%)–30 malignancies among them	6 breast carcinoma 6 BCC 4 vulvar adenocarcinoma 4 endometrial carcinoma 3 pancreatic carcinoma 3 lung cancer 3 stomach cancer 1 thyroid cancer	NA

(continued on next page)

Table 2
(*continued*)

Studies	Total No. of Patients	No. of Patients Affected (%)	Malignancy	Chronology with EMPD Diagnosis
Piura et al,[57] 1999	5	1 (20%)	Apocrine gland adenocarcinoma	NA
Parker et al,[39] 2000	76	21 (28%)	13 underlying adenocarcinoma 3 cervical carcinoma 2 breast carcinoma 1 endometrial cancer 1 ovarian carcinoma 1 adenocarcinoma (unknown origin)	NA Within 3 mo
Zollo & Zeitouni,[40] 2000	22	7 (32%)	1 thigh histiofibrosarcoma 4 breast carcinoma 1 pancreas carcinoma 1 multiple (follicular thyroid, breast, cecal carcinoma)	NA
Pierie et al,[5] 2003	19	NA	3 breast carcinoma 1 BCC 1 renal cell carcinoma 1 rectal carcinoma 1 vulvar adenocarcinoma 1 bladder carcinoma 1 hepatocellular carcinoma	Synchronous

Abbreviations: BCC, basal cell carcinoma; NA, not applicable; SCC, squamous cell carcinoma; TCC, transitional cell carcinoma.

and validated in EMPD. In particular, a few questions need to be addressed. Is there evidence for increased survival in patients who have undergone ELND? At what level, if any, of dermal invasion does the risk for lymphatic spread become relevant? Is there a survival advantage for SLNB with or without CLND compared with standard surgical excision only? Akin to the studies on melanoma,

Table 3
Reported series/cases of underlying malignancy with male genitalia EMPD

Studies	Total No. of Patients	No. of Patients Affected (%)	Malignancy	Chronology with EMPD Diagnosis
Chanda[8] 1985	18	2 (11%)	1 prostatic carcinoma 1 hypernephroma	Within 1 y
		2 (11%)	1 prostatic carcinoma 1 bladder carcinoma	>1 y before or after
Chang et al,[58] 1996	22	1 (4%)	1 gall bladder carcinoma	5 y after
Zollo & Zeitouni,[40] 2000	6	3 (50%)	2 prostatic carcinoma 1 oropharynx carcinoma	NA
Park et al,[59] 2001	6	0	—	—
Lai et al,[60] 2002	33	7 (21%)	7 underlying adnexal carcinoma	NA
		3 (9%)	1 prostate carcinoma 1 rectosigmoid carcinoma 1 prostate carcinoma	Synchronous Metasynchronous
Yang et al,[61] 2005	36	1 (3%)	1 renal cell carcinoma	17 mo after
Wang et al,[62] 2008	130	0	—	—

Male genitalia defined as penis, scrotum, or groin.
Abbreviation: NA, not applicable.

Table 4
Reported series or cases of underlying malignancy with EMPD (site nonspecified)

Studies	Total No. of Patients	No. of Patients Affected (%)	Malignancy	Chronology with EMPD Diagnosis
Helwig & Graham,[63] 1963	38	13 (34%)	13 underlying adnexal carcinoma	NA
		10 (26%)	4 rectal adenocarcinoma 2 breast adenocarcinoma 1 mucinous adenocarcinoma of urethra 3 BCC of face	NA
Tsutsumida et al,[64] 2003	34	5 (15%)	1 thyroid cancer 1 prostate cancer 1 gastric cancer 1 hepatocellular carcinoma/ colon cancer 1 lung/prostate cancer	NA
Chiu et al,[65] 2007	11 males	0 (0%)	—	—
Yoon et al,[66] 2008	28	8 (28%)	1 bladder cancer 1 lung cancer 1 sigmoid cancer + early gastric cancer	NA
			1 rectal cancer	5 y after
			1 gastric GIST + colorectal adenoma	Synchronous
			3 colorectal adenomas	Synchronous
Hatta et al,[4] 2008	76	0	—	—

Abbreviations: BCC, basal cell carcinoma; GIST, gastric gastrointestinal stromal tumor; NA, not applicable.

might there a place for SLNB in the prognosis of minimally invasive disease? An approach to SLNB is outlined in **Fig. 5**, based on current knowledge.

Another aspect of investigations worth mentioning is ^{18}F-fluorodeoxyglucose-positron emission tomography (FDG-PET) and its ability to potentially detect subclinical nodal metastases. A

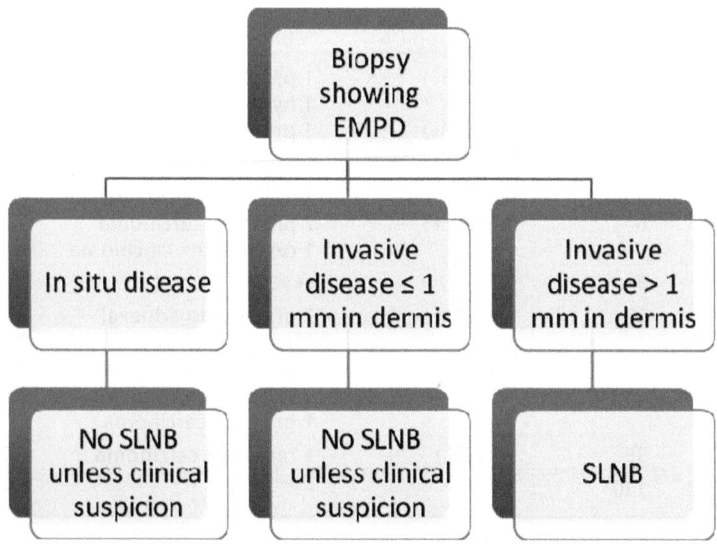

Fig. 5. Approach to SLNB.

case series[77] evaluating seven male patients with penoscrotal EMPD showed that PET scans failed to detect primary lesions when tumor thickness was less than 0.5 mm and only detected those greater than 2 cm. Interestingly, three out of those detected four cases had dermal invasion. An analysis of three cases[78] demonstrated that PET scans were less sensitive than SLNB at detecting micrometastases as nodal involvement less than or equal to 10 mm was not discovered. However, these series comprise only a total of 10 patients and neither institution used integrated PET or CT scans, the combination of which complements each modality's strengths.[79]

APPROACH TO CONFIRMED DIAGNOSIS OF EMPD

As much of the discussion above has summarized, the literature still remains vague regarding precise risk for internal malignancy and standard investigations to perform. However, as with any initial disease diagnosis, thorough history and review of systems are paramount. The need for a complete physical examination, including a full skin examination; palpation for enlarged lymph nodes and hepatosplenomegaly; and clinical breast and digital rectal examinations, cannot be overly emphasized and constitute a baseline. A summary of the investigations performed on EMPD at the authors' institution is listed below.

Approach to EMPD investigations

- History and review of systems
- Complete cutaneous examination
- Evaluate lymph nodes, liver, and spleen
- Breast examination
- Mammography
- Gynecologic examination, including colposcopy, PAP smear, and pelvic ultrasound
- Urologic evaluation, including cystoscopy with or without uroscan
- Colonoscopy with or without CT abdomen
- Serum CEA (if invasive EMPD).

For patients with vulvar EMPD, a reasonable initial work-up includes screening for GU and GI tract involvement as well as breast disease. Our approach consists of a complete pelvic examination (including Pap smear and colposcopy[80]), cystoscopy with or without CT scan urogram, abdominopelvic ultrasound with or without CT scan, mammography, and colonoscopy. A serum CEA level could also be obtained if the disease were found to be invasive.

For patients with perianal EMPD, we usually screen primarily for associated GI and GU system neoplasms with upper and lower endoscopy with or without CT scan, cystoscopy with or without CT urogram, and mammogram (if female). Serum CEA and prostate-specific antigen levels are also options.

Men with penoscrotal lesions of EMPD do not seem to have as high prevalence of associated internal malignancies as that seen in other locations, especially with Asian men.[8,58,60,61] Nonetheless, GU malignancies tend to be seen more commonly and we often perform baseline screening with colonoscopy and cystoscopy with or without CT urogram. In addition, serum prostate-specific antigen and CEA levels may be added to the panel.

Unfortunately, there are no published guidelines regarding need and frequency of follow-up in cases of primary and secondary EMPD. In addition, no consensus exists pertaining to subsequent internal malignancy screening if the initial one is negative. Based on the literature and the experience at the authors' institution, a reasonable approach to an initially diagnosed primary noninvasive EMPD would be a clinical evaluation twice a year for the first 3 years then once yearly thereafter. Internal malignancy screening may be directed toward particular signs or symptoms thereafter. In secondary EMPD, a closer follow-up three to four times a year is warranted, with repeat yearly screening directed to site of lesion.

TREATMENT

Surgery is still considered the mainstay of treatment for patients with EMPD. Over the years, many therapeutic modalities have been attempted on patients with EMPD in an effort to reduce the significant morbidity associated with the often-radical surgical treatments performed. Because of the rarity of this condition, experience in its management is limited. Consequently, reported studies reviewing or proposing treatment options are often retrospective and include few patients, thus leaving surgeons to tailor treatment according to each patient's situation. Until 1990, surgery was performed with wide local excision 2 to 3 cm beyond the clinical margins and down to 0.5 cm of subcutaneous tissue. Surgical procedures included wide local excision, simple or radical vulvectomy.[40,81–89]

Faced with a high recurrence rate ranging from 30% to 60% and often mutilating surgical procedures, margin status gained interest.[90–93] Perioperative identification of margins was attempted with the use of frozen sections or fluorescein.[94] Intraoperative frozen section studies revealed high rates of false-negative margins (approaching

Table 5
Imiquimod cream treatment regimens

Authors	EMPD Location	Primary or Secondary	Previous Treatments	Regimen	Response to Treatment
Zampogna et al,[115] 2002	Scrotum (case 1) Perineum and inguinal area (case 2)	Primary Noninvasive (cases 1 and 2)	Electrodessication and curettage (case 1) None (case 2)	Nightly for 6 nights, then 4 d of rest then every other day for 16 wk (case 1) Nightly for 3wk, then every other day for 7.5 wk (case 2)	No recurrence after 1 y (case 1) No recurrence after 4 mo (case 2)
Berman et al,[116] 2003	Scrotum and right groin	Primary with dermal microinvasion	None	Daily for 6 wk	No recurrence after 6 mo
Qian et al,[117] 2003	Scrotum	Primary Noninvasive	MMS × 2 Photodynamic therapy × 2	3 times weekly for 6 wk	No recurrence after 14 mo
Wang et al,[118] 2003	Vulva	Primary, noninvasive		Nightly for 6 nights, then 4 d rest, then 2–3 times per wk for 5 wk	Resolution 2 wk after treatment
Moyal-Barracco et al,[119] 2005	Vulva and perianal (17 cases)	Primary, noninvasive	Surgery[8] Laser[1]	Twice weekly for 36 applications (modified in relation to side effects)	4 PR 5 CR (1 recurred at 10 mo follow-up)
Mirer et al,[120] 2006	Intergluteal fold, anal margin and right major labium	Primary Noninvasive	None	5 days per wk first mo Every other day 2 m Twice weekly for 3–4 mo	No recurrence after 1 y

Badgwell & Rosen,[121] 2006	Thigh	Primary Noninvasive	None	Twice weekly for 16 wk	No recurrence after
Ye at al,[122] 2006	Scrotum	Primary Noninvasive	Large surgical excision	-Nightly for 6 wk then every other day for 4 wk -Combination 5-FU 5% cream AM, retinoic acid afternoon and imiquimod HS × 12 d	-Residual EMPD post imiquimod treatment -No recurrence after 2 y
Vereecken et al,[123] 2007	Perianal	Primary Noninvasive	3 local resections	Nightly application × 3 mo	No recurrence after 1 y
Hatch & Davis,[124] 2008	Vulva (2 cases)	Primary Noninvasive	*Case 1*: none *Case 2*: radical vulvectomy 2 y prior	*Case 1*: Every other day × 26 applications, then daily applications for total 11 wk; combined with betamethasone. Daily tx continued for total of 11 wk, then once weekly. *Case 2*: daily for 5 wk then every other day for 28 wk, alternating with clobetasol cream. Continued once weekly.	*Case 1*: No recurrence after 12 mo *Case 2*: No recurrence after 6 mo

Abbreviations: AM, morning; CR, complete response; PR, partial response; HS, at bedtime; TX, treatment.

40%), limited use in the presence of multicentric disease,[54,55] as well as little effect on disease outcome.[40,83,85–88] Kodama and colleagues[56] reported a lower recurrence rate in patients by using intraoperative frozen sections, but all patients in this study subsequently underwent complete vulvectomy from repeated resections. Preti and colleagues[85] reported a 15% to 62% risk of recurrence after surgical treatment of EMPD and little effect of margin status on this outcome.

Routine frozen sections, by processing technique, sample only 0.1% of the surgical margin. Consequently, Mohs micrographic surgery (MMS) was attempted with the goal of obtaining complete tumor-free margins while preserving unaffected tissue and reducing the need for mutilating surgery.[40,91,95–99] O'Connor and colleagues'[95] retrospective review of 95 patients treated at the Mayo Clinic included a report on 12 patients treated with MMS. After a mean follow-up of 24 months, MMS had a local recurrence rate of 8% as opposed to 22%, after a 65-month follow-up, for the 83 patients who underwent wide local excision. Time to recurrence has been reported at an average of 2.5 years and sometimes even several years after initial surgery.[96] In a retrospective study by Hendi and colleagues,[97] recurrence rate after MMS was 16% for primary EMPD and 50% for recurrent EMPD. Patients included in this study were both male and female. EMPD location included male genitalia, female genitalia, groin, perianal, and axillary regions. The mean margin to clear all tumors was 2.5 cm, whereas margins of 5 cm were needed to obtain microscopically clear margins in 97% of cases. The Geisinger-experience retrospective study on MMS and EMPD reported 10 patients (9 primary and 1 recurrent) treated by MMS with no recurrence after a mean follow-up period of 34 months.[98]

High recurrence rates associated with EMPD have been attributed to subclinical extension and multifocal disease. To remedy this situation, several adjuvant techniques have been studied to help uncover the extent of tumor spread and precise location of disease. Multiple scouting biopsies[99] have been advocated and reported by several investigators using various techniques. Preoperative knowledge of lesion size and extent provides for better preparatory surgical and reconstructive planning, but requires additional interventions and delays time to surgery. Despite this, tumor-free margins cannot be established with certainty because of the occurrence of false-negative biopsies, often stemming from sampling errors or simply from the multifocal nature of EMPD. A study by Coldiron and colleagues[96] evaluated recurrence of EMPD after MMS versus conventional excision using fixed or frozen margins. They combined results from their own experience with those from a written survey of members of the American College of Micrographic Surgery and compared these with cases selected from the literature that had undergone conventional surgery. They reported a recurrence rate of 23% for MMS versus 33% for conventional excision with margin control.

Laser treatment of EMPD gained interest in the hopes that it would provide a conservative approach to eradicate the disease while preserving vulvar anatomy and sexual function. Already used to treat vulvar intraepithelial neoplasia, several surgeons began exploring this option to treat vulvar intraepithelial Paget's disease. CO2 and Nd: YAG lasers have been reported useful in the treatment of EMPD.[100–102] Though operative and hospitalization times are shorter, the procedure can be quite painful for a considerable period of time, prompting certain patients to defer a subsequent treatment. Another major drawback is the lack of histologic evidence for noninvasive disease or clear surgical margins. Whereas some investigators reported success with laser treatment,[100–102] several reports noted significant recurrence after the use of laser surgery in this condition.[40,83,103] Reasons for high recurrence rates (reaching up to 67%) after a 2-year follow-up included the use of laser therapy in more extensive lesions, multifocality of the tumor, and perhaps an overly superficial ablation by laser (up to the reticular dermis in all studies) when compared with surgical removal.[83]

Photodynamic therapy (PDT) has been used successfully to treat several cutaneous neoplasms. Visible light will activate the photosensitizing agent, generating reactive oxygen species and selectively destroy neoplastic tissue. In EMPD, both topical (Δ-aminolevulinic acid [ALA]) and systemic (porfimer sodium [PDT]) have been studied.[104–108] PDT has been used alone or in combination with other treatment modalities, including conventional surgery, laser, radiation therapy, and chemotherapy. Many regimens have been attempted with 20% ALA compounds. Variations on a similar theme can be noted in the route of administration (topical or intralesional), duration of ALA application and selected light source used to irradiate tumor (argon dye laser, excimer dye laser, halogen lamp, red lamp). Topical ALA, able to reach epidermal and appendageal disease, appears to offer an excellent cosmetic outcome. However, questions arise regarding its ability to reach all neoplastic cells.

Intravenous administration of porfimer sodium alleviates this concern, especially when treating a large lesion. However, this treatment might generate a more severe local reaction leading to a longer healing time. Conclusions are difficult to draw concerning PDT treatment efficacy as follow-up times, treatment parameters and tumor invasiveness vary considerably between reported cases. Also, many patients treated with PDT were initially approached with another modality. Though prospective studies are needed, PDT can be considered a useful option especially when treating inoperable patients or EMPD in difficult anatomic locations.

The use of CO2 laser on lesions delineated by prior photodynamic diagnosis has been reported,[109,110] the objective being to better delineate tumor margins before laser surgery. Investigators reported the use of ALA 20% in an ointment base applied topically for 6 hours under occlusive foil. After removal of the ointment, the area was illuminated under Wood light and biopsied at several sites, with EMPD found in all areas. Finally, the fluorescent area was vaporized with CO2 laser, reaching a depth of 2 mm and extending 1 cm beyond the fluorescent area. At follow-up, residual tumor was visualized with PDT and was vaporized once again. The subsequent 14-month follow-up showed no recurrence.

Less aggressive measures using topical therapies have long been considered and attempted in patients with EMPD.[111–113] In particular, various treatment regimens using 5-fluorouracil (5-FU) have been tried over the last several years, mostly in combination therapy, before surgery[114] or after surgery, to evaluate residual disease[113] and rarely as a single agent. In certain cases requiring a less invasive approach, 5-FU has been reported effective in clearing lesions. However, investigators caution against the use of 5-FU as monotherapy as it has been reported to clear clinical but not pathologic disease. Haberman and colleagues[111] described using 5-FU 1% cream daily for 12 weeks in a patient with perianal and scrotal EMPD. Though clinical lesions cleared, biopsy specimens following treatment showed persistent disease, which was a similar finding reported by Kawatsu and Miki[112] Alternatively, Eliezri and colleagues[114] reported the use of 5-FU twice daily for 10 days, applied to an area 5 cm beyond the clinical lesion, before MMS to help delineate areas of subclinical EMPD. Its use as an adjunct before MMS proved useful in planning the surgical intervention but could not completely delineate EMPD margins as was proven after pathologic review.

Imiquimod cream, a low-molecular-weight imidazoquinoline amine, has shown some interesting results and multiple case reports have surfaced over the course of the last decade detailing various treatment regimens (**Table 5**). Most patients were treated thrice weekly for an average of 3 months. In most studies with imiquimod 5% cream, biopsies were done immediately after treatment and several months later[115–125] with both clinical and pathologic clearance of EMPD frequently reported. These results contrast with the 5-FU response, where clinical resolution was noted without pathologic cure.

This biologic response modifier enhances both innate and acquired immune function and is known to stimulate cytokines, specifically interferon-alpha (IFN-α) and tumor necrosis factor-alpha (TNF-α), at the site of application. Response to treatment would seem to go beyond a simple destructive effect by actually stimulating a specific immune response to tumor cells. Side effects reported with treatment range from moderate-to-severe local irritation to flu-like symptoms, nausea, and vomiting.

Imiquimod can be considered an alternative to surgery, an adjunct before or after surgery, and even part of a therapeutic combination with other treatment modalities.[122] Though only case reports or case series have been published thus far, results seem promising.

Topical bleomycin has also been attempted in the treatment of vulvar EMPD. Four cases of recurrent EMPD of the vulva reported by Watring and colleagues[126] were treated with topical bleomycin 3.5% in an ointment base twice daily for 2 weeks with a rest period of 4 to 6 weeks and a maximum of four cycles. All achieved complete clinical remission of the disease but one patient experienced a recurrence 30 months later requiring retreatment with a single course of topical bleomycin. Side effects were limited to treated areas.

Case reports and case series on the use of radiotherapy in EMPD have surfaced with interesting results. Used as an initial treatment mostly in selected patient groups (ie, the elderly or those unfit to undergo conventional surgery), cases of large EMPD lesions or EMPD located in functionally delicate anatomic areas for surgery, radiotherapy has also been reported in combination with surgery or following a recurrence. Described treatment techniques, including beam type, beam energy, and total doses, differ between publications. Initial reports suggested a high recurrence rate,[127,128] whereas later[128–136] ones seem to present more encouraging results. Acute and chronic radiation toxicity can occur.

In locally advanced or metastatic EMPD, many anecdotal reports have been published but no study has evaluated the efficacy of a predefined chemotherapeutic regimen. Reported treatments include 5-FU, 5-FU/mitomycin C, carboplatin/5-FU, low-dose 5-FU/cisplatin, low-dose mitomycin C/etoposide/cisplatin, mitomycin/epirubicin/vincristine/cisplatin/5-FU, and docetaxel.[137–141] Though certain cases have demonstrated some measurable response, conclusions cannot be drawn. Most reported regimens were inspired by treatments used for visceral adenocarcinoma.

SUMMARY

From the many articles reviewed above, readers have probably come to the likely conclusion that extramammary Paget's disease, despite having first been described over 100 years ago, still remains a largely confusing and relatively rare disease. Multiple retrospective reviews covering all topics, from prognostic factors to internal malignancy associations to various treatment modalities, have been published over the last few decades and have elucidated certain issues. However, it is clear that randomized controlled trials are needed to adequately evaluate lymph node involvement and compare therapeutic strategies, so that standardization may be attempted and initial treatment protocols elaborated to determine the best combination of greatest efficacy with least morbidity.

ACKNOWLEDGMENTS

Contributors include Christina Lam and Deana Funaro for article conception and design, drafting of manuscript, and critical revision of manuscript; and Deana Funaro for article supervision.

REFERENCES

1. Curtin JP, Rubin SC, Jones WB, et al. Paget's disease of the vulva. Gynecol Oncol 1990;39:374–7.
2. Lloyd J, Flanagan AM. Mammary and extramammary Paget's disease. J Clin Pathol 2000;53(10):742–9.
3. Shepherd V, Davidson EJ, Davies-Humphreys J. Extramammary Paget's disease. BJOG 2005;112:273–9.
4. Hatta N, Yamada M, Hirano T, et al. Extramammary Paget's disease: treatment, prognostic factors and outcome in 76 patients. Br J Dermatol 2008;158(2):313–8.
5. Pierie JP, Choudry U, Muzikansky A, et al. Prognosis and management of extramammary Paget's disease and the association with secondary malignancies. J Am Coll Surg 2003;196:45–50.
6. Fanning J, Lambert HC, Hale TM, et al. Paget's disease of the vulva: prevalence of associated vulvar adenocarcinoma, invasive Paget's disease, and recurrence after surgical excision. Am J Obstet Gynecol 1999;180(1 Pt 1):24–7.
7. Kanitakis J. Mammary and extramammary Paget's disease. J Eur Acad Dermatol Venereol 2007;21(5):581–90.
8. Chanda JJ. Extramammary Paget's disease: prognosis and relationship to internal malignancy. J Am Acad Dermatol 1985;13(6):1009–14.
9. Goldblum JR, Hart WR. Perianal Paget's disease: a histologic and immunohistochemical study of 11 cases with and without associated rectal adenocarcinoma. Am J Surg Pathol 1998;22(2):170–9.
10. Neuhaus IM, Grekin RC. Mammary and extramammary Paget disease. Fitzpatrick's dermatology in general medicine. 7th edition. McGraw-Hill Professional; 2007.
11. Liegl B, Leibl S, Gogg-Kamerer M, et al. Mammary and extramammary Paget's disease: an immunohistochemical study of 83 cases. Histopathology 2007;50(4):439–47.
12. Kuan SF, Montag AG, Hart J, et al. Differential expression of mucin genes in mammary and extramammary Paget's disease. Am J Surg Pathol 2001;25(12):1469–77.
13. Yoshii N, Kitajima S, Yonezawa S, et al. Expression of mucin core proteins in extramammary Paget's disease. Pathol Int 2002;52:390–9.
14. Moll I, Moll R. Cells of extramammary Paget's disease express cytokeratins different from those of epidermal cells. J Invest Dermatol 1985;84(1):3–8.
15. Battles OE, Page DL, Johnson JE. Cytokeratins, CEA and mucin histochemistry in the diagnosis and characterization of extramammary Paget's disease. Am J Clin Pathol 1997;108(1):6–12.
16. Smith KJ, Tuur S, Corvette D, et al. Cytokeratin 7 staining in mammary and extramammary Paget's disease. Mod Pathol 1997;10(11):1069–74.
17. Lundquist K, Kohler S, Rouse RV. Intraepidermal cytokeratin 7 expression is not restricted to Paget cells but is also seen in Toker cells and Merkel cells. Am J Surg Pathol 1999;23(2):212–9.
18. Nowak MA, Guerriere-Kovach P, Pathan A, et al. Perianal Paget's disease: distinguishing primary and secondary lesions using immunohistochemical studies including gross cystic disease fluid protein-15 and cytokeratin 20 expression. Arch Pathol Lab Med 1998;122(12):1077–81.
19. Goldblum JR, Hart WR. Vulvar Paget's disease: a clinicopathologic and immunohistochemical study of 19 cases. Am J Surg Pathol 1997;21(10):1178–87.
20. Mori O, Hachisuka H, Sasai Y. Immunohistochemical demonstration of EMA, CEA, and keratin on mammary and extramammary Paget's disease. Acta Histochem 1989;85(1):93–100.

21. Helm HK, Goellner JR, Peters MS. Immunohistochemical stains in Extramammary Paget's disease. Am J Dermatopathol 1992;14(5):402–7.
22. Diaz de Leon E, Carcangiu ML, Prieto VG, et al. Extramammary Paget disease is characterized by the consistent lack of estrogen and progesterone receptors but frequently expresses androgen receptor. Am J Clin Pathol 2000;113(4):572–5.
23. Liegl B, Horn HC, Moinfar F. Androgen receptors are frequently expressed in mammary and extramammary Paget's disease. Mod Pathol 2005;18(10): 1283–8.
24. Tanskanen M, Jahkola T, Asko-Seljavaara S, et al. HER2 oncogene amplification in extramammary Paget's disease. Histopathology 2003;42(6): 575–9.
25. Horn LC, Purz S, Krumpe C, et al. COX-2 and Her-2/neu are overexpressed in Paget's disease of the vulva and the breast: results of a preliminary study. Arch Gynecol Obstet 2008;277(2):135–8.
26. Plaza JA, Torres-Cabala C, Ivan D, et al. HER-2/neu expression in extramammary Paget disease: a clinicopathologic and immunohistochemistry study of 47 cases with and without underlying malignancy. J Cutan Pathol 2009;36(7):729–33.
27. Aoyagi S, Akiyama M, Shimizu H. High expression of Ki-67 and cyclin D1 in invasive extramammary Paget's disease. J Dermatol Sci 2008;50(3): 177–84.
28. Ellis PE, Fong LF, Rolfe KJ, et al. The role of p53 and Ki67 in Paget's disease of the vulva and the breast. Gynecol Oncol 2002;86(2):150–6.
29. Zhang C, Zhang P, Sung CJ, et al. Overexpression of p53 is correlated with stromal invasion in extramammary Paget's disease of the vulva. Hum Pathol 2003;34(9):880–5.
30. Yanai H, Takahashi N, Omori M, et al. Immunohistochemistry of p63 in primary and secondary vulvar Paget's disease. Pathol Int 2008;58(10): 648–51.
31. Yamada Y, Matsumoto T, Arakawa A, et al. Evaluation using a combination of lymphatic invasion on D2-40 immunostain and depth invasion is a strong predictor for nodal metastasis in extramammary Paget's disease. Pathol Int 2008;58:114–7.
32. Brown HM, Wilkinson EJ. Uroplakin-III to distinguish primary vulvar Paget disease from Paget disease secondary to urothelial carcinoma. Hum Pathol 2002;33:545–8.
33. Willman JH, Golitz LE, Fitzpatrick JE. Vulvar clear cells of Toker: precursors of extramammary Paget's disease. Am J Dermatopathol 2005;27(3): 185–8.
34. Chiba H, Kazama T, Takenouchi T, et al. Two cases of vulval pigmented extramammary Paget's disease: histochemical and immunohistochemical studies. Br J Dermatol 2000;142:1190–4.
35. Chilukuri S, Page R, Reed JA, et al. Ectopic extramammary Paget's disease arising on the cheek. Dermatol Surg 2002;28(5):430–3.
36. Cohen MA, Hanly A, Poulos E, et al. Extramammary Paget's disease presenting on the face. Dermatol Surg 2004;30(10):1361–3.
37. Onishi Y, Ohara K. Ectopic extramammary Paget's disease affecting the upper abdomen. Br J Dermatol 1996;134:958–61.
38. Gonzalez-Castro J, Iranzo P, Palou J, et al. Extramammary Paget's disease involving the external ear. Br J Dermatol 2002;138(5):914–5.
39. Parker LP, Parker JR, Bodurka-Bevers D, et al. Paget's disease of the vulva: pathology, pattern of involvement and prognosis. Gynecol Oncol 2000; 77:183–9.
40. Zollo JD, Zeitouni NC. The Roswell Park Cancer Institute experience with extramammary Paget's disease. Br J Dermatol 2000;142(1):59–65.
41. Feuer GA, Shevchuk M, Calanog A. Vulvar Paget's disease: the need to exclude an invasive lesion. Gynecol Oncol 1990;38:81–9.
42. Williams SL, Rogers LW, Quan SH. Perianal Paget's disease: report of 7 cases. Dis Colon Rectum 1976; 19(1):30–40.
43. Beck DE, Fazio VW. Perianal Paget's disease. Dis Colon Rectum 1987;30:263–6.
44. Berardi R, Lee S, Chen H. Perianal extramammary Paget's disease. Surg Gynecol Obstet 1988;167: 359–66.
45. Armitage NC, Jass JR, Richman PI, et al. Paget's disease of the anus: a clinicopathologic study. Br J Surg 1989;76(1):60–3.
46. Goldman S, Ihre T, Lagerstedt U, et al. Perianal Paget's disease: report of 5 cases. Int J Colorectal Dis 1992;7(3):167–9.
47. Marchesa P, Fazio VW, Oliart S, et al. Long-term outcome of patients with perianal Paget's disease. Ann Surg Oncol 1997;4(6):475–80.
48. Sarmiento JM, Wolff BG, Burgart LJ, et al. Paget's disease of the perianal region—An aggressive disease? Dis Colon Rectum 1997;40:1187–94.
49. McCarter MD, Quan SHQ, Busam K, et al. Long-term outcome of perianal Paget's disease. Dis Colon Rectum 2003;46:612–6.
50. Tulchinsky H, Zmora O, Brazowski E, et al. Extramammary Paget's disease of the perianal region. Colorectal Dis 2003;6:206–9.
51. Minicozzi A, Borzellino G, Momo R, et al. Perianal Paget's disease: presentation of 6 cases and literature review. Int J Colorectal Dis 2010;25(1): 1–7.
52. Taylor PT, Stenwig JT, Klausen H. Paget's disease of the vulva. Gynecol Oncol 1975;3:46–60.
53. Breen JL, Smith CI, Gregori CA. Extramammary Paget's disease. Clin Obstet Gynecol 1978;21(4): 1107–15.

54. Gunn RA, Gallager HS. Vulvar Paget's disease: a topographic study. Cancer 1980;46:590–4.
55. Fishman DA, Chambers SK, Schwartz PE, et al. Extramammary Paget's disease of the vulva. Gynecol Oncol 1995;56:266–70.
56. Kodama S, Kaneko T, Saito M, et al. A clinicopathologic study of 30 patients with Paget's disease of the vulva. Gynecol Oncol 1995;56:63–70.
57. Piura B, Rabinovich A, Dgani R. Extramammary Paget's disease of the vulva: report of 5 cases and review of the literature. Eur J Gynaecol Oncol 1999;20(2):98–101.
58. Chang YT, Liu HN, Wong CK. Extramammary Paget's disease: a report of 22 cases in Chinese males. J Dermatol 1996;23(5):320–4.
59. Park S, Grossfeld GD, Mcaninch JW, et al. Extramammary Paget's disease of the penis and scrotum: excision, reconstruction and evaluation of occult malignancy. J Urol 2001;166:2112–7.
60. Lai YL, Yang WG, Tsay PK, et al. Penoscrotal extramammary Paget's disease: a review of 33 cases in a 20-year experience. Plast Reconstr Surg 2003; 112(4):1017–23.
61. Yang WJ, Kim DS, Im YJ, et al. Extramammary Paget's disease of penis and scrotum. Urology 2005;65(5):972–5.
62. Wang Z, Lu M, Dong GQ, et al. Penile and scrotal Paget's disease: 130 Chinese patients with long-term follow-up. BJU Int 2008;102:485–8.
63. Helwig EB, Graham JH. Anogenital (extramammary) Paget's disease: a clinicopathological study. Cancer 1963;16:387–403.
64. Tsutsumida A, Yamamoto Y, Minakawa H, et al. Indications for lymph node dissection in the treatment of extramammary Paget's disease. Dermatol Surg 2003;29(1):21–4.
65. Chiu TW, Wong PS, Ahmed K, et al. Extramammary Paget's disease in Chinese males: a 21-year experience. World J Surg 2007;31:1941–6.
66. Yoon SN, Park IJ, Kim HC, et al. Extramammary Paget's disease in Korea: its association with gastrointestinal neoplasms. Int J Colorectal Dis 2008;23:1125–30.
67. Kohler S, Smoller BR. Gross cystic disease fluid protein-15 reactivity in extramammary Paget's disease with and without associated internal malignancy. Am J Dermatopathol 1996;18(2): 118–23.
68. Zhu Y, Ye DW, Yao XD, et al. Clinicopathological characteristics, management and outcome of metastatic penoscrotal extramammary Paget's disease. Br J Dermatol 2009;161:577–82.
69. Cochran AJ, Essner R, Rose DM, et al. Principles of sentinel lymph node identification: background and clinical implications. Langenbecks Arch Surg 2000;385:252–60.
70. Fine BA, Fowler LJ, Valente PT, et al. Minimally invasive Paget's disease of the vulva with extensive lymph node metastases. Gynecol Oncol 1995;57: 262–5.
71. Morton DL, Wen DR, Wong JH, et al. Technical details of intraoperative lymphatic mapping for early stage melanoma. Arch Surg 1992;127(4): 392–9.
72. Hatta N, Morita R, Yamada M, et al. Sentinel lymph node biopsy in patients with extramammary Paget's disease. Dermatol Surg 2004;30(10): 1329–34.
73. Ewing T, Sawicki J, Ciaravino G, et al. Microinvasive Paget's disease. Gynecol Oncol 2004;95: 755–8.
74. Baron M, Hitzel A, Sartor A, et al. Paget's disease of the vulva: interest of sentinel lymph node analysis. Gynecol Obstet Fertil 2006;34:619–21.
75. Tsujino Y, Mizumoto K, Matsuzaka Y, et al. Fluorescence navigation with indocyanine green for detecting sentinel nodes in extramammary Paget's disease and squamous cell carcinoma. J Dermatol 2009;36:90–4.
76. Kudo G, Toyama H, Hasegawa K, et al. Sentinel lymph node navigation surgery in Paget's disease of the vulva. Clin Nucl Med 2002;27(2):909–10.
77. Cho SB, Yun M, Lee MG, et al. Variable patterns of positron emission tomography in the assessment of patients with extramammary Paget's disease. J Am Acad Dermatol 2005;52(2):353–5.
78. Aoyagi S, Sato-Matsumura KC, Shimizu H. Staging and assessment of lymph node involvement by 18F-Fluorodeoxyglucose-Positron Emission Tomography in invasive extramammary Paget's disease. Dermatol Surg 2005;31(5):595–8.
79. Poeppel TD, Krause BJ, Heusner TA, et al. PET/CT for the staging and follow-up of patients with malignancies. Eur J Radiol 2009;70(3):382–92.
80. Mai Gu, Ghafari S, Lin F. Pap smears of patients with extramammary Paget's disease of the vulva. Diagn Cytopathol 2004;32(6):353–7.
81. Garzetti GG, Bertani A, Tranquilli AL, et al. Paget's disease of the vulva: advantages of demolitive surgery. Eur J Gynaecol Oncol 1992;13(Suppl 1): 74–7.
82. Petkovic S, Jeremic K, Vidakovic S, et al. Paget's disease of the vulva—a review of our experience. Eur J Gynaecol Oncol 2006;27(6):611–2.
83. Louis-Sylvestre C, Haddad B, Paniel BJ. Paget's disease of the vulva: results of different conservative treatments. Eur J Obstet Gynecol Reprod Biol 2001;99:253–5.
84. Maclean AB, Makwana M, Ellis PE, et al. The management of Paget's disease of the vulva. J Obstet Gynaecol 2004;24(2):124–8.
85. Preti M, Micheletti B, Ghiringhello B, et al. La malattia di Paget vulvare. Minerva Ginecol 2000;52:203–11.

86. Bergen S, DiSaia PJ, Liao SY, et al. Conservative management of extramammary Paget's disease of the vulva. Gynecol Oncol 1989;33:151–6.
87. Tebes S, Cardosi R, Hoffman M. Paget's disease of the vulva. Am J Obstet Gynecol 2002;187(2):281–4.
88. Molinie V, Paniel BJ, Lessana-Leibowitch M, et al. Maladie de Paget vulvaire: 36 cas. Ann Dermatol Venereol 1993;120:522–7.
89. Black D, Tornos C, Soslow RA, et al. The outcomes of patients with positive margins after excision for intraepithelial Paget's disease of the vulva. Gynecol Oncol 2007;104:547–50.
90. Abide JM, Nahai F, Bennett RG. The meaning of surgical margins. Plast Reconstr Surg 1984;73(3): 492–7.
91. Mohs FE, Blanchard L. Microscopically controlled surgery for extramammary Paget's disease. Arch Dermatol 1979;115:706–8.
92. Stacy D, Burrell MO, Franklin EW. Extramammary Paget's disease of the vulva and anus: use of intraoperative frozen-section margins. Am J Obstet Gynecol 1986;155(3):519–23.
93. Murata Y, Kumano K. Extramammary Paget's disease of the genitalia with clinically clear margins can be adequately resected with 1 cm margin. Eur J Dermatol 2005;15(3):168–70.
94. Misas JE, Cold CJ, Hall FW. Vulvar Paget's disease: fluorescein-aided visualizaton of margins. Obstet Gynecol 1991;77:156–9.
95. O'Connor WJ, Lim KK, Zalla MJ, et al. Comparison of Mohs micrographic surgery and wide local excision for extramammary Paget's disease. Dermatol Surg 2003;29(7):723–7.
96. Coldiron BM, Goldsmith BA, Robinson JK. Surgical treatment of extramammary Paget's disease. Cancer 1991;67(4):933–8.
97. Hendi A, Brodland DG, Zitelli JA. Extramammary Paget's disease: surgical treatment with Mohs micrographic surgery. J Am Acad Dermatol 2004; 51(5):767–73.
98. Thomas CJ, Wood GC, Marks VJ. Mohs micrographic surgery in the treatment of rare aggressive cutaneous tumors: the Geisinger experience. Dermatol Surg 2007;33(3):333–9.
99. Appert DL, Otley CC, Phillips PK, et al. Role of multiple scouting biopsies before Mohs micrographic surgery for extramammary Paget's disease. Dermatol Surg 2005;31(11 Pt 1):1417–22.
100. Valentine BH, Arena B, Green E. Laser ablation of recurrent Paget's disease of vulva and perineum. J Gynecol Surg 1992;8(1):21–4.
101. Weese D, Murphy J, Zimmern PE. Nd:YAG laser treatment of extramammary Paget's disease of the penis and scrotum. J Urol (Paris) 1993;99(5):269–71.
102. Ewing TL. Paget's disease of the vulva treated by combined surgery and laser. Gynecol Oncol 1991;43:137–40.
103. Choi JB, Yoon ES, Yoon DK, et al. Failure of carbon dioxide laser treatment in three patients with penoscrotal extramammary Paget's disease. BJU Int 2001;88:297–8.
104. Shieh S, Dee AS, Cheney RT, et al. Photodynamic therapy for the treatment of extramammary Paget's disease. Br J Dermatol 2002;146:1000–5.
105. Henta T, Itoh Y, Kobayashi M, et al. Photodynamic therapy for inoperable vulvar Paget's disease using δ-aminolaevulinic acid: successful management of a large skin lesion. Br J Dermatol 1999; 141:347–9.
106. Mikasa K, Watanabe D, Kondo C, et al. 5-Aminolevulinic acid-based photodynamic therapy for the treatment of two patients with extramammary Paget's disease. J Dermatol 2005;32:97–101.
107. Runfola MA, Weber TK, Rodriguez-Bigas MA, et al. Photodynamic therapy for residual neoplasms of the perianal skin. Dis Colon Rectum 2000;43(4): 499–502.
108. Li L, Deng Y, Zhang L, et al. Treatment of perianal Paget's disease using photodynamic therapy with assistance of fluorescence examination: case report. Lasers Med Sci 2009;24:981–4.
109. Becker-Wegerich PM, Fritsch C, Schulte KW, et al. Carbon dioxide laser treatment of extramammary Paget's disease guided by photodynamic diagnosis. Br J Dermatol 1998;138:169–72.
110. Fukui T, Watanabe D, Tamada Y, et al. Photodynamic therapy following carbon dioxide laser enhances efficacy in the treatment of extramammary Paget's disease. Acta Derm Venereol 2009; 89:150–4.
111. Haberman HF, Goodall J, Llewellyn M. Extramammary Paget's disease. Can Med Assoc J 1978; 118:161–2.
112. Kawatsu T, Miki Y. Triple extramammary Paget's disease. Arch Dermatol 1971;104:316–9.
113. Del Castillo LF, Garcia C, Schoendorff C, et al. Spontaneous apparent clinical resolution with histologic persistence of a case of extramammary Paget's disease: response to topical 5-FU. Cutis 2000;65:331–3.
114. Eliezri YD, Silvers DN, Horan DB. Role of preoperative topical 5-FU in preparation for Mohs micrographic surgery of extramammary Paget's disease. J Am Acad Dermatol 1987;17(3): 497–505.
115. Zampogna JC, Flowers FP, Roth WI, et al. Treatment of primary cutaneous extramammary Paget's disease with topical imiquimod monotherapy: two case reports. J Am Acad Dermatol 2002;47(4): S229–35.
116. Berman B, Spencer J, Villa A, et al. Successful treatment of extramammary Paget's disease of the scrotum with imiquimod 5% cream. Clin Exp Dermatol 2003;28(Suppl 1):36–8.

117. Qian ZQ, Zeitouni NC, Shieh S, et al. Successful treatment of extramammary Paget's disease with imiquimod. J Drugs Dermatol 2003;2:73–6.
118. Wang LC, Blanchard A, Judge DE, et al. Successful treatment of recurrent extramammary Paget's disease of the vulva with topical imiquimod 5% cream. J Am Acad Dermatol 2003;49(4):769–70.
119. Moyal-Barracco M, Berville-Levy S, Rouzier R, et al. Traitement par imiquimod de la maladie de Paget vulvaire et péri-anale: étude pilote de 17 cas. Ann Dermatol Venereol 2005;132(9):S11–2.
120. Mirer E, El Sayed F, Ammoury A, et al. Treatment of mammary and extramammary Paget's skin disease with topical imiquimod. J Dermatolog Treat 2006; 17(3):167–71.
121. Badgwell C, Rosen T. Treatment of limited extent extramammary Paget's disease with 5 percent imiquimod cream. Dermatol Online J 2006;12(1):22.
122. Ye JN, Rhew DC, Yip F, et al. Extramammary Paget's disease resistant to surgery and imiquimod monotherapy but responsive to imiquimod combination topical chemotherapy with 5-FU and retinoic acid: a case report. Cutis 2006;77:245–50.
123. Vereecken P, Awada A, Ghanem G, et al. A therapeutic approach to perianal extramammary Paget's disease: topical imiquimod can be useful to prevent or defer surgery. Med Sci Monit 2007;13(6):CS75–7.
124. Hatch KD, Davis JR. Complete resolution of Paget disease of the vulva with imiquimod cream. J Low Genit Tract Dis 2008;12(2):90–4.
125. Denehy T, Taylor RR, McWeeney DT, et al. Successful immune modulation therapy with topical imiquimod 5% cream in the management of recurrent extramammary Paget's disease of the vulva. Gynecol Oncol 2006;101(1 Suppl 1):S88–9.
126. Watring WG, Roberts JA, Lagasse LD, et al. Treatment of recurrent Paget's disease of the vulva with topical bleomycin. Cancer 1978;41:10–1.
127. Balducci L, Crawford ED, Smith GF, et al. Extramammary Paget's disease: an annotated review. Cancer Invest 1988;6:293–303.
128. Brierley JD, Stockdale AD. Radiotherapy: an effective treatment for extramammary Paget's disease. Clin Oncol (R Coll Radiol) 1991;3:3–5.
129. Moreno-Arias GA, Conill C, Castells-Mas A, et al. Radiotherapy for genital extramammary Paget's disease in situ. Dermatol Surg 2001;27(6):587–90.
130. Guerrieri M, Back MF. Extramammary Paget's disease: role of radiation therapy. Australas Radiol 2002;46:204–8.
131. Burrows NP, Jones DH, Hudson PM, et al. Treatment of extramammary Paget's disease by radiotherapy. Br J Dermatol 1995;132:970–2.
132. Luk NM, Yu KH, Yeung WK, et al. Extramammary Paget's disease: outcome of radiotherapy with curative intent. Clin Exp Dermatol 2003;28:360–3.
133. Besa P, Rich TA, Delclos L, et al. Extramammary Paget's disease of the perineal skin: role of radiotherapy. Int J Radiat Oncol Biol Phys 1992;24:73–8.
134. Yanagi T, Kato N, Yamane N, et al. Radiotherapy for extramammary Paget's disease: histopathological findings after radiotherapy. Clin Exp Dermatol 2007;32:506–8.
135. Perniciaro C, Buskirk SJ. Extramammary Paget's disease treated with radiotherapy. J Dermatolog Treat 1993;4:164–5.
136. Kwan WH, Teo PM, Ngar YK, et al. Perineal Paget's disease: effective treatment with fractionated high dose rate brachytherapy. Clin Oncol (R Coll Radiol) 1995;7:400–1.
137. Kariya K, Tsuji T, Schwartz RA. Trial of low-dose 5-FU/Cisplatin therapy for advanced extramammary Paget's disease. Dermatol Surg 2004;30(2Pt2):341–4.
138. Beleznay KM, Levesque MA, Gill S. Response to 5-FU in metastatic extramammary Paget disease of the scrotum presenting as pancytopenia and back pain. Curr Oncol 2009;16(5):81–3.
139. Watanabe Y, Hoshiai H, Ueda H, et al. Low-dose mitomycin C, etoposide, and cisplatin for invasive vulvar Paget's disease. Int J Gynecol Cancer 2002;12:304–7.
140. Yamazaki N, Yamamoto A, Wada T, et al. A case of metastatic extramammary Paget's disease that responded to combination chemotherapy. J Dermatol 1999;26:311–6.
141. Mochitomi Y, Sakamoto R, Gushi A, et al. Extramammary Paget's disease/carcinoma successfully treated with a combination chemotherapy: report of two cases. J Dermatol 2005;32:632–7.

Index

Note: Page numbers of article titles are in **boldface** type.

Dermatol Clin 28 (2010) 827–833
doi:10.1016/S0733-8635(10)00152-X

United States Postal Service

Statement of Ownership, Management, and Circulation
(All Periodicals Publications Except Requestor Publications)

1. Publication Title	2. Publication Number	3. Filing Date
Dermatologic Clinics of North America	0 0 0 - 7 0 5	9/15/10
4. Issue Frequency	**5. Number of Issues Published Annually**	**6. Annual Subscription Price**
Jan, Apr, Jul, Oct	4	$296.00

7. Complete Mailing Address of Known Office of Publication (*Not printer*) (*Street, city, county, state, and ZIP+4®*)

Elsevier Inc.
360 Park Avenue South
New York, NY 10010-1710

Contact Person: Stephen Bushing
Telephone (Include area code): 215-239-3688

8. Complete Mailing Address of Headquarters or General Business Office of Publisher (*Not printer*)

Elsevier Inc., 360 Park Avenue South, New York, NY 10010-1710

9. Full Names and Complete Mailing Addresses of Publisher, Editor, and Managing Editor (*Do not leave blank*)

Publisher (*Name and complete mailing address*)

Kim Murphy , Elsevier, Inc., 1600 John F. Kennedy Blvd. Suite 1800, Philadelphia, PA 19103-2899

Editor (*Name and complete mailing address*)

Carla Holloway, Elsevier, Inc., 1600 John F. Kennedy Blvd. Suite 1800, Philadelphia, PA 19103-2899

Managing Editor (*Name and complete mailing address*)

Catherine Bewick, Elsevier, Inc., 1600 John F. Kennedy Blvd. Suite 1800, Philadelphia, PA 19103-2899

10. Owner (*Do not leave blank. If the publication is owned by a corporation, give the name and address of the corporation immediately followed by the names and addresses of all stockholders owning or holding 1 percent or more of the total amount of stock. If not owned by a corporation, give the names and addresses of the individual owners. If owned by a partnership or other unincorporated firm, give its name and address as well as those of each individual owner. If the publication is published by a nonprofit organization, give its name and address.*)

Full Name	Complete Mailing Address
Wholly owned subsidiary of	4520 East-West Highway
Reed/Elsevier, US holdings	Bethesda, MD 20814

11. Known Bondholders, Mortgagees, and Other Security Holders Owning or Holding 1 Percent or More of Total Amount of Bonds, Mortgages, or Other Securities. If none, check box → ☐ None

Full Name	Complete Mailing Address
N/A	

12. Tax Status (*For completion by nonprofit organizations authorized to mail at nonprofit rates*) (*Check one*)
The purpose, function, and nonprofit status of this organization and the exempt status for federal income tax purposes:
☐ Has Not Changed During Preceding 12 Months
☐ Has Changed During Preceding 12 Months (*Publisher must submit explanation of change with this statement*)

PS Form 3526, September 2007 (Page 1 of 3 (Instructions Page 3)) PSN 7530-01-000-9931 **PRIVACY NOTICE**: See our Privacy policy in www.usps.com

13. Publication Title: Dermatologic Clinics of North America

14. Issue Date for Circulation Data Below: July 2010

15. Extent and Nature of Circulation		Average No. Copies Each Issue During Preceding 12 Months	No. Copies of Single Issue Published Nearest to Filing Date
a. Total Number of Copies (*Net press run*)		1161	1200
b. Paid Circulation (By Mail and Outside the Mail)	(1) Mailed Outside-County Paid Subscriptions Stated on PS Form 3541. (*Include paid distribution above nominal rate, advertiser's proof copies, and exchange copies*)	333	296
	(2) Mailed In-County Paid Subscriptions Stated on PS Form 3541 (*Include paid distribution above nominal rate, advertiser's proof copies, and exchange copies*)		
	(3) Paid Distribution Outside the Mails Including Sales Through Dealers and Carriers, Street Vendors, Counter Sales, and Other Paid Distribution Outside USPS®	215	205
	(4) Paid Distribution by Other Classes Mailed Through the USPS (e.g. First-Class Mail®)		
c. Total Paid Distribution (*Sum of 15b (1), (2), (3), and (4)*) →		548	501
d. Free or Nominal Rate Distribution (By Mail and Outside the Mail)	(1) Free or Nominal Rate Outside-County Copies Included on PS Form 3541	95	101
	(2) Free or Nominal Rate In-County Copies Included on PS Form 3541		
	(3) Free or Nominal Rate Copies Mailed at Other Classes Through the USPS (e.g. First-Class Mail)		
	(4) Free or Nominal Rate Distribution Outside the Mail (Carriers or other means)		
e. Total Free or Nominal Rate Distribution (Sum of 15d (1), (2), (3) and (4)		95	101
f. Total Distribution (Sum of 15c and 15e) →		643	602
g. Copies not Distributed (See instructions to publishers #4 (page #3)) →		518	598
h. Total (Sum of 15f and g)		1161	1200
i. Percent Paid (15c divided by 15f times 100) →		85.23%	83.22%

16. Publication of Statement of Ownership

☐ If the publication is a general publication, publication of this statement is required. Will be printed in the **October 2010** issue of this publication. ☐ Publication not required

17. Signature and Title of Editor, Publisher, Business Manager, or Owner

Stephen R. Bushing – Fulfillment/Inventory Specialist

Date: September 15, 2010

I certify that all information furnished on this form is true and complete. I understand that anyone who furnishes false or misleading information on this form or who omits material or information requested on the form may be subject to criminal sanctions (including fines and imprisonment) and/or civil sanctions (including civil penalties).

PS Form 3526, September 2007 (Page 2 of 3)

Printed and bound by CPI Group (UK) Ltd, Croydon, CR0 4YY
03/10/2024
01040359-0018